Moderate Sedation/Analgesia

Core Competencies for Practice

Second Edition

Michael Kost, CRNA, MS, MSN

Program Director
Frank J. Tornetta School of Anesthesia at Montgomery Hospital
1301 Powell Street
Norristown, Pennsylvania

Assistant Professor
La Salle University School of Nursing
1900 West Olney Avenue
Philadelphia, Pennsylvania

President
Specialty Health Education, Inc.
P. O. Box 992
Blue Bell, Pennsylvania

With 104 illustrations

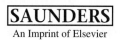
An Imprint of Elsevier

SAUNDERS
An Imprint of Elsevier

11830 Westline Industrial Drive
St. Louis, Missouri 63146

MODERATE SEDATION/ANALGESIA: ISBN 0-7216-0324-6
CORE COMPETENCIES FOR PRACTICE
Copyright © 2004, Elsevier Inc. All rights reserved.

NOTICE

Anesthesia is an ever-changing field. Standard safety precautions must be followed, but as new research and clinical experience broaden our knowledge, changes in treatment and drug therapy may become necessary or appropriate. Readers are advised to check the most current product information provided by the manufacturer of each drug to be administered to verify the recommended dose, the method and duration of administration, and contraindications. It is the responsibility of the licensed prescriber, relying on experience and knowledge of the patient, to determine dosages and the best treatment for each individual patient. Neither the publisher nor the author assumes any liability for any injury and/or damage to persons or property arising from this publication.

Previous edition copyrighted 1998.

Library of Congress Cataloging-in-Publication Data
Kost, Michael.
    Moderate sedation/analgesia : core competencies for practice/Michael Kost.–2nd ed.
        p. ; cm.
    Rev. ed. of: Manual of conscious sedation/ Michael Kost. ©1998.
    Available for continuing education credit.
    Includes bibliographical references and index.
    ISBN 0-7216-0324-6
        1. Conscious sedation. 2. Intravenous anesthesia. I. Kost, Michael. Manual of conscious sedation. II. Title.
    [DNLM: 1. Conscious Sedation–Nurses' Instruction. 2. Anesthesia, Intravenous–Nurses' Instruction. WO 200 K86ma 2004]
    RD85.C64K673 2004
    617.9′62–dc22
                                                                        2003066742

Executive Editor: Michael Ledbetter
Senior Developmental Editor: Lisa P. Newton
Publishing Services Manager: Catherine Jackson
Project Manager: Anne Gassett Konopka
Design Manager: Teresa McBryan
Cover Art: Paula Ruckenbrod

Printed in the United States of America

Last digit is the print number: 9 8 7 6 5 4 3 2 1

Moderate
Sedation/Analgesia

Core Competencies for Practice

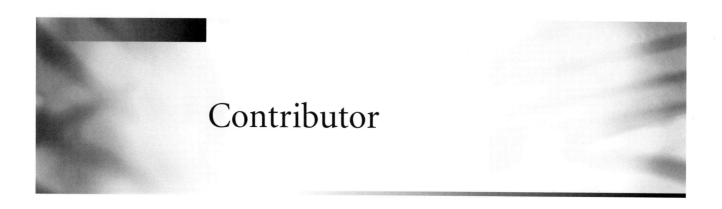

Contributor

Krista Bragg, CRNA, MSN
Staff Nurse Anesthetist
Children's Hospital of Pittsburgh
Pittsburgh, Pennsylvania
Adjunct Faculty
University of Pittsburgh
School of Nursing
Pittsburgh, Pennsylvania
(author of Chapter 10, Pediatric Patient Care)

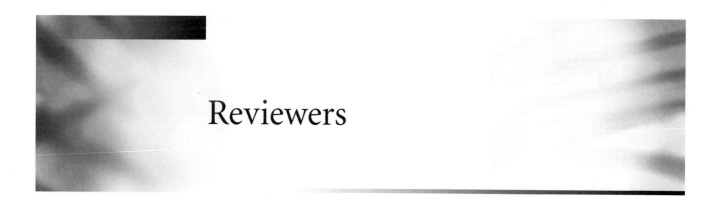

Reviewers

Loraine Hopkins-Pepe, MSN, RN, CCRN
Elkins Park Hospital
Clinical Educator, Staff Development
MossRehab Einstein at Elkins Park
Elkins Park, PA

John M. O'Donnell, CRNA, MSN
Director, University of Pittsburgh
School of Nursing Anesthesia Program
Secondary Appointment, University of Pittsburgh
School of Dental Medicine
Adjunct Assistant Professor, Florida International University
Pittsburgh, PA

About the Author

Michael Kost, CRNA, MS, MSN, is program director of the Frank J. Tornetta School of Anesthesia at Montgomery Hospital, Norristown, Pennsylvania. He is president of Specialty Health Education, Inc., Blue Bell, Pennsylvania, a healthcare company that specializes in educational and consulting services to healthcare facilities and organizations. He received his bachelor of science in nursing from Widener University, Chester, Pennsylvania, CRNA certificate from the Montgomery Hospital School of Anesthesia, and a master of science in anesthesia from Saint Joseph's University, Philadelphia, Pennsylvania. He received his master of science in nursing as a clinical specialist in gerontology from Gwynedd Mercy College, Gwynedd Valley, Pennsylvania. He has presented to national and local chapters of professional organizations and is a frequent lecturer and author on sedation, ambulatory anesthesia, perianesthesia care, and pharmacology topics. He is the author of *Manual of Conscious Sedation*, W. B. Saunders (1998) and the *Sedation Clinical Competency CD-ROM Program*, Specialty Health Education, Inc. (2004).

my wife, Nancy
For her continued support and understanding

John, Eric, Rebecca
For their encouragement

SJN and all the physicians and nurses at the
Children's Hospital of Philadelphia Oncology Unit
Thank You!

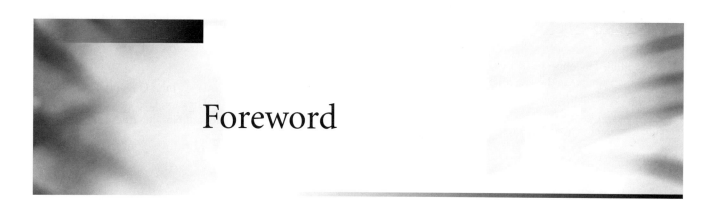

Foreword

"The man who can make hard things easy is the educator."
RALPH WALDO EMERSON (1803-1882)

In his new edition, *Moderate Sedation/Analgesia: Core Competencies for Practice, 2nd edition*, Michael Kost clearly outlines the process of sedation/analgesia care for non-anesthesia health-care providers against a regulatory and professional standards backdrop. This text remains the definitive resource for all non-anesthesia practitioners working in this rapidly expanding area of clinical practice.

Over the past few years, the utilization of moderate sedation (procedural sedation) has grown significantly, particularly in moving outside of the controlled operating room setting into diverse clinical areas. Physicians, nurses, and other healthcare providers now participate in the procedural sedation process as a primary component of their professions. Moderate sedation/analgesia is now a patient expectation and a valuable diagnostic or therapeutic adjunct for a wide array of tests and treatments. The primary benefits of sedation/analgesia remain anxiolysis, amnesia, and analgesia. It is incumbent upon all non-anesthesia clinicians practicing in this specialty to recognize that sedation/analgesia is associated with a variety of inherent risks. ***The underlying theme of this text continues to focus on patient safety as the first consideration in any sedation situation.*** This core curriculum provides a template for the necessary educational preparation, development of resources, and an understanding of the required credentialing and regulatory needs associated with the administration of sedation/analgesia. It may be used as the cornerstone for sedation/analgesia education and credentialing programs.

Questions regarding training, resources, regulation, policy, procedure, and patient care implementation continue to arise on a daily basis. Mr. Kost responded to the need for a comprehensive yet practical reference by publishing the *Manual of Conscious Sedation* in 1998. This most recent edition, based on a core curriculum approach, is a valuable educational resource tool for both daily use and as a means for periodic evaluation. The concise, easily understandable format targets an audience of clinicians who are *actually engaged* in the administration of sedation/analgesia. The text is also a resource for administrators developing sedation policy and procedures and competency programs. This new core curriculum will serve as an educational resource for experienced clinicians and as a valuable guide for healthcare providers new to sedation/analgesia practice.

The addition of a pediatric sedation chapter by a pediatric anesthesia specialist increases the value and utility of the text. A chapter on Pediatric Sedation by Krista Bragg, CRNA, MSN (Children's Hospital of Pittsburgh) adds insight into the specific patient care requirements for safe sedation care of children. The pediatric chapter is critical, as it imparts many of the specific skills and knowledge required for pediatric sedation secondary to the pharmacokinetic, pharmacodynamic, and developmental variations associated with pediatric sedation care.

In summary, Michael Kost, CRNA, MS, MSN, has done an outstanding job once again in compiling and writing this definitive resource in the area of sedation practice for use by non-anesthesia healthcare professionals. Administrators, educators, students, and clinicians will find this text to be an incredibly valuable resource in approaching the challenges inherent in the administration of sedation/analgesia (conscious sedation).

John O'Donnell, CRNA, MSN
Director, University of Pittsburgh
School of Nursing Anesthesia Program

Preface

The administration of sedation/analgesia is common practice in a variety of clinical settings. The increased use of sedatives, hypnotics, analgesics, and in some cases, anesthetic agents outside the operating room proper has produced a demand for highly educated, clinically competent non-anesthesia providers. This text will focus on the preprocedural, procedural, and postprocedural aspects of sedation/ analgesia patient care. Its concise format is designed to function as an educational resource tool and a means for periodic self-evaluation. *Moderate Sedation/Analgesia: Core Competencies for Practice, 2nd edition* is a comprehensive text that incorporates the latest information available on the practice of sedation/analgesia by non-anesthesia providers. Written for clinicians engaged in the administration of sedation/ analgesia, it also functions as a practical guide for clinicians in a wide variety of settings.

Each chapter is preceded with learning objectives. The Joint Commission on Accreditation of Healthcare Organizations Standards for Operative or Other High-Risk Procedures and/or the Administration of Moderate or Deep Sedation or Anesthesia, and the American Society of Anesthesiologists Task Force on Sedation and Analgesia by Non-Anesthesiologists Practice Guidelines for Sedation and Analgesia are also presented in appropriate chapters. All chapters are followed with a Learner Self-Assessment section to assist the reader in achieving maximal educational benefit. Post-Test Questions are also presented at the conclusion of each chapter. ***In addition, continuing education credit is available for each chapter. For information on obtaining continuing education credit from Specialty Health Education, Inc., please see details printed on the inside front cover.***

The book is written in three units. Unit I addresses presedation patient care issues. Chapter 1 focuses on the goals, definitions, and practice standards and guidelines associated with sedation practice. Chapter 2 combines comprehensive presedation patient assessment strategies related to organ systems, pathophysiologic disease processes, recommended treatment strategies, and appropriate patient selection strategies.

Unit II features a variety of comprehensive aspects associated with sedation patient care. The administration of sedative, hypnotic, and analgesic medications requires a thorough understanding of the pharmacokinetic and pharmacodynamic effects of each medication. Chapters 3, 4, and 5 feature a concise review of pharmacologic concepts, medication classifications, techniques of administration, and specific medication pharmacologic profiles. Specific requirements associated with procedural patient care are presented in Chapter 6.

Respiratory complications associated with the administration of sedation/analgesia are featured in Chapter 7. A comprehensive review of airway anatomy, airway evaluation, and emergency airway management strategies provides the learner with a systematic approach to crisis management in the event of respiratory depression or arrest. Intravenous insertion techniques, complications of intravenous therapy, and profiles of intravenous solutions are richly illustrated in Chapter 8.

Presedation, procedural care, and postprocedural geriatric patient care issues are comprehensively presented in Chapter 9. Chapter 10, Pediatric Patient Care, was authored by Krista Bragg, CRNA, MSN, a pediatric anesthesia specialist. The pediatric chapter focuses on all aspects associated with pediatric sedation care.

Unit III encompasses the monitoring requirements and postsedation aspects of patient care. Postprocedure care, documentation, discharge planning, and recovery scoring mechanisms are reviewed and available for easy reference in Chapter 11. Risk management strategies and educational issues associated with providing and maintaining a sedation educational program are provided for educators and individual participants alike. Figures and tables in Chapter 12 address sedation position description, credentialing, and departmental documentation issues related to the administration of sedation. The appendices provided in the text complement a variety of aspects associated with sedation patient care.

Finally, it is my hope that the information presented in this text enriches the learner's fundamental knowledge of sedation patient care and contributes to enhanced vigilance and ultimately to decreased morbidity and mortality.

ACKNOWLEDGMENTS

Sincere thanks to Michael Ledbetter, executive editor, Lisa P. Newton, senior developmental editor, and Anne Gassett, project manager, all of Elsevier, for their continued support and guidance throughout this entire project. To Diane Quinley, administrative assistant, Specialty Health Education, Inc., for her continued support and dedication.

With sincere thanks to the reviewers and contributor for their attention to detail, recommendations, and editorial comment.

Michael Kost, CRNA, MS, MSN

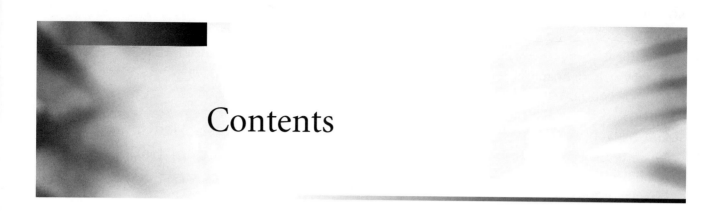

Contents

Unit Two
PROCEDURAL PATIENT CARE

CHAPTER 3
Pharmacologic Concepts, 70

CHAPTER 4
Sedation/Analgesia Medication and Techniques of Administration, 81

CHAPTER 5
Sedation/Analgesia Pharmacologic Profile, 99

CHAPTER 6
Procedural Patient Monitoring, 127

CHAPTER 7
Airway Management and Management of Respiratory Complications, 164

APPENDICES

CHAPTER 1

Goals, Definitions, Practice Standards, and Guidelines

CORE COMPETENCIES

At the completion of this chapter, the learner shall:

◆ Identify JCAHO standards and intents related to the administration of sedation by qualified providers.

◆ Define minimal sedation, moderate sedation, deep sedation, and general anesthesia.

◆ Identify five goals and objectives of moderate sedation/analgesia.

◆ State the clinical endpoints of moderate sedation/analgesia.

◆ List the regulatory, statutory, and recommended practice guidelines associated with the administration of sedation.

◆ Identify the applicable standards and intents promulgated by the Joint Commission on Accreditation of Healthcare Organizations as they relate to the administration of sedation/ analgesia by healthcare providers.

◆ Compare and contrast practice standards, practice guidelines, and position statements related to sedation care.

Joint Commission on Accreditation of Healthcare Organizations Standards for Operative or Other High-Risk Procedures and/or the Administration of Moderate or Deep Sedation or Anesthesia

Operative or other procedures and the administration of sedation or anesthesia often occur simultaneously. However, procedures do occur without sedation, and sedation or anesthesia is administered for noninvasive procedures (hyperbaric treatment, CT scan, MRI). Therefore, the following standards address both operative or other procedures and/or the administration of moderate or deep sedation or anesthesia.

Whenever an operative or other procedure is conducted, whether or not sedation or anesthesia is administered, appropriate patients must be involved in planning for and providing care to the patient. All procedures carry risk, but that risk is increased when sedation or anesthesia is administered.

The standards for sedation and anesthesia care apply when patients in any setting, receive, for any purpose, by any route, the following:

• General, spinal, or other major regional sedation and anesthesia or

• Sedation (with or without analgesia) that, in the manner used, may be reasonably expected to result in the loss of protective reflexes

Because sedation is a continuum, it is not always possible to predict how an individual patient receiving sedation will respond. Therefore, each hospital develops specific, appropriate protocols for the care of patients receiving sedation. These protocols are consistent with professional standards and address at least the following:

- *Sufficient qualified individuals present to perform the procedure and to monitor the patient throughout administration and recovery*
- Appropriate equipment for care and resuscitation
- Appropriate monitoring of vital signs—heart and respiratory rates and oxygenation
- Documentation of care
- Monitoring of outcomes

Definitions of four levels of sedation and anesthesia include the following:

- **Minimal sedation (anxiolysis)**

    A drug-induced state during which patients respond normally to verbal commands. Although cognitive function and coordination may be impaired, ventilatory and cardiovascular functions are unaffected.

- **Moderate sedation/analgesia ("conscious sedation")**

    A drug-induced depression of consciousness during which patients respond purposefully to verbal commands, either alone or accompanied by light tactile stimulation. No interventions are required to maintain a patent airway, and spontaneous ventilation is adequate. Cardiovascular function is usually maintained.

- **Deep sedation/analgesia**

    A drug-induced depression of consciousness during which patients cannot be easily aroused but respond purposefully after repeated or painful stimulation. The ability to independently maintain ventilatory function may be impaired. Patients may require assistance in maintaining a patent airway and spontaneous ventilation may be inadequate. Cardiovascular function is usually maintained.

- **Anesthesia**

    Consists of general anesthesia and spinal or major regional anesthesia. It does *not* include local anesthesia. General anesthesia is a drug-induced loss of consciousness during which patients are not arousable, even by painful stimulation. The ability to independently maintain ventilatory function is often impaired. Patients often require assistance in maintaining a patent airway, and positive pressure ventilation may be required because of depressed spontaneous ventilation or drug-induced depression of neuromuscular function. Cardiovascular function may be impaired.

© Joint Commission: Standards for Operative or Other High-Risk Procedures and/or the Administration of Moderate or Deep Sedation or Anesthesia, January, 2004. Reprinted with permission.

The administration of sedation for surgical, therapeutic, and diagnostic procedures has gained widespread popularity over the past decade.[1-5] Not only has the number of procedures requiring the administration of sedation increased, the variety of procedures in the surgical and diagnostic caseload has also increased. A list of the more common surgical, therapeutic, and diagnostic procedures conducted with sedation is presented in Box 1-1. The rationale for the proliferation of the administration of sedation is varied. Technologic advances have made it possible to perform a multitude of procedures outside the confines of the conventional operating room environment. In addition, as healthcare reimbursement continues to evolve, a critical review of practice patterns has ensued. As healthcare continues to focus on efficiency coupled with an increase in outpatient procedures, the administration of sedation/analgesia by non-anesthesia providers offers a desirable alternative for specific therapeutic and diagnostic procedures. The use of sedation/analgesia has increased the demand for **qualified** providers. Healthcare providers have responded to this demand through implementation of educational programs, definition of clinical competencies, and promulgation of practice standards and guidelines.[6-8]

Pharmacologic advances have also contributed to the increased use of sedation/analgesia for specific patient populations. The introduction of intravenous medications with shorter half-lives, no active metabolites, and minimal cumulative effects has increased the margin of safety and efficacy associated with the administration of sedation. Monitoring

---

BOX 1-1

Common Minor Surgical, Therapeutic, and Diagnostic Procedures by Specialty Using Sedation/Analgesia*

Burns
- Dressing changes

Cardiology
- Angioplasty
- Cardiac catheterization
- Cardioversion
- Electrophysiologic ablation
- Insertion of invasive lines
- Insertion of internal defibrillator
- Pacemaker insertion
- Transesophageal echocardiography
- Vascular access

Cosmetic Surgery
- Blepharoplasty
- Chemical peel
- Dermabrasion
- Liposuction
- Otoplasty
- Rhinoplasty
- Rhytidectomy
- Skin laser enhancement

Gastroenterology
- Colonoscopy
- Endoscopy
- Endoscopic retrograde cholangiopancreatography (ERCP)
- Liver biopsy

General Surgery
- Hernia repair
- Incision and drainage
- Lipoma excision
- Superficial biopsies

Gynecology
- Dilatation and curettage (D & C)
- Dilatation and evacuation (D & E)

- Cone biopsy
- Hysteroscopy
- Incision and drainage
- In vitro fertilization
- Laparoscopy
- Lesion fulguration

Ophthalmology
- Blepharoplasty
- Cataract extraction
- Lens implant

Oral Surgery
- Dental caries
- Odontectomy
- Periodontal

Orthopedics
- Arthroscopy
- Closed fracture reduction
- Hand surgery
- Joint manipulation

Pulmonology
- Bronchoscopy
- Endotracheal intubation
- Chest tube insertion

Radiology
- Arteriography
- Computed tomography
- Embolization
- Interventional radiology procedures
- Localization and biopsy
- Magnetic resonance imaging

Urology
- Cystoscopy
- Lithotripsy
- Vasectomy

*This is not an all-inclusive list.

---

advances have also had a significant impact on the delivery of sedation and analgesia. The advent of pulse oximetry introduced into clinical practice in the 1980s produced the ability to assist the clinician in the diagnosis of hypoxic states. This ability has greatly enhanced the margin of safety associated with administration of sedation/analgesia.

> The increased use of sedation/analgesia is associated with pharmacologic and clinical monitoring advances coupled with changes in the healthcare reimbursement structure.

DEFINITIONS

It is important to define the combination of amnestic, anxiolytic, and analgesic medications used to achieve a state

of sedation. The term *conscious sedation* was first described by Dr. C. R. Bennett. In a paper entitled "Conscious Sedation in Dental Practice," he presented information related to the administration of intravenous sedative medications in conjunction with local anesthetics.[9] The technique used sedative and analgesic medications combined with local anesthetics in the affected area. In this way, the patients maintained their protective airway reflexes and were provided a minimally depressed level of consciousness.

As outlined in Table 1-1, it is important for the healthcare practitioner providing sedation services to recognize that sedation and analgesia comprise a continuum. This continuum consists of four levels of sedation and anesthesia. The *JCAHO Standards for Operative or other High-Risk Procedures and/or the Administration of Moderate or Deep*

TABLE 1-1

Continuum of Sedation as Adopted by the ASA House of Delegates, October 13, 1999

	MINIMAL SEDATION (ANXIOLYSIS)	MODERATE SEDATION/ ANALGESIA (CONSCIOUS SEDATION)	DEEP SEDATION/ ANALGESIA	GENERAL ANESTHESIA
Responsiveness	Normal response to verbal stimulation	Purposeful* response to verbal or tactile stimulation	Purposeful* response following repeated or painful stimulation	Unarousable even with painful stimulus
Airway	Unaffected	No intervention required	Intervention may be required	Intervention often required
Spontaneous Ventilation	Unaffected	Adequate	May be inadequate	Frequently inadequate
Cardiovascular Function	Unaffected	Usually maintained	Usually maintained	May be impaired

*Reflex withdrawal from a painful stimulus is not considered a purposeful response.
Adopted by the American Society of Anesthesiologists House of Delegates, October 13, 1999. *American Society of Anesthesiologists, Newsletter*, May 2002, Volume 66, Number 5. Reprinted with permission.

Sedation or Anesthesia and the *Practice Guidelines for Sedation and Analgesia by Non-Anesthesiologists* utilize the definitions and terminology in the "Continuum of Depth of Sedation, Definition of General Anesthesia, and Levels of Sedation/Analgesia," which was approved by the House of Delegates of the American Society of Anesthesiologists on October 13, 1999.[8,10-11] These definitions include:

◆ Minimal sedation (anxiolysis)
◆ Moderate sedation/analgesia (conscious sedation)
◆ Deep sedation/analgesia
◆ General anesthesia

Minimal sedation (anxiolysis) is a drug-induced state during which patients respond normally to verbal commands. Although cognitive function and coordination may be impaired, ventilatory and cardiovascular functions are unaffected.

Moderate sedation/analgesia ("conscious sedation") is a drug-induced depression of consciousness during which patients respond purposefully to verbal commands, either alone or accompanied by light tactile stimulation. No interventions are required to maintain a patent airway, and spontaneous ventilation is adequate. Cardiovascular function is usually maintained.

Deep sedation/analgesia is a drug-induced depression of consciousness during which patients cannot be easily aroused but respond purposefully following repeated or painful stimulation. The ability to independently maintain ventilatory function may be impaired. Patients may require assistance in maintaining a patent airway, and spontaneous ventilation may be inadequate. Cardiovascular function is usually maintained.

Anesthesia consists of general anesthesia and spinal or major regional anesthesia. It does *not* include local anesthesia. General anesthesia is a drug-induced loss of consciousness during which patients are not arousable, even by painful stimulation. The ability to independently maintain ventilatory function is often impaired. Patients often require assistance in maintaining a patent airway, and positive-pressure ventilation may be required because of depressed spontaneous ventilation or drug-induced depression of neuromuscular function. Cardiovascular function may be impaired.

> It is important that healthcare practitioners recognize sedation occurs on a continuum. Patient response to pharmacologic agents varies based on the medication administered, dosage, technique of administration, and the presence of concomitant disease states.

GOALS AND OBJECTIVES

The continuum of sedation identified in Table 1-1 represents the defined levels of sedation and anesthesia outlined. The response to the administration of moderate sedation/analgesia depends on individual patient response, the total dose of medication administered, and the patient's physiologic status. Varied patient response or the overzealous administration of sedation and analgesic agents may result in a state of deep sedation or general anesthesia. **Deep sedation or general anesthesia predisposes the patient to an increased incidence of respiratory depression, decreased response to the hypoxic drive, and cardiovascular depression.**

> To avoid complications, it is imperative for all healthcare practitioners who participate in the administration of sedation services to recognize that unresponsiveness and unconsciousness are not the objectives of moderate sedation/analgesia.

Pharmacologic medications used to achieve a state of sedation/analgesia include:

◆ **Benzodiazepines:** amnesia, anxiolysis
◆ **Opioids, dissociative agents:** analgesia
◆ **Sedative/hypnotics:** anxiolysis

Combinations of these carefully titrated medications provide the clinician the ability to perform therapeutic, diagnostic, and minor surgical procedures while the patient is maintained in an altered level of consciousness. **The administration and combination of benzodiazepines, opioids, and sedative/hypnotics may produce profound synergistic effects.** These synergistic effects may lead to a state of deep sedation or general anesthesia. As early as 1990, Bailey reported in *Anesthesiology* more than 80 deaths directly attributed to the administration of conscious sedation with benzodiazepines specifically when combined with an opioid.[12] This demonstrated synergism combined with preexisting medical conditions and varied patient response may lead to the development of hypoxemia, apnea, deep sedative states, or general anesthesia. To prevent the development of an unconscious state during diagnostic or surgical procedures, it is important to understand the pharmacokinetic and pharmacodynamic profile of the pharmacologic agents used to produce the sedate state (see Chapters 4 and 5). The clinician must also appreciate the potency and synergistic action of combined medications used during procedural patient care.

> Healthcare professionals providing sedation services must possess an in-depth understanding of the pharmacodynamic and pharmacokinetic profile of each sedative, opioid, or hypnotic that they administer, respectively.

The objectives of moderate sedation/analgesia listed in Box 1-2 were initially presented in 1985 by Scammon, Klein, and Choi.[13] The primary goal of moderate sedation/analgesia is to allay patient fear and anxiety associated with the proposed procedure. The goal of sedation techniques is to use

---

BOX 1-2

Objectives of Sedation

1. **Maintain adequate sedation with minimal risk.** The patient's ability to communicate is preserved. Physiologic monitoring is employed, and emergency resuscitation is on hand.
2. **Relieve anxiety and produce amnesia.** These objectives are accomplished by means of good preoperative communication and instruction and low levels of visual and auditory stimuli.
3. **Provide relief from pain and other noxious stimuli.** Opioids are given to supplement local or topical anesthetics and to block pain sensations remote from the operative site.

From Scammon FL, Klein SL, Choi WW: Conscious sedation for procedures under local or topical anesthesia. *Ann Otol Rhinol Laryngol.* 1985;94:21.

---

the *least* amount of sedation while providing for patient comfort. Additional goals of moderate sedation/analgesia include:

◆ Mood alteration
◆ Enhanced patient cooperation
◆ Elevation of pain threshold
◆ Stable vital signs
◆ Amnesia
◆ Rapid recovery

LEGAL SCOPE OF PRACTICE

An understanding of the continuum of sedation and of sedation definitions is required for healthcare providers to maintain compliance with legal scope-of-practice issues in many jurisdictions. As healthcare providers respond to the increased number of procedures that require sedation services, they must be cognizant of legal scope-of-practice issues. Legal scope-of-practice issues related to nursing are delegated and administered through state boards of nursing. Individual state statutes define the practice of nursing. As registered nurses have become more involved in the administration of sedation services and patient monitoring, scope-of-practice issues have been raised in many states.

In the late 1980s, the demand for registered nurses to participate in the administration of conscious sedation procedures and the monitoring of patients receiving these services increased dramatically.[14] In response, registered nurses concerned with legal scope-of-practice issues contacted their individual state boards of nursing to inquire about the conscious sedation practice patterns that were developing in their institutions. Responses from state boards of nursing varied in their position regarding the administration of sedation and the monitoring of patients receiving it. Some state boards have adopted formal position or policy statements that delineate the responsibility of professional registered nurses engaged in the administration of sedation. Many state boards of nursing have enacted formal policy statements that define and identify prescriptive responsibilities and requirements of the registered nurse participating in the administration of sedation services. Some state boards of nursing have not taken formal action on the issue. A few select state boards of nursing may not have statutory authority to enact such legislation, whereas some continue to gather information on the issue. Registered nurses must be aware of their state board of nursing requirements associated with the clinical practice of sedation (Advanced Cardiac Life Support [ACLS] course completion, monitoring requirements, intravenous access, etc.). An example of a state board of nursing policy statement related to conscious sedation is identified in Box 1-3, which features the Pennsylvania Board of Registered Nursing policy statement related to the administration of sedation by registered nurses.

> Registered nurses providing sedation should periodically contact their state board of nursing to determine if there are any updates or changes to sedation policy statements.

BOX 1-3

Pennsylvania Code
Title 49. Professional and Vocational
Standards
Department of State
Chapter 21. State Board of Nursing
Conscious Sedation

49 § 21.413 Pt. I
As used in this subsection, "conscious sedation" is defined as a minimally depressed level of consciousness in which the patient retains the ability to independently and continuously maintain an airway and respond appropriately to physical stimulation and verbal commands. The registered nurse who is not a certified registered nurse anesthetist may administer intravenous conscious sedation medications, under § 21.14, during minor therapeutic and diagnostic procedures, when the following conditions exist:

(1) The specific amount of intravenous conscious sedation medications has been ordered in writing by a licensed physician and a licensed physician is physically present in the room during administration.
(2) Written guidelines specifying the intravenous medications that the registered nurse may administer in a particular setting are available to the registered nurse.
(3) Electrocardiogram, blood pressure, and oximetry equipment are used for both monitoring and emergency resuscitation purposes pursuant to written guidelines which are provided for minimum patient monitoring. Additional emergency resuscitation equipment is immediately available.
(4) The patient has a patent intravenous access.
(5) The registered nurse involved in direct patient care has completed a course in advanced cardiac life support (ACLS) or pediatric cardiac life support, which establishes competency in airway management and resuscitation appropriate to the age of the patient.
(6) The registered nurse possesses the knowledge, skills and abilities related to the management of patients receiving intravenous conscious sedation with evaluation of competence on a periodic basis. This includes, but is not limited to, arrhythmia detection, airway management, and pharmacologic action of drugs administered. This includes emergency drugs.
(7) The registered nurse managing the care of the patient receiving intravenous conscious sedation medication may not have other responsibilities during the procedure. The registered nurse may not leave the patient unattended or engage in tasks that would compromise continuous monitoring.
(8) The registered nurse monitors the patient until the patient is discharged by a qualified professional authorized to discharge the patient in accordance with established criteria of the facility.

Reprinted with permission of the Pennsylvania State Board of Nursing.

Physicians may be subject to statutory authority related to the administration of sedation and the monitoring of patients receiving it. As early as 1991, the state of New Jersey enacted legislation that required "all physicians wishing to perform intravenous conscious sedation in the hospital setting to be credentialed by the Department of Anesthesia within that institution."[15] The purpose of this legislation was to increase physician awareness of the medications used for conscious sedation procedures. It is also a mechanism to enhance the physician's understanding of monitoring modalities used during performance of the diagnostic procedure.

JOINT COMMISSION ON ACCREDITATION OF HEALTHCARE ORGANIZATIONS

The mission of the JCAHO is to improve the quality of care provided to the public. Healthcare organizations may apply for and undergo a full accreditation survey every 3 years. The accreditation process focuses on an assessment of an organization's compliance with standards developed by the JCAHO. The new *Standards for Additional Special Procedures: Standards for Operative or other High-Risk Procedures and/or the Administration of Moderate or Deep Sedation or Anesthesia* (Comprehensive Accreditation Manual for Hospitals) became effective in January 2004.[8] **These standards for sedation and anesthesia care apply when patients receive, in any setting, for any purpose, by any route, moderate or deep sedation as well as general, spinal, or other major regional anesthesia.** *The JCAHO Standards for the Administration of Moderate or Deep Sedation or Anesthesia* apply to patients receiving moderate sedation/analgesia (conscious sedation), deep sedation/analgesia, and anesthesia. These standards **DO NOT** apply to patients receiving minimal sedation (anxiolysis). For years institutions have struggled with their definitions and terminology in what actually constituted minimal sedation (anxiolysis). Some facilities utilized policies and procedures that limited the administration of anxiolysis to specific medications, quantity of medication administered, and routes of administration (oral/rectal). The JCAHO has clearly rectified this situation by stating that the *JCAHO Standards for the Administration of Moderate or Deep Sedation or Anesthesia* "apply when patients receive, in any setting, for any purpose, by any route, moderate or deep sedation as well as general anesthesia, spinal, or other major regional anesthesia."[14] Therefore, former misconceptions associated with "intent" of sedation, "credentialing" of the sedation provider, or "specific medications" utilized to achieve a sedate state are not the factors that "trigger" application of the *JCAHO Standards for the Administration of Moderate or Deep Sedation or Anesthesia*. The *Standards for Moderate and Deep Sedation and Anesthesia* include:

Standard PC.13.20

Operative or other procedures and/or the administration of moderate or deep sedation or anesthesia are planned.

Standard PC.13.30

Patients are monitored during the procedure and/or administration of moderate or deep sedation or anesthesia.

Standard PC.13.40

Patients are monitored immediately after the procedure and/or administration of moderate or deep sedation or anesthesia.

> It is important that hospital administrators/managers furnish the personnel and support required to provide appropriate presedation, procedural, and postsedation care in accordance with the requirements outlined in *the JCAHO Standards for the Administration of Moderate or Deep Sedation or Anesthesia.*

The entire content (JCAHO Standards, Rationales, Elements of Performance and Scoring) of the *JCAHO Standards* (Comprehensive Accreditation Manual for Hospitals) related to sedation and anesthesia are provided in Appendix B.

One aspect of complying with the JCAHO standards is effective policy and procedure development. Comprehensive hospital policies and procedures related to the administration of sedation services must provide the same level of care for patients throughout the institution. In an attempt to improve quality patient care and promote the safe administration of sedation/analgesia by qualified persons, these policies and procedures must encompass promulgated standards, recommended practice guidelines, and position statements published by professional organizations. These policies and procedures must also adhere to state statutory law. Policies and procedures delineated in relation to the administration of sedation and analgesia must address the following:

◆ Knowledge of anatomy, physiology, cardiac arrhythmia recognition, and complications related to the administration of intravenous sedation.
◆ Knowledge of the pharmacokinetic and pharmacodynamic principles associated with sedation medications.
◆ Demonstrated competence and training in presedation assessment, planning of sedation, and monitoring of physiologic parameters, including respiratory rate, oxygen saturation, blood pressure, cardiac rate and rhythm, and patient level of consciousness.
◆ An understanding of the principles of oxygen delivery and the ability to use an oxygen-delivery device.
◆ The ability to rapidly assess, diagnose, and intervene in the event of an untoward reaction associated with the administration of sedation and analgesic medications.
◆ Proven skill in airway management.
◆ Accurate documentation of the medications administered.
◆ Postsedation monitoring and discharge planning.
◆ Competency validation for training and education mechanisms.

The American Society of Anesthesiologist's **Sedation Model Policy** featured in Box 1-4, provides the clinician and institution with a template on which to build its sedation/analgesia policies.

PROFESSIONAL ORGANIZATIONS

As identified in Figure 1-1 on p. 12, scope of practice issues include practice standards, practice guidelines, and position statements promulgated by professional organizations related to the administration of sedation. **Practice standards** are the highest mandate for clinical behavior. A standard represents behaviors that must be exercised by the practitioner. Standards allow for little variation in performance behavior that cannot be justified by clear and compelling rationale. An example of practice standards include the JCAHO's *Standards for the Administration of Moderate or Deep Sedation or Anesthesia.*[8]

Practice guidelines provide behavior and critical decision-making recommendations that are commonly accepted within a professional discipline. Practice guidelines are not mandated recommendations; however, they may eventually evolve into standards. An example of practice guidelines featured in Appendix A include *Practice Guidelines for Sedation and Analgesia by Non-Anesthesiologists, an Updated Report by the American Society of Anesthesiologists Task Force on Sedation and Analgesia by Non-Anesthesiologists.*[11]

Position statements utilize less forceful criteria than practice guidelines or standards. They generally represent emerging trends on a given topic, address economically driven practice modalities, or discuss procedural policies. In July 1991, the Nursing Organizations Liaison Forum in Washington, D.C., adopted a position statement for the management of patients receiving intravenous conscious sedation for short-term therapeutic, diagnostic, or surgical procedures titled "Endorsement of Position Statement on the Role of the Registered Nurse (RN) in the Management of Patients Receiving Intravenous Conscious Sedation for Short-Term, Therapeutic, Diagnostic, or Surgical Procedures"[16] (see Appendix C). This position statement has been endorsed by 23 professional nursing organizations. Professional organizations involved in the development of the position statement are listed in Box 1-5 on p. 12. A variety of additional professional organizations have also promulgated practice guidelines or position statements related to the management of patients receiving sedation and analgesia. A review of the literature reveals that there are numerous standards, practice guidelines, position statements, and recommendations related to sedation management.[8,11,16]

Despite promulgated standards, protocols, practice guidelines, and position statements there continues to be lack of continuity in the training, education, and clinical competency requirements for healthcare practitioners engaged in the administration and management of patients receiving sedation/analgesia. A recent survey entitled "The Administration of Conscious Sedation by Non-Anesthesia Personnel" utilized a questionnaire to effectively address the clinical and didactic preparation of nurses who deliver conscious sedation.[17] The questionnaire was developed by a multidisciplinary task force composed of anesthetists, gastroenterologists, and

BOX 1-4

ASA Sedation Model Policy

Subject:
Sedation and analgesia (a.k.a. conscious sedation) for diagnostic, therapeutic, and invasive procedures.

Purpose:
To establish appropriate standards for administering and monitoring sedation and analgesia.

Policy:
Sedation and analgesia for diagnostic, therapeutic, and invasive procedures shall be practiced throughout the hospital in accordance with the following guidelines.

Definitions:
1. Levels of Sedation
Sedation occurs in a dose-related continuum, is variable, and depends on each patient's response to various drugs. The definitions listed below progress on a continuum from a high state of consciousness to unconsciousness. **This policy addresses only practices for sedation and analgesia (a.k.a. conscious sedation).**

   A. Analgesia and Anxiolysis: Diminution or elimination of pain and anxiety in a conscious patient. The patient is easily awakened by normal or softly spoken verbal commands and is oriented when awake. All vital signs are stable, there is **no significant risk** of losing protective reflexes, and the patient is able to maintain pre-procedure mobility.

   B. Sedation and Analgesia: A state of depressed level of consciousness in which a patient is able to maintain a patent airway independently and continuously and can be aroused by physical stimuli. These patients are unable to hold a conversation but respond to commands by appropriate action or brief verbalization. Patients receiving chloral hydrate **alone** up to 75 mg/kg may require more vigorous stimulation. Patients undergoing sedation and analgesia have a **small risk** of unexpectedly progressing to deep sedation and losing protective reflexes.

   C. Deep Sedation: A medically controlled state of depressed consciousness or unconsciousness from which the patient is **not** easily aroused by physical stimuli. Patients undergoing deep sedation have a **significant risk** of partial or complete loss of protective reflexes, including the inability to consistently maintain a patent airway independently and the inability to respond purposefully to physical stimulation or verbal commands. Loss of gag reflex, inability to maintain oral secretions, and loss of swallowing reflex may occur.

2. Other Definitions
   A. Pediatric Patient: All patients from birth through 17 years of age.

   B. Licensed Independent Practitioner (LIP): A physician or dentist who has a current license to practice and is approved to administer sedation. This does not include Advanced Registered Nurse Practitioners (ARNPs) or Physician Assistants (PAs).

   C. Diagnostic Procedure: This includes, but is not limited to diagnostic radiology, including computed tomography, nuclear magnetic resonance imaging, and echocardiography.

   D. Therapeutic Procedure: This includes, but is not limited to orthopedic manipulations, radiation therapy, and hyperbaric medicine.

   E. Invasive Procedure: A procedure involving puncture or incision of the skin or insertion of an instrument or foreign material into the body including, but not limited to, percutaneous aspiration and/or biopsy, cardiac or diagnostic catheterization, endoscopy, transesophageal echocardiography, angioplasty, central venous catheter placement, and percutaneous placement of long-term intravenous catheters (PICC).

Applicability:
This policy applies to the use of sedation and analgesia in all hospital departments and areas except as stated below:

1. This policy does not apply to patients who have an anesthesiologist providing sedation because anesthesiologists are governed by the standards of care established by the Department of Anesthesiology. This includes patients receiving monitored anesthesia care (MAC), deep sedation, and general anesthesia.

2. This policy does not apply to patients in the Intensive Care Unit (ICU) or Post Anesthesia Care Unit (PACU) under a 1:2 nurse to patient ratio who are mechanically ventilated or whose cardiovascular and respiratory status are continuously monitored by the same monitoring devices as specified per this policy. These patients are excluded because their care always includes continuous, close attention to their cardiorespiratory status and because vital signs are documented according to ICU protocol based on patient acuity.

3. This policy does not cover patients who receive anxiolytic or analgesic agents that are **administered routinely** to alleviate pain and agitation (e.g., sedation for treatment of insomnia, postoperative analgesia) because they are not at significant risk.

Continued

BOX 1-4—cont'd

Pre-Sedation Protocol:

1. *Factors Affecting Candidacy for Sedation*
   A. Candidates for sedation and analgesia shall be in good general medical health and have adequate ventilatory reserve. For patients who have significant medical problems (e.g., severe systemic disease, morbid obesity, sleep apnea, upper or lower structural airway abnormalities), consideration shall be given for consultation with an anesthesiologist or an attending physician specializing in the primary disease process affecting the patient.
   B. Infants with a history of apnea, those born prematurely (less than 37 weeks' gestation) who are less than 60 weeks' post-conceptual age, or full-term newborns less than 44 weeks' post-conceptual age should be monitored for 12 hours following sedation and analgesia. The degree of monitoring post procedure is determined by measures of appropriate discharge criteria from the unit in which the procedure occurred.
   C. **Patients will not receive sedation and analgesia unless they can be reasonably expected to meet preselected discharge criteria specified in the Postoperative Management section, part 4, below.**
   D. **Satisfactory arrangements for transportation after the procedure must be made before the patient is sedated.**

2. *Pre-Sedation Assessment*
   A. A pre-sedation assessment is required prior to administration of sedation and analgesia. The pre-sedation assessment will be documented in the patient's medical record (see example of generic form attached). The pre-sedation assessment must be reviewed with respect to the patient's condition immediately **prior to** administration of sedation and analgesia by the LIP supervising the sedation who will sign the pre-sedation assessment form.
   B. A pre-sedation assessment includes but is not limited to:
      1. Physical status assessment (review of systems, vital signs, airway, cardiopulmonary reserve)
      2. Past and present drug history including drug allergies
      3. Previous adverse experience with sedation and analgesia as well as with regional and general anesthesia
      4. Results of relevant diagnostic studies
      5. History of tobacco, alcohol, and substance use/abuse
      6. Verification of patient NPO status
      7. Plan and choice of sedation
      8. Transportation arrangements for patients who are expected to be discharged from the facility
   C. Multiple Administration of Sedation and Analgesia

   In patients who are undergoing procedures that require sedation and analgesia multiple times per day or single/multiple times on successive days, the initial pre-anesthesia assessment is sufficient as long as the physician performing the procedure determines through subsequent evaluation of the patient that no change has occurred in the patient's clinical status that would alter the outcome of administration of sedation and analgesia. A short note shall be placed in the patient's medical record stating that an evaluation of the patient's clinical status was performed prior to subsequent administration of sedation and analgesia.

3. *Consent for Sedation*
   A. The patient or the patient's parent/legal representative must be informed about the risks and benefits and must consent to the proposed sedation plan.
   B. Documentation of informed consent will be included in the medical record. This may be included with consent for the procedure.

4. *NPO Guidelines*
   A. Verification of NPO status in adult patients shall occur before the start of sedation and analgesia, and the patient shall be NPO for at least 4 hours prior to the procedure unless the physician has weighed the benefits for a shorter NPO period and it is documented in the medical record.
   B. Verification of NPO status in pediatric patients shall occur before the start of sedation and analgesia. For elective procedures, the child shall receive no solids or nonhuman milk for **4 hours** before sedation unless the risk of nutritional deprivation outweighs the benefit of NPO in the estimation of the physician.
      Small amounts of clear liquids or human milk are acceptable up to **2 hours** before sedation and analgesia. Children at risk for regurgitation or aspiration (e.g., known gastroesophageal reflux, extreme obesity) may benefit from pharmacologic therapy to reduce gastric volume and increase gastric pH before sedation or from a longer NPO period of time prior to the procedure. If delayed gastric emptying is present, an Anesthesiology or gastrointestinal consult should be considered before sedation and analgesia.
   C. Certain radiologic procedures require the administration of oral fluids in conjunction with sedation and analgesia. Risk of aspiration during these procedures must be weighed against the benefits of sedation and analgesia.

Continued

BOX 1-4—cont'd

Equipment:
Equipment must be available that is appropriate for the size of the child or adult being sedated and must be checked before sedation and analgesia are given. Minimum equipment in the area of the sedated patient **must include:**
1. A self-inflating positive-pressure oxygen delivery system capable of administering oxygen at a 10 L/min flow rate for at least 60 minutes or a flow-inflating resuscitation bag system (i.e., Mapleson-D). Note: A full E-cylinder (2200 psi) holds about 600 L of oxygen.
2. Appropriate sizes of airway management equipment (e.g., masks, oral airways, endotracheal tubes, and laryngoscopes). Note: May be on the resuscitation cart.
3. A suction apparatus with catheters and Yankauer-type rigid suction device.
4. Monitors including those capable of measuring:
   A. Oxygenation (pulse oximeter)
   B. Blood pressure (automated or manual device)
   C. Heart rate
5. Emergency resuscitation cart or kit as approved by the Hospital Code Blue Committee including a defibrillator and ECG device.
6. Telephone or other device capable of summoning assistance in an emergency.

Sedation Management:
1. *Monitoring and Documentation of the Procedure*
   A. Baseline vital signs shall be recorded in the sedation record before administering sedation and analgesia.
   B. During sedation, the following vital signs shall be monitored and documented in the sedation record at **5-minute intervals:**
      1. Heart rate: continuous monitoring. This must be done by ECG in all patients with cardiac or pulmonary disease and may be monitored by pulse oximetry in all other patients.
      2. Respiratory rate
      3. Oxygen saturation (pulse oximeter): continuous monitoring
      4. Blood pressure
   C. The patient's general appearance and responses to stimulation are extremely important parameters and should be assessed and documented periodically. Additionally, special attention should be paid to the positioning of the patient after sedation and analgesia because airway obstruction and peripheral neurologic injury can occur.
   D. Alternative monitors may be used and alternative vital signs measured in situations when:
      1. The use of conventional monitors would be unsafe, as in hyperbaric atmospheres, in water, or in an MRI.
      2. The use of conventional monitors would preclude imaging procedures because they would:
         a. distort the image or,
         b. stimulate movement and produce artifact (e.g., BP cuffs in children, verbal stimulation or responses during head CT or MRI).
   In these situations, alternative vital sign(s) shall be measured and documented in the sedation record.

2. *Staff Qualifications*
   A. The person monitoring sedation and analgesia cannot be the same person who performs the procedure unless the procedure is itself that of monitoring (i.e., EEG).
   B. The person(s) administering and monitoring sedation and analgesia shall:
      1. Be familiar with the effects of the drugs used.
      2. Know how to recognize airway obstruction and correct it.
      3. Know how to monitor required parameters, how to recognize abnormalities in the required parameters, and how to intervene.
      4. Be able to manage ventilation with a self-inflating bag valve mask (see equipment section).
   C. A person who can initiate cardiopulmonary resuscitation shall be available in the immediate area.
   D. Privileges
      1. LIPs who order sedation and analgesia shall apply for privileges to do so from the office of the Chief of Staff.

3. *Medications*
   A. Drugs which can be incrementally dosed are preferred. Special attention should be paid to calculate dosage on a weight basis (mg/kg) instead of using fixed dosages.
   B. Pharmacologic antagonists, including naloxone and flumazenil, should be immediately available in the sedation suite or in the emergency cart.
   C. All IV sedation and analgesia should be performed at the location of the procedure.
   D. All drugs administered for sedation and analgesia shall have dose and time of administration recorded.

Continued

BOX 1-4—cont'd

4. Intravenous Access
IV access is required for patients receiving IV sedation and analgesia, and personnel must be proximally available to secure IV access in patients receiving sedation and analgesia by other routes of administration (e.g., PO, IM, PR, intranasal) in case of emergency.

Post-Procedure Management (Procedure Area, Recovery Area, or Inpatient Unit Area):
Post-sedation recovery management may be done either in a designated special care area or on an inpatient unit as long as the following criteria are met:

1. Equipment
Suction, positive-pressure oxygen delivery system, airway management equipment, monitoring equipment, and resuscitation equipment equivalent to that used in the sedation area shall be immediately available.

2. Monitoring
A. Post-procedure Monitoring
Vital signs including blood pressure, heart rate, respiratory rate, and oxygen saturation shall be taken and documented at **15-minute** intervals (or more often as needed).
B. Discontinuation of Monitoring
Monitoring shall be continued until post-sedation discharge criteria have been met (see section 4, Discharge Criteria).

3. Transfer/Transport
Conditions for transporting patients who have undergone sedation and analgesia are as follows:
A. A patient recovering from sedation and analgesia may be transferred to another unit prior to discharge criteria being met, if the unit receiving the patient provides the same level of post-procedure care monitoring and arrangements have been made with the nursing staff.
B. Report should be given to the unit nursing staff including any significant complications which occurred during or following the sedation. The nurse responsible for the patient should review the record of the procedure and sedation. This report should include the patient's pre-sedation medical history, sedation administered, observed side effects or complications, and use, if any, of pharmacologic antagonists. Post-procedure orders should be written by the responsible physician, including appropriate monitoring requirements.
C. During transport of a patient **under sedation and analgesia** (i.e., patient has not met discharge criteria), the patient shall be accompanied by a person who can initiate cardiopulmonary resuscitation and has appropriate qualifications and equipment for monitoring sedation en route as defined in the Sedation Management section of the policy.

4. Discharge Criteria
A. **All** of the following criteria must be met prior to discontinuation of post-procedure monitoring or discharge from the facility with a responsible person. Definition: A responsible person is someone who can receive and understand instructions, stay with the patient, and call for assistance as instructed.
   1. Patient is easily awakened by normal or softly spoken verbal commands.
   2. Patient is oriented when awake as appropriate for age.
   3. All vital signs are stable.
   4. There is **no significant risk** of losing protective reflexes.
   5. Patient is able to maintain pre-procedure mobility **with minimal assistance as appropriate for the procedure.**
   6. Minimal nausea and/or dizziness.
B. For all adult patients to be discharged from the facility without a responsible person the following criteria must be met prior to discharge:
   1. Patient **remains awake** without stimulus for 30 minutes.
   2. Patient is oriented as appropriate for age.
   3. All vital signs are stable.
   4. There is **no significant risk** of losing protective reflexes.
   5. Patient is able to maintain pre-procedure mobility **without assistance.**
   6. No nausea and/or dizziness.
   7. Satisfactory transportation arrangements have been indicated by the patient that do not require the patient to operate a motor vehicle.
C. The person responsible for the patient (or the adult patient if meeting *criteria specified in B*) shall receive written instructions prior to discharge from the facility that include:
   1. Information about expected behavior following sedation.
   2. Instructions for eating.

Continued

BOX 1-4—cont'd

3. Warning signs of complications.
4. Special instructions in case of emergency.
5. A telephone number to contact the medical service responsible for the patient's care that is available 24 hours per day.
6. A notation shall be placed in the medical record that instructions were received and understood by a responsible person or adult patient (if meeting criteria specified in B).

Quality Assessment and Improvement:
Ongoing quality assessment and improvement is the responsibility of the service administering sedation and analgesia. Quality assessment and sedation and analgesia policy indicator compliance will be monitored quarterly and reported to the individual units, unit directors, and Department Chairs responsible for administration of sedation and analgesia.

Reprinted with permission: from American Society of Anesthesiologists, Park Ridge, IL; website: www.asahq.org.

representatives involved in postsedation care, critical care, and risk management. Six hundred questionnaires were mailed directly to inpatient and outpatient healthcare providers and registered nurses who administer conscious sedation. The 275 responses represent a 47% rate of return. Practice settings of respondents featured in Figure 1-2 included critical care units (adult/pediatric); emergency departments; gastroenterology offices; radiology units; short-procedure units; operating room suites, and ambulatory care units. The size of the facilities surveyed in which respondents practice is highlighted in Figure 1-3. The results of the survey identify current trends in the educational preparation of nurses who administer conscious sedation.

Results with respect to statutory regulations and position statements revealed 66% of the nurses surveyed were aware that their state boards of nursing had position statements or practice guidelines regarding conscious sedation. However,

58% of those who were aware of the existence of this information reported that they had never read the practice guidelines promulgated by their respective state boards. Of the respondents who reported knowledge of state board of nursing practice standards, 65% worked in settings where the practice guidelines were not available. This is an alarmingly high rate when one considers that state boards of nursing define the legal scope of practice issues related to the administration of sedation and analgesia by registered nurses. Often, the guidelines promulgated by state boards of nursing are very prescriptive as to duties to be assumed by the sedation nurse. Guidelines in some states require administration of the first dose of sedation/analgesia medication by the physician, physician presence during the administration of additional medication, specific monitoring requirements, and basic and advanced cardiac life-support requirements for nurses administering and participating in the management of patients receiving sedation/analgesia.

FIGURE 1-1 Relationship among clinical practice standards, practice guidelines, and position statements. (From Foster S, Callahan M. *Professional Study and Resource Guide for CRNA.* Park Ridge, IL, AANA Publishing; 2001:257.)

BOX 1-5

Professional Nursing Organizations Liaison Forum, Washington, DC, July 1991

American Association of Critical Care Nurses (AACN)
American Association of Nurse Anesthetists (AANA)
American Nurses Association (ANA)
Association of Operating Room Nurses (AORN)
Association of Pediatric Oncology Nurses (APON)
American Society of Postanesthesia Nurses (ASPAN)
American Society of Pain Management Nurses (ASPMN)
American Society of Plastic and Reconstructive Surgical Nurses (ASPRN)
Emergency Nurses Association (ENA)
Intravenous Nurses Society, Inc. (INS)
National Flight Nurses Association (NFNA)
Nursing Pain Association (NPA)
Oncology Nurses Society (ONS)
Society of Gastroenterology Nurses and Associates (SGNA)

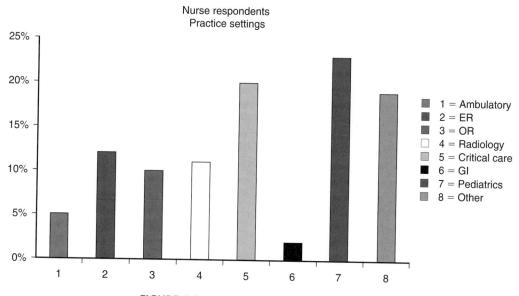

FIGURE 1-2 Nurse respondents practice settings.

The total hours of clinical and didactic instruction received by survey respondents before administering sedation/analgesia are highlighted in Figure 1-4; the numbers are surprisingly low. **The fact that so few hours of educational training and preparation are incorporated into the clinical and didactic education of nurses seems supportive of the recommendation of a standardized core curriculum (Box 1-6) related to the preparation of healthcare providers participating in the administration and management of patients receiving sedation/analgesia.** A standardized *core curriculum* provides consistent educational preparation through in-services, learning modules, and didactic/clinical workshops.

> A standardized "core curriculum" provides sedation educators and practitioners with a mechanism to assure entry-level competence in providing quality patient care.

As Dr. Charles Cote succinctly states, "rather than wasting time establishing and publishing new guidelines and protocols, it would be more useful to devote our energies toward developing scientifically documented safer methods for sedation and **programs to educate the practitioner about the pharmacology and pharmacodynamics of the drug used.**"[18]

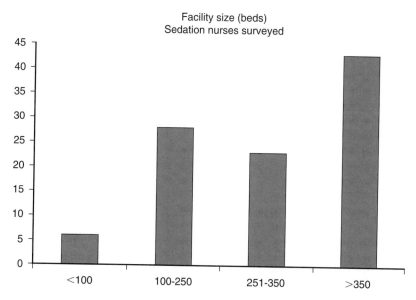

FIGURE 1-3 Facility size (beds) sedation nurses surveyed.

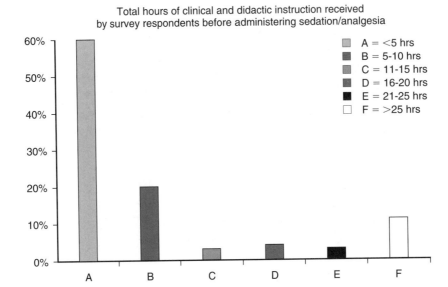

Total hours of clinical and didactic instruction received
by survey respondents before administering sedation/analgesia

A = <5 hrs
B = 5-10 hrs
C = 11-15 hrs
D = 16-20 hrs
E = 21-25 hrs
F = >25 hrs

FIGURE 1-4 Totals hours of clinical and didactic instruction received by survey respondents before administering sedation/analgesia.

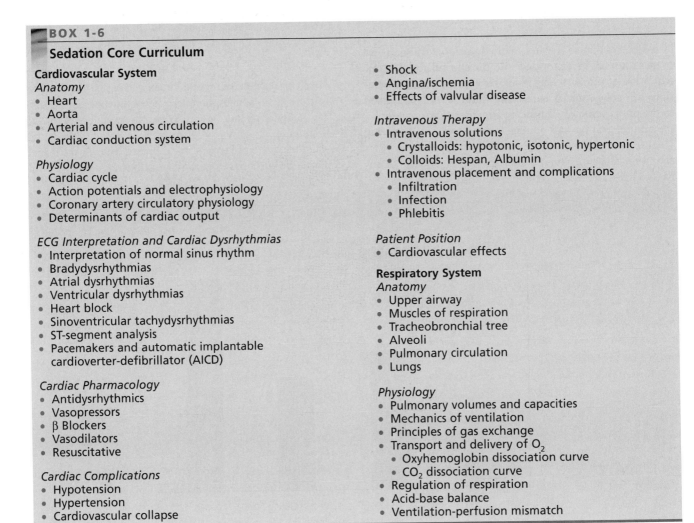

BOX 1-6

Sedation Core Curriculum

Cardiovascular System
Anatomy
- Heart
- Aorta
- Arterial and venous circulation
- Cardiac conduction system

Physiology
- Cardiac cycle
- Action potentials and electrophysiology
- Coronary artery circulatory physiology
- Determinants of cardiac output

ECG Interpretation and Cardiac Dysrhythmias
- Interpretation of normal sinus rhythm
- Bradydysrhythmias
- Atrial dysrhythmias
- Ventricular dysrhythmias
- Heart block
- Sinoventricular tachydysrhythmias
- ST-segment analysis
- Pacemakers and automatic implantable cardioverter-defibrillator (AICD)

Cardiac Pharmacology
- Antidysrhythmics
- Vasopressors
- β Blockers
- Vasodilators
- Resuscitative

Cardiac Complications
- Hypotension
- Hypertension
- Cardiovascular collapse

- Shock
- Angina/ischemia
- Effects of valvular disease

Intravenous Therapy
- Intravenous solutions
  - Crystalloids: hypotonic, isotonic, hypertonic
  - Colloids: Hespan, Albumin
- Intravenous placement and complications
  - Infiltration
  - Infection
  - Phlebitis

Patient Position
- Cardiovascular effects

Respiratory System
Anatomy
- Upper airway
- Muscles of respiration
- Tracheobronchial tree
- Alveoli
- Pulmonary circulation
- Lungs

Physiology
- Pulmonary volumes and capacities
- Mechanics of ventilation
- Principles of gas exchange
- Transport and delivery of O_2
  - Oxyhemoglobin dissociation curve
  - CO_2 dissociation curve
- Regulation of respiration
- Acid-base balance
- Ventilation-perfusion mismatch

Continued

BOX 1-6—cont'd

Pharmacologic Effects on Pulmonary Mechanics
- Respiratory depression/obstruction
  - Hypercarbia
  - Hypoxemia
  - Respiratory insufficiency
- Laryngospasm
- Bronchospasm
- Aspiration pneumonitis

Pulmonary Disease
- Asthma
- Bronchitis
- Snoring, stridor, obstructive sleep apnea
- Obesity

Oxygen Delivery Devices
- Oxygen tanks and hospital pipelines
- Nasal cannula
- Face mask
  - Partial rebreather
  - Nonrebreather
  - Venturi mask
- Face tent
- Ambu bag
- Mapleson system
- T-Piece or Brigg's
- Mechanical ventilation

Patient Position
- Pulmonary effects

Airway Management and Assessment
Airway Assessment
- Mallampati classification
- Abnormal anatomy
  - Hypognathic (recessed) jaw
  - Hypergnathic (protruding) jaw
  - Deviated trachea
  - Large tongue
  - Short, thick neck
  - Protruding teeth
  - High arched palate
  - Small mouth opening
  - Limited range of motion
  - Arthritis

Airway Management
- Mechanical methods to relieve obstruction
  - Head tilt
  - Chin lift
  - Jaw thrust
  - Nasal airway
  - Oral airway
  - Endotracheal intubation
- Pharmacologic methods to relieve respiratory depression
  - Romazicon (Flumazenil)
  - Narcan (Naloxone)
- Methods to relieve laryngospasm
  - Positive-pressure ventilation
  - Succinylcholine (Anectine)
- Methods to relieve bronchospasm
  - Inhaled bronchodilators
  - β_2-adrenergic agonists

- Sympathomimetics
- Methylxanthines
- Corticosteroids

Total Patient Care Considerations
Presedation Assessment
Goals of Presedation Patient Assessment
Patient Selection
Medical History and Sedation Considerations
- Cardiovascular assessment
  - Coronary artery disease
  - Myocardial infarction
  - Presence of dysrhythmias
  - Pacemakers
  - Defibrillators
  - Automatic implantable cardioverter-defibrillator
- Pulmonary assessment
  - Chronic obstructive pulmonary disease: asthma, bronchitis
  - Obstructive sleep apnea
- Hepatic assessment
  - Enzyme induction
  - Hepatitis
  - Cirrhosis
- Renal assessment
  - Renal insufficiency
  - Dialysis
- Neurologic assessment
  - Convulsive disorders
  - Stroke
  - Carotid artery and vertebral disease
  - Peripheral nervous system assessment
- Endocrine assessment
  - Diabetes
  - Thyroid disease
  - Adrenal cortical disease: Cushing's disease, Addison's disease, Conn's syndrome, hypoaldosteronism
- Adrenal medulla disease:
- Pheochromocytoma
- Gastrointestinal assessment
  - Gastroesophageal reflux
  - Ulcer disease

Anesthesia and Surgical History
Medication Evaluation
Allergies
- Anaphylactic reaction
- Anaphylactoid reaction
- Latex allergy

Presedation Laboratory Data Clinical Considerations
Dentition Evaluation and Implications
Social History
- Tobacco use
- Drug abuse/intake
- Opioid abuse
- Stimulant medications
- Benzodiazepine abuse
- Marijuana abuse
- Herbal use

Continued

BOX 1-6—cont'd

Pregnancy Status
- Cardiovascular effects
- Pulmonary effects
- Gastrointestinal effects
- Procedural management implications

NPO Status
- NPO instructions
- NPO compliance

Informed Consent
ASA Physical Status Classification System
- ASA 1-3

Presedation Patient Instructions
- NPO
- Time of arrival
- Responsible adult
- Procedure specific requirements

Focused Physical Examination
- Vital signs
- Airway
- Heart
- Lungs

Procedural Care
- Patient monitoring
  - Electrocardiogram
  - Blood pressure
  - Pulse oximetry
  - Level of consciousness
  - End-tidal carbon dioxide
  - Bispectral index monitoring
- Administration of medications
  - Oxygen
  - Sedatives
  - Analgesics
  - Hypnotics
- Healthcare practitioner/nursing care
  - Subjective/objective patient assessment
  - Complications

Post-Sedation Patient Care
- Purpose
- Patient assessment
  - Patient monitoring
  - Vital signs every 5 minutes
- Objective numerical discharge scoring
  - Activity, respiration, circulation, level of consciousness, oxygen saturation, dressing, pain, ambulation, fasting, urine output
- Post-sedation teaching and discharge instructions
- Patient discharge and post-sedation follow-up
  - Presence of competent caregiver

Sedation Pharmacology
Definitions
- Minimal sedation (anxiolysis)
- Moderate sedation/analgesia (formerly conscious sedation)
- Deep sedation/analgesia
- General anesthesia

Goals and Objectives
Benzodiazepines
- Pharmacokinetics
- Pharmacodynamics
- Clinical considerations
  - Diazepam (Valium)
  - Midazolam (Versed)
  - Lorazepam (Ativan)

Opioids
- Pharmacokinetics
- Pharmacodynamics
- Clinical considerations
  - Altentanil (Alfenta)
  - Morphine sulfate
  - Meperidine (Demerol)
  - Hydromorphone (Dilaudid)
  - Fentanyl (Sublimaze)

Sedative/Hypnotics
- Pharmacokinetics
- Pharmacodynamics
- Clinical considerations
  - Propofol (Diprivan)

Dissociative Anesthetics
- Pharmacokinetics
- Pharmacodynamics
- Clinical considerations
  - Ketamine (Ketalar)

Butyrophenones
- Pharmacokinetics
- Pharmacodynamics
- Clinical considerations
  - Droperidol (Inapsine)

Local Anesthetics
- Pharmacokinetics
- Pharmacodynamics
- Clinical considerations
  - Ester
    - Chloroprocaine (Nesacaine)
    - Cocaine
    - Procaine (Novocain)
    - Tetracaine (Pontocaine)
  - Amides
    - Bupivacaine (Marcaine)
    - Etidocaine (Duranest)
    - Lidocaine (Xylocaine)
    - Mepivicaine (Carbocaine)
    - Prilocaine (Citanest)
    - Benzocaine (Hurricaine, Americaine)
    - Ropivacaine

Pharmacologic Antagonists
- Pharmacokinetics
- Pharmacodynamics

Continued

BOX 1-6—cont'd

- Clinical considerations
  - Romazicon (Flumazenil)
  - Naloxone Hydrochloride (Narcan)

Techniques of Administration
- Titration to clinical effect technique
- Bolus technique
- Continuous infusion technique

Specific Patient Populations
Geriatrics and Pediatrics
- Defined
- Terminology

Systems Review and Sedation Considerations
- Cardiovascular
- Respiratory
- Renal
- Hepatic
- Central nervous system
- Thermoregulation

Pharmacokinetic and Pharmacodynamic Considerations
- Dosage requirements/alterations
- Clinical considerations

Airway Considerations
- Anatomic

Psychological Well-Being
Legal Scope of Practice
Practice Standards
- Joint Commission on Accreditation of Healthcare Organizations Standards *for Additional Special Procedures: Standards for Operative or other High-Risk Procedures and/or the Administration of Moderate or Deep Sedation or Anesthesia*

Practice Guidelines
- American Society of Anesthesiologists Task Force on Sedation and Analgesia by Non-Anesthesiologists. Practice Guidelines for Sedation and Analgesia by Non-Anesthesiologists. *Anesthesiology.* 2002;96(4)

Position Statements
- American Nurses Association
- Specialty organizations

Risk Management and Performance Improvement
- Quality defined
- Performance improvement process

Implementation of Sedation Educational Program
- Policy development
- Educational process
- Administrative/management support
- Competency assessment

SUMMARY

The administration of sedation/analgesia for diagnostic, therapeutic, or surgical procedures is a highly specialized skill. Clinicians engaged in the art and science of administering sedation and analgesia must be trained to recognize the fine line between a tranquil amnestic patient and an unconscious, unresponsive patient. To satisfactorily achieve the objectives of sedation/analgesia and provide adequate sedation with minimal risk, educational preparation and competency validation should be focused on:

- Cardiovascular anatomy and physiology
- Respiratory anatomy and physiology
- Airway assessment and management
- Presedation, procedural, and postsedation patient care
- Pharmacology
- Legal scope of practice issues

To maximize patient safety during sedation/analgesia these objectives must be achieved. Topical areas will be highlighted throughout this text.

LEARNER SELF-ASSESSMENT

In order to achieve maximal educational benefit from this chapter, please complete the Learner Self-Assessment below. This self-assessment tool provides the ability to identify areas requiring additional review. Reference material for each question is provided in Appendix F.

1. Healthcare practitioner considerations associated with **JCAHO Standards** related to the administration of sedation by qualified personnel include:

2. As outlined in the **"Continuum of Sedation,"** the following states of sedation and anesthesia are defined as:
   a. Minimal sedation

   b. Moderate sedation/analgesia

   c. Deep sedation/analgesia

   d. Anesthesia

3. The **goals and objectives** associated with the administration of moderate sedation/analgesia include:
   a.

   b.

   c.

   d.

   e.

4. The **clinical endpoints** associated with a state of "moderate sedation" include:
   a.

   b.

5. Identify specific **legal scope-of-practice issues** related to the administration of sedation/analgesia by non-anesthesia personnel as they relate to:
   a. Practice standards

   b. Practice guidelines

   c. Position statements

POST-TEST QUESTIONS

Please note: If you are applying for CE credit, you must contact Specialty Health Education, Inc. @ 800-694-8041 for a CE Application Packet.

1. Which of the following is NOT an objective of moderate sedation? _____
   A. Guard the patient's safety and welfare
   B. Maintain adequate sedation with minimal risk
   C. Allay patient fear and anxiety
   D. Produce an unconscious patient

2. A drug-induced depression of consciousness during which patients respond purposefully to verbal commands, either alone or accompanied by light tactile stimulation, no interventions are required to maintain a patent airway, spontaneous ventilation is adequate, and cardiovascular function is usually maintained is defined as which of the following states of sedation? _____
   A. Minimal sedation
   B. Moderate sedation
   C. Deep sedation
   D. General anesthesia

3. Which of the following states of sedation was formerly defined as conscious sedation? _____
   A. Minimal sedation
   B. Moderate sedation
   C. Deep sedation
   D. General anesthesia

4. Which of the following characteristics best describes a patient in a state of "deep sedation?" _____
   A. Ventilation = adequate; cardiovascular function usually maintained
   B. Ventilation = unaffected; cardiovascular function unaffected
   C. Ventilation = may be inadequate, cardiovascular function usually maintained
   D. Airway = unaffected; responsiveness is normal response to verbal stimulation

5. Which of the following states may predispose the patient to an increased incidence of respiratory depression, decreased response to the hypoxic drive, and cardiovascular depression? _____

   A. General anesthesia
   B. Deep sedation
   C. Moderate sedation
   D. Minimal sedation

6. Cardiovascular function may be impaired in which of the following states according to the "Continuum of Sedation?" _____
   A. General anesthesia
   B. Deep sedation
   C. Moderate sedation
   D. Minimal sedation

7. Which of the following is the highest mandate for clinical behavior? _____
   A. Position statements
   B. Practice guidelines
   C. Practice standards
   D. Hospital policy

8. Guides to provide behavior and critical decision making that are commonly accepted within a professional discipline include _____.
   A. Position statements
   B. Practice guidelines
   C. Practice standards
   D. Hospital policy

9. The "Endorsement of Position Statements on the Role of the Registered Nurse in the Management of Patients Receiving IV Conscious Sedation for Short-Term Therapeutic, Diagnostic, or Surgical Procedures" is an example of a _____.
   A. Practice standard
   B. Practice guideline
   C. Position statement
   D. Hospital policy

10. The term *conscious sedation* was initially described in the _____ literature.
   A. Gastroenterology
   B. Pediatric
   C. Critical care
   D. Dental

REFERENCES

1. Mokhashi M, Hawes R.: Struggling toward easier endoscopy. *Gastrointest Endosc.* 1998;48:432-440.
2. Murphy M. Sedation. *Ann Emerg Med.* 1996;27:461-463.
3. Nurses uneasy about IV sedation for long cases. *OR Manager.* 2000;16(3):1-3.
4. Robins E, Bozadjian E. Developing a competency based program for conscious sedation. *Crit Care Nurs Clin North Am.* 1997;9:273-279.
5. Kortbawi P. Developing a conscious sedation program: From policy development through quality improvement. *Gastroenterol Nurs.* 1997;20:34-41.
6. Association of Operating Room Nurses. *Standards, Recommended Practices and Guidelines.* Denver: AORN; 2002:185-194.
7. American Nurses Association. *Policy Statement on Conscious Sedation.* Washington, DC: The Association, 1991.
8. *Standards for Additional Special Procedures: Standards for Operative or other High-Risk Procedures and/or the Administration of Moderate or Deep Sedation or Anesthesia.* Comprehensive Accreditation Manual for Hospitals: The Official Handbook. Joint Commission on Accreditation of Healthcare Organizations. Oakbrook Terrace, IL, 2004.
9. Bennett C. *Conscious Sedation in Dental Practice,* 2nd ed. St. Louis: CV Mosby, 1978.
10. American Society of Anesthesiologists. *Continuum of Depth of Sedation: Definitions of General Anesthesia and Levels of Sedation/Analgesia.* Park Ridge, IL, ASA House of Delegates, October 13, 1999.
11. American Society of Anesthesiologists. Practice guidelines for sedation and analgesia by non-anesthesiologists. *Anesthesiology.* 2002;96:1004-1017.
12. Bailey P, Pace N, Ashburn M, et al. Frequent hypoxemia and apnea after sedation with midazolam and fentanyl. *Anesthesiology.* 1990;73:826.
13. Scammon F, Klein S, Choi W. Conscious sedation for procedures under local or topical anesthesia. *Ann Otol Rhinol Laryngol.* 1985;92:21.
14. Gunn I. The many issues regarding intravenous conscious sedation. *Specialty Nursing Forum.* 1990;2:3.
15. Nemiroff M. IV conscious sedation: Essential techniques of monitoring. *Trends Health Care Law Ethics.* 1993;8:1.
16. Endorsement of position statement on the role of the registered nurse (RN) in the management of patients receiving IV conscious sedation. Washington, DC: American Nurses Association, 1991.
17. Kost M, Brown D, Dezayas B. The administration of conscious sedation by non-anesthesia personnel. *Anesthesia Today.* 11(2):2000.
18. Coté C. Sedation protocols: Why so many variations? *Pediatrics.* 94(3):1995.

CHAPTER 2

Presedation Assessment and Patient Selection

At the completion of this chapter, the learner shall:

◆ Identify JCAHO standards and intents related to presedation patient assessment.

◆ Identify "Practice Guidelines for Sedation and Analgesia by Non-Anesthesiologists" related to presedation patient assessment.

◆ List the goals of presedation patient assessment.

◆ Identify two methods utilized to calculate ideal body weight.

◆ State the components of the patient's medical history and its impact on procedural care.

◆ List specific physiologic alterations in the cardiovascular, pulmonary, hepatic, renal, neurologic, and endocrine systems identified in the presedation patient assessment and their implications for procedural patient care.

◆ State the implications for the sedation plan of care based on the patient's past surgical/anesthesia history.

◆ List the treatment protocol for an allergic reaction.

◆ Identify the sedation patient population that requires presedation laboratory testing.

◆ State the sedation patient care considerations associated with positive findings on social history including:

• Tobacco use

• Alcohol consumption

• Substance abuse

• Herbal product use

• Pregnancy

◆ State the current recommended NPO guidelines for sedation patients.

◆ Define assault and battery as it relates to informed consent.

◆ Utilize the ASA Physical Status Classification System to assign a numerical summary assessment at the conclusion of the presedation patient interview.

Joint Commission on Accreditation of Healthcare Organizations Standards for Operative or Other High-Risk Procedures and/or the Administration of Moderate or Deep Sedation or Anesthesia

Standard PC.13.20

Operative or other procedures and/or the administration of moderate or deep sedation or anesthesia are planned.

Rationale for PC.13.20

Because the response to procedures is not always predictable and sedation-to-anesthesia is a continuum, it is not always possible to predict how an individual patient will respond. Therefore, qualified individuals are trained in professional standards and techniques to manage patients in the case of a potentially harmful event.

Elements of Performance for PC.13.20

1. Sufficient numbers of qualified staff are available* to evaluate the patient, perform the procedure, monitor, and recover the patient.

2. Individuals administering moderate or deep sedation and anesthesia are qualified† and have the appropriate credentials to manage patients at whatever level of sedation or anesthesia is achieved, either intentionally or unintentionally.

3. A registered nurse supervises perioperative nursing care.

4. Appropriate equipment to monitor the patient's physiologic status is available.

5. Appropriate equipment to administer intravenous fluids and drugs, including blood and blood components, is available as needed.

6. Resuscitation capabilities are available.

Before operative and other procedures or the administration of moderate or deep sedation or anesthesia:

7. Patient acuity is assessed to plan for the appropriate level of postprocedure care.

8. ***Preprocedural education, treatments, and services are provided according to the plan for care, treatment, and services.***

9. The site, procedure, and patient are accurately identified and clearly communicated before surgery.

10. ***A presedation or preanesthesia assessment is conducted.***

11. ***Before sedating or anesthetizing a patient, a licensed independent practitioner with appropriate clinical privileges plans or concurs with the planned anesthesia.***

12. ***The patient is reevaluated immediately before moderate or deep sedation and before anesthesia induction.***

---

*For hospitals providing obstetric or emergency operative services, this means they can provide anesthesia services as required by law and regulation.

†**Qualified** The individuals providing moderate or deep sedation and anesthesia have at a minimum had competency-based education, training, and experience in the following:
1. Evaluating patients before moderate or deep sedation and anesthesia.
2. Performing the moderate or deep sedation and anesthesia, including rescuing patients who slip into a deeper-than-desired level of sedation or analgesia. This includes the following:
   a. *Moderate* sedation – are qualified to rescue patients from deep sedation and are competent to manage a compromised airway and to provide adequate oxygenation and ventilation.
   b. *Deep* sedation – are qualified to rescue patients from general anesthesia and are competent to manage an unstable cardiovascular system as well as a compromised airway and inadequate oxygenation and ventilation.

© Joint Commission: Standards for Operative or Other High-Risk Procedures and/or the Administration of Moderate or Deep Sedation or Anesthesia, January, 2004. Reprinted with permission.

Practice Guidelines for Sedation and Analgesia by Non-Anesthesiologists

American Society of Anesthesiologists Task Force on Sedation and Analgesia by Non-Anesthesiologists

Recommendations. Clinicians administering sedation/analgesia should be familiar with sedation-oriented aspects of the patient's medical history and how these might alter the patient's response to sedation/analgesia. These include: (1) abnormalities of the major organ systems; (2) previous adverse experience with sedation/analgesia as well as regional and general anesthesia; (3) drug allergies, current medications, and potential drug interactions;

(4) time and nature of last oral intake; and (5) history of tobacco, alcohol, or substance use or abuse. Patients presenting for sedation/analgesia should undergo a focused physical examination, including vital signs, auscultation of the heart and lungs, and evaluation of the airway. (Example I, "Airway Assessment Procedures for Sedation and Analgesia" [see Chapter 7]). Preprocedure laboratory testing should be guided by the patient's underlying medical condition and the likelihood that the results will affect the management of sedation/analgesia. These evaluations should be confirmed immediately before the sedation is initiated.

Recommendation. Whenever possible, appropriate medical specialists should be consulted before the administration of sedation to patients with significant underlying conditions. The choice of specialists depends on the nature of the underlying condition and the urgency of the situation. For severely compromised or medically unstable patients (e.g., anticipated difficult airway, severe obstructive pulmonary disease, coronary artery disease, or congestive heart failure), or if it is likely that sedation to the point of unresponsiveness will be necessary to obtain adequate conditions, practitioners who are not trained in the administration of general anesthesia should consult an anesthesiologist.

From American Society of Anesthesiologists Task Force on Sedation and Analgesia by Non-Anesthesiologists. Practice guidelines for sedation and analgesia by non-anesthesiologists. *Anesthesiology.* 2002;96(4):1006, 1013. Reprinted with permission.

PRESEDATION PATIENT ASSESSMENT

The goals of a thorough presedation assessment include:
1. Identify presedation risk factors.
2. Assure each patient's physiologic condition is optimized before the procedure.
3. Reduce patient anxiety through education and communication.
4. Ensure adequate presedation planning and patient education.
5. Obtain informed consent.
6. Optimize patient care, satisfaction, and comfort.
7. Evaluate the patient's health status, determining if any presedation investigation or specialty consultations are required.
8. Formulate a sedation plan.
9. Communicate patient management issues between providers.

Presedation assessment must be conducted in an unhurried, reassuring atmosphere. Adequate time must be allotted to alleviate the patient's anxiety while allowing sufficient time to gather data and answer the patient's questions. When feasible, presedation assessment should be conducted several days before the proposed procedure. This assessment is best conducted in conjunction with the healthcare provider who will participate in the administration of sedation. Emergent cases may preclude the clinician's ability to obtain a presedation assessment in a relaxed atmosphere. Nonetheless, a complete assessment is still required before the administration of sedation. The assessment should be documented in the patient's record.

Thorough presedation assessment allows the clinician time to gather additional data, order indicated laboratory and diagnostic tests, and implement a sedation plan. The presedation assessment period should attempt to identify patient risk factors that may lead to complications while affording the clinician the opportunity to assure that the patient is in the best physical condition for the planned procedure. A comprehensive presedation assessment begins with a review of the medical record. Pertinent information recorded in the patient record offers insight into the patient's overall health status as well as an opportunity to review the patient's past medical history. In some surgicenters, clinics, or physician offices, previous hospital records are not readily available. Therefore, the patient as the medical historian is relied on to give an accurate past medical history.

In the presence of a well-documented past medical history recorded in the patient's record, the provider may use the presedation assessment period to confirm information with the patient. Patients with a significant medical history may require additional laboratory tests and screening before the procedure. By performing a presedation assessment several days before the scheduled procedure, the provider may order indicated tests, obtain specialty consultation, and request previous hospital records for review. To ensure that all presedation assessments are performed in a consistent manner and avoid the omission of key information, many clinicians follow a prescribed format when interviewing the patient. Components of this prescribed format are outlined in Box 2-1.

Initial presedation assessment starts with a review of the planned procedure. By asking the patient to confirm the planned procedure, the clinician is assured that the patient is aware of the scheduled procedure. Some patients may not be able to specifically repeat the name of the procedure or diagnostic examination. However, a basic understanding of the procedure and the anatomic area should be confirmed to ensure that the patient has been advised by the physician as to the nature of the planned intervention.

BOX 2-1

Components of Presedation Patient Assessment

- Patient age, height, weight
- Proposed procedure
- Attending physician or service

Medical History
Cardiac
- Hypertension
- Coronary artery disease
- Angina
- Exercise tolerance
- Myocardial infarction
- Cardiac dysrhythmia
- Presence of pacemaker/AICD
- Valvular heart disease

Pulmonary
- Dyspnea
- Exercise tolerance
- Asthma
- Bronchitis
- Obstructive sleep apnea
- Tobacco use

Hepatic
- Enzyme induction
- Hepatitis
- Cirrhosis
- Ascites

Renal
- Renal insufficiency
- Renal failure
- Dialysis

Neurologic
- Cerebrovascular insufficiency
- Carotid artery and vertebral basilar disease
- Stroke
- Convulsive disorders
- Headaches
- Syncope
- Peripheral nervous system assessment

Endocrine
- Diabetes
- Hyper/hypothyroidism
- Adrenal disease

Gastrointestinal
- Nausea
- Vomiting
- Recent weight loss
- Hiatal hernia

Hematology
- Anemia
- Aspirin, NSAID use
- Excessive bleeding

Musculoskeletal
- Arthritis
- Back pain
- Joint pain

Surgical History
- Anesthesia complications (nausea, vomiting, delayed emergence)
- Diagnostic procedures
- Family anesthesia history
- Operations

Medications
- Name
- Dosage
- Patient compliance

Allergies
- Anaphylactic
- Anaphylactoid
- Side effects

Laboratory Data
- Additional laboratory profiles
- Chest radiograph
- Electrocardiogram
- Electrolytes

Dentition
- Capped teeth
- Loose/chipped teeth

Social History
- Tobacco use
- Alcohol use
- Illicit drug use
- Herbal use
- Possibility of pregnancy

NPO Status
- Instructions
- Liquids
- Solids

Informed Consent
- Patient questions answered
- Written consent obtained
- Patient instructions given

ASA Physical Status Classification
- ASA Risk 1-3

Name of presedation evaluator and date

Completion of the presedation assessment must be confirmed before the administration of any sedative agents, and the patient should be reassessed immediately before the commencement of the procedure.

PATIENT SELECTION
Age

The patient's age should be noted on the presedation assessment form. Although chronologic age does not necessarily correlate with physiologic age, it should be noted.

Appreciation of the patient's functional age is far more important than the chronologic age. It is equally important to ascertain the psychologic state of the patient at the time of the presedation assessment. Psychologic characteristics and the anxiety level of the patient are assessed throughout the entire presedation process. During the initial phase of the presedation assessment some patients may interject and ask, "What are you going to do to me?" or "What are you going to give me?" It is important to reiterate to the patient that once you conclude your assessment you will answer questions related to the patient's upcoming plan of care. **It is premature to comment or recommend a sedation plan before a complete and thorough presedation assessment has been conducted.**

Height and Weight

It is important to record an accurate height and weight before the planned procedure. Body mass index offers a useful way to calculate a patient's ideal body weight.

BMI = (Weight in kg)/(Height in meters)²

Example:

$$70 \text{ kg}/1.7 \text{ m}^2 = 70 \text{ kg}/2.89 \text{ m} = 24 \text{ kg/m}^2$$

Interpretation:

Overweight: 25-29.9 kg/m²
Obese: 30-35 kg/m²
Morbidly obese: 35 kg/m²

Another method utilized to calculate body weight is ideal body weight. Actual patient weight is compared with ideal body weight. Obesity = 20% excess of ideal body weight when using the IBW formula.

Ideal Body Weight (IBW)
IBW (male): 105 pounds + 6 pounds
for each inch > 5 feet
IBW (female): 100 pounds + 5 pounds
for each inch > 5 feet

Assessment of ideal body weight is important because obesity has a significant impact on the cardiovascular, pulmonary, gastrointestinal, endocrine, and hepatic systems. Obesity is defined as body weight greater than ideal weight. The multisystemic effects of obesity are listed in Table 2-1. **To avoid the development of deep sedation states, dosage requirements for sedative medications should be based on ideal body weight and NOT the patient's actual weight.**

At times, management of the obese patient's airway during the administration of sedation may be challenging. Because of an increase in body mass and redundant oropharyngeal airway tissue, the patient must not be allowed to progress into a state of deep sedation. **Heightened vigilance in titration of medications is required for this patient population.** Obese patients are prone to pulmonary aspiration secondary to increased gastric volume and gastric reflux and may benefit from presedation administration

of H_2 blockers (ranitidine, famotidine) and gastric stimulants (metoclopramide). These medications are discussed in the presedation gastrointestinal assessment section of this chapter. Because of the significant challenges associated with management of obese patients, presedation concerns may require consultation with a member of the anesthesia care team. Diagnostic tests indicated for the obese patient may include a complete blood cell count, a radiograph of the chest, and a baseline electrocardiogram to rule out ventricular hypertrophy. Unless there is a specific contraindication, it is prudent to administer supplemental oxygen to all obese patients for sedation procedures. Postoperative administration of oxygen therapy should continue until the patient has fully recovered and there are no clinical signs of hypoxia.

> A plan of minimal sedation is indicated when non-anesthesia clinicians are requested to provide administration of sedation/analgesia to obese patients.

MEDICAL HISTORY: ORGAN SYSTEM ASSESSMENT
Cardiovascular System

The purpose of the presedation cardiac assessment includes:

- Assessment for the presence of preexisting cardiovascular disease
- Assessment for disease severity, stability, and prior treatment
- Identification of comorbid states
  - Diabetes, chronic obstructive pulmonary disease (COPD)
- Identification of the type of procedure to be performed
  - Assessment of inherent procedural risks
- Identification of interventions that will decrease the incidence of complications

TABLE 2-1
Multisystemic Effects of Obesity

PULMONARY	CARDIOVASCULAR	GASTROINTESTINAL
Chest wall mass ↑	Cardiac output ↑	Intra-abdominal
CO₂ production ↑	Hypertension	pressure ↑
Functional	Pulmonary	Intragastric
residual	hypertension	pressure ↑
capacity ↓↓	Stroke volume ↑	Risk of aspiration ↑
Pulmonary		
compliance ↓		
Total oxygen		
consumption ↑		
Work of		
breathing ↑		

Hypertension

Hypertension is defined as a systolic blood pressure greater than 140 mm Hg or a diastolic blood pressure greater than 90 mm Hg or more on at least two occasions measured at least 1 to 2 weeks apart.[1] Classification of systemic blood pressure for adults is identified in Table 2-2. End organs affected by hypertension include the heart, brain, and kidneys. The heart is predisposed to hypertrophic changes secondary to increased vascular resistance associated with the hypertensive state. Hypertensive damage to the intracerebral vasculature may result in hemorrhage or stroke. End-organ renal damage secondary to hypertension reduces glomerular filtration rate and renal blood flow. Systemic hypertension is a significant risk factor for the development of ischemic heart disease and is a major cause of congestive heart failure, cerebrovascular accident, arterial aneurysm, and end-stage renal disease.[2] Healthcare provider concerns associated with caring for the hypertensive patient include:

♦ Duration of hypertension (when initially diagnosed)
♦ Effectiveness of prescribed treatment plan (diet, salt restriction, medication use)
♦ Identification of medication and dosage used to treat hypertension
♦ Identification of the patient's presedation anxiety level

Unfortunately, it is estimated that fewer than one third of the patients with systemic hypertension in the United States are aware of their condition or are being adequately treated.[3]

Presedation assessment of the hypertensive patient should initially include documentation of the patient's baseline blood pressure. It is equally important to assess the patient's level of compliance with the prescribed treatment plan. During this portion of the cardiovascular assessment, dietary compliance (salt restriction, weight reduction) and antihypertensive medication efficacy assessment should be ascertained. This includes an accurate assessment and identification of medications used to treat hypertension. Common antihypertensive medications, associated side effects, and specific considerations are highlighted in Table 2-3. **To maintain a consistent plasma level of antihypertensive medications, current recommendations include administration of antihypertensive medications up to and including the day of the scheduled procedure.** It is not uncommon for patients presenting for their procedure to be hypertensive on initial presedation blood pressure screening. Presedation anxiety increases catecholamine release. At times this patient population is normotensive when presedation assessment is performed several days before the procedure and hypertensive on the day of the procedure. Management of patients in this group includes thorough patient preparation for the procedure, reassurance, and administration of the patient's morning antihypertensive medication. Once an intravenous line is established, the administration of small doses of a benzodiazepine may reduce the patient's anxiety level with a resultant decrease in blood pressure. If the blood pressure does not return to the patient's baseline or if the diastolic blood pressure remains elevated, it may be prudent to cancel the procedure. In this situation, referral of the patient to a specialist (cardiologist, internist) for further evaluation and improved blood pressure control before the procedure is recommended. Additional complications of poorly controlled hypertension include altered baroreceptor response, wide fluctuations of blood pressure during the procedure, and intravascular volume depletion.

> Hypertensive patients should receive presedation medication instructions before the planned procedure.

Coronary Artery Disease

It is vitally important to assess for the presence of myocardial ischemia in patients presenting for sedation services. Myocardial ischemia occurs when there is an imbalance between coronary blood flow and myocardial consumption. The imbalance in this supply and demand phenomenon results in the development of myocardial ischemia. Risk factors for the development of coronary artery disease and myocardial ischemia include:

♦ Male gender
♦ Increased age
♦ Hypercholesterolemia
♦ Systemic hypertension
♦ Cigarette smoking
♦ Diabetes mellitus
♦ Obesity
♦ Sedative lifestyle
♦ Family history of myocardial ischemia

When evaluating patients for coronary artery disease, it is important to ascertain a history of chest pain. Questions

TABLE 2-2

Classification of Systemic Blood Pressure for Adults*

CATEGORY	SYSTOLIC BLOOD PRESSURE (mm Hg)	DIASTOLIC BLOOD PRESSURE (mm Hg)
Optimal	<120	<80
Normal	<130	<85
High normal	130-139	85-89
Systemic hypertension		
Stage 1 (mild)	140-159	90-99
Stage 2 (moderate)	160-179	100-109
Stage 3 (severe)	≥180	≥110

*Adults are defined as individuals 18 years of age and older.
From Stoelting R, Dierdorf S. *Anesthesia and Co-Existing Disease.* 4th ed. New York: Churchill Livingstone; 2002:94. Adapted from The Sixth Report of the Joint National Committee on Prevention, Detection, Evaluation and Treatment of High Blood Pressure (JNC VI). *Arch Intern Med.* 1997;157:2413-20.

TABLE 2-3

Common Antihypertensive Medications

DRUGS	SIDE EFFECTS	SPECIAL CONSIDERATIONS
Diuretics		
Thiazides	Hypokalemia Hyperuricemia Glucose intolerance Hypercholesterolemia Hypertriglyceridemia Sexual dysfunction Alkalosis	May enhance digitalis toxicity. May precipitate acute gout. May be ineffective in renal failure. May decrease lithium clearance.
Loop diuretics	Same as for thiazide	Effective in renal failure. May precipitate gout or enhance digitalis toxicity. Hypnotratemia especially in elderly patients.

Potassium-sparing drugs
    Amiloride
    Spironolactone
	Hyperkalemia
	Sexual dysfunction
	Gynecomastia	

Adrenergic Antagonists		
Beta-Adrenergic Antagonists	Bradycardia Bronchospasm Congestive heart failure Hypertriglyceridemia Mask hypoglycemia Sedation Sexual dysfunction	Do not use in patients with asthma or COPD. Do not use in patients with CHF, sick sinus syndrome, or heart block. Use cautiously in patients with diabetes mellitus and peripheral vascular disease. Abrupt discontinuation may result in rebound sympathetic nervous system stimulation.
Centrally Acting Drugs		
Methyldopa	Drowsiness Dry mouth Fatigue	Rebound hypertension may occur when abruptly discontinued. May cause liver damage. May cause hemolytic anemia (Coombs' test). Decreases anesthetic requirements.
Reserpine	Fatigue Nasal congestion Sexual dysfunction	Do not use in patients with a history of mental depression. Decreases anesthetic requirements.
Clonidine	Sedation Bradycardia Xerostomia	Decreases anesthetic requirements. Abrupt discontinuation may result in rebound hypertension. May be an analgesic alone or in combination with neuraxial opioids.
Alpha-Adrenergic Antagonists		
Prazosin	First-dose syncope Orthostatic hypotension Fluid retention	Use cautiously in elderly patients. Elicitation of reflex tachycardia is unlikely. Hypotension during neuraxial blockade may be exaggerated as compensatory vasoconstriction is blocked.
Combined Alpha and Beta-Adrenergic Antagonists		
Labetalol	Bronchospasm Orthostatic hypotension Fatigue	Use cautiously in patients with asthma or COPD. Use cautiously in patients with CHF, sick sinus syndrome, or heart block. May precipitate angina pectoris in patients with ischemic heart disease.
Vasodilators Hydralazine Minoxidil	Tachycardia Headache Fluid retention	May precipitate angina pectoris in patients with ischemic heart disease. Lupus syndrome may occur.

Continued

TABLE 2-3		
Common Antihypertensive Medications—cont'd		
DRUGS	SIDE EFFECTS	SPECIAL CONSIDERATIONS
	Sodium retention Positive antinuclear antibody Hypertrichosis	May cause or aggravate pleural effusion.
Angiotensin-Converting Enzyme Inhibitors Benazepril Captopril Enalapril Lisinopril Moexipril	Cough Rhinorrhea Angioedema Rash Hyperkalemia Proteinuria Loss of taste	May be associated with hemodynamic instability and hypotension during general anesthesia especially if large fluid shifts are associated with the surgical procedure. May cause neutropenia in patients with autoimmune collagen disease. May cause reversible acute renal failure in patients with renal artery stenosis. May cause fetal toxicity. NSAIDs may antagonize antihypertensive effects.
Angiotensin II Receptor Antagonists Irbesartan Losartan Valsartan	Dizziness	May be associated with hypotension following the induction of anesthesia. May cause reversible acute renal failure in patients with renal artery stenosis. May cause fetal toxicity.
Calcium Channel-Blocking Drugs Verapamil	CHF Hypotension Heart block Syncope Hepatic dysfunction Bradycardia	Use cautiously in patients with CHF or heart block.

CHF, Congestive heart failure; *COPD,* chronic obstructive pulmonary disease; *NSAIDs,* nonsteroidal anti-inflammatory drugs.
From Stoelting R, Dierdorf S. *Anesthesia and Co-Existing Disease.* 4th ed. New York: Churchill Livingstone; 2002:97; adapted from Oparil S, Calhoun DA: High blood pressure. *Sci Am Med.* 2000;1-16.

used by the practitioner to elicit a history of coronary artery disease are listed in Box 2-2. In addition to the questions outlined in Box 2-2, patients must describe their chest pain. Factors to be considered include:

◆ Character
◆ Frequency
◆ Location
◆ Duration
◆ Radiation
◆ Methods of relief

Physical assessment of the patient with coronary artery disease includes assessment of skin color, presence of jugular venous distention, peripheral edema, assessment of baseline blood pressure, and auscultation of heart sounds. An electrocardiogram (ECG) may reveal normal sinus rhythm, the presence of dysrhythmias, or signs of previous infarction. Previous ECGs should be available for comparison. Postoperative monitoring must also be continued until the patient is fully recovered and demonstrates no signs of cardiovascular instability.

Patients with coronary artery disease should receive their prescribed nitrates, calcium channel blockers, beta blockers, and antihypertensive medications before the scheduled procedure.

Myocardial Infarction

Presedation assessment of patients with previous myocardial infarction must identify the length of time elapsed since the last myocardial infarction. Questioning to elicit a history of angina, precipitating factors and cardiovascular instability, or shortness of breath is required. If the patient admits to a history of angina, mechanisms of relief must be ascertained.

BOX 2-2

Assessment of Coronary Artery Disease

• Do you have a history of angina, chest tightness, or heaviness?
• Do you ever have indigestion not associated with eating?
• Have you ever had coronary artery bypass or heart surgery?
• Do you ever get short of breath?
• Have you ever been told you have an abnormal ECG?
• Have you ever felt skipped beats?
• Describe your daily activities and exercise

Classic studies reveal that in patients with a history of myocardial infarction, reinfarction may occur at a rate as high as 30% if surgery is performed within the first 3 months after the infarction. This incidence decreases to 15% when surgery is performed within the 3- to 6-month post-infarction period. The incidence of reinfarction decreases to approximately 5% after 6 months.[4,5] **If reinfarction does occur, the mortality rate is approximately 50%.**[6] **It is common practice to delay elective operations for up to 6 months after an acute myocardial infarction.**[7] In addition, patients with a history of myocardial ischemia or recent myocardial infarction scheduled for elective therapeutic, surgical, or diagnostic procedures benefit from aggressive hemodynamic monitoring, prompt pharmacologic treatment of systemic hypotension, and treatment of tachycardia.[8-10]

Cardiac Dysrhythmias

Cardiac dysrhythmias may be caused by:

- Effects of medications administered
- Hypoxemia
- Hypercarbia
- Electrolyte abnormalities
- Alterations of the autonomic nervous system
- Procedural manipulations
- Presedation patient anxiety
- Hypovolemia
- Hypotension

In most patients with normal cardiac reserve, dysrhythmias are generally well tolerated. Patients with limited cardiac reserve, however, may not tolerate even the most benign dysrhythmias. Newly diagnosed dysrhythmias or those that impair myocardial performance require further evaluation and consultation. Cardiac dysrhythmias and treatment protocols are featured in Chapter 6, Procedural Patient Monitoring.

Pacemakers

Presedation assessment of the patient with a pacemaker must initially evaluate the rationale for the device (e.g., sick sinus syndrome, syncope). Pacemakers are frequently inserted because of bradyarrhythmias. The clinician must recognize not only the indication for placement but also the pacemaker's default rhythm. Electrocautery is sensed by demand pacemakers and may result in asystole or inhibition of firing. Before electrocautery is used, the clinician should have the pacemaker programming device available for conversion to a fixed pacemaker rate. Many of the currently used pacemakers are capable of conversion to a fixed rate in the presence of electrocautery. However, for pacemakers without this capability, the technique of converting to a fixed rate should be demonstrated to the attending physician and healthcare provider before the planned procedure. Common permanent pacemaker modes are featured in Table 2-4. The grounding plate should be placed the greatest possible distance from the pacemaker and lead. During the use of bipolar electrocautery, it is important to monitor pulsatile flow with a pulse oximeter. Because electrocautery interferes with ECG monitoring, adequacy of pulsatile flow is ensured with pulse oximetry pulsatile display. **Therefore, pacemaker considerations associated with the procedural care of the patient presenting for sedation include:**

- Obtain thorough patient history to assess for pacemaker dependency, symptoms, and reoccurrence of symptoms.
- Obtain pacemaker information before the start of the procedure (manufacturer).

TABLE 2-4

Common Permanent Pacemaker Modes

CODE	INDICATION	FUNCTION	PERIOPERATIVE MANAGEMENT
VVI	Bradycardia without the need for preserved atrioventricular conduction	Demand ventricular pacing	Magnet use may be helpful and converts to asynchronous pacing usually at 72 beats per minute.
VVIR	Bradycardia without the need for preserved atrioventricular conduction; chronotropic incompetence	Allows a somewhat physiologic response to exercise	Pacemaker may sense perioperative changes (e.g., temperature and respiratory rate) as related to exercise or unpredictable response to magnet placement; suggest postoperative interrogation.
DDD	Bradycardia when AV synchrony can be preserved	Provides more physiologic response; maintains AV concordance	Unpredictable response to magnet placement; suggest postoperative interrogation.
DDDR	Patients requiring physiologic response of heart rate (i.e., chronotropic incompetence)	Provides increased physiologic response to exercise; maintains AV concordance	Pacemaker may sense perioperative changes (e.g., temperature and respiratory rate) as related to exercise or unpredictable response to magnet placement; suggest postoperative interrogation.

From Faust R. *Anesthesiology Review.* 3rd ed. Philadelphia: Churchill Livingstone; 2002:341.

◆ Program rate-adaptive off and/or predict implications during the procedure.
◆ Consider programming to be asynchronous.
◆ Ensure that a pacemaker magnet is available.
◆ Ensure that an alternate pacing modality is available.
◆ Ensure that intravenous chronotropes are available.
◆ A cardiology consultation probably is not needed if the patient is asymptomatic and recent evaluations of the generator are satisfactory. Generator interrogation is always advisable.

Defibrillators (Automatic Internal Defibrillators)

Patients with ventricular tachycardia or fibrillation unresponsive to pharmacologic therapy may be treated with automatic implantable cardioverter-defibrillators (AICD or ICD). There are approximately nine companies producing 126 models of AICDs.[11] These defibrillators deliver a 25- to 30-joule discharge to convert the patient from a life-threatening dysrhythmia.[12] **Presedation consultation with the cardiologist should address postinsertion follow-up, battery strength, status of the pulse generator, and the cardiologist's suggestions for procedural care.** If electrocautery use is planned, the generator may be disabled with a magnet. As with pacemakers, magnet behavior in many ICDs can be altered by programming. Most devices will suspend tachyarrhythmia detection (and thus therapy) when a magnet is appropriately placed to activate the reed switch. However, device interrogation and calling the manufacturer remain the most reliable way to determine magnet response. The AICD may be reactivated at the conclusion of the procedure. While the AICD is disabled, an external defibrillator must be immediately available in the clinical setting. In many facilities external defibrillator "hands free" pads are placed to ensure patient safety.

Valvular Heart Disease

Prophylactic antibiotics are indicated for patients with valvular heart disease, ventricular/atrial septal defects, intravascular shunts, and previous endocarditis. Antibiotics are given to protect against the development of endocarditis after bacteremic events. Blood-borne bacteria may lodge on damaged valve leaflets, resulting in bacterial endocarditis. Procedures associated with bacteremia include instrumentation of the gallbladder, gastrointestinal/genitourinary tract, and oropharynx. Recommendations for prevention of bacterial endocarditis are listed in Box 2-3.

Completion of the presedation cardiac evaluation should incorporate the findings of the patient's history, physical examination, and a review of laboratory data. Patients with a recent myocardial infarction, unstable angina, poor exercise tolerance, cardiac dysrhythmias, dyspnea, fatigue, coronary artery disease, or hypertension may require cardiac consultation. When indicated, additional cardiac testing (e.g., stress test, echocardiogram, or cardiac catheterization) may reveal valuable information that will alter presedation

and procedural management of the sedation patient. The American College of Cardiology/American Heart Association Task Force has updated its *Guidelines for Perioperative Cardiovascular Evaluation for Noncardiac Surgery* featured in Figure 2-1. Adequate time must be allotted to ensure that the patient is hemodynamically stable and in optimum cardiovascular condition before the planned procedure.

Pulmonary Assessment

Sedative and analgesic medications interfere with the regulation of spontaneous pulmonary ventilation. Patterns of respiration are featured in Figure 2-2. Prevention of respiratory complications, including respiratory failure, atelectasis, and hypoxia, require careful presedation assessment and planning. Presedation pulmonary assessment must address the type, severity, and reversibility of preexisting pulmonary disease. Symptoms of pulmonary disease must be ascertained by the clinician before the anticipated procedure. Pulmonary symptoms that predispose the patient to increased risk include:
◆ Chronic cough
◆ Sputum production
◆ Rhinitis
◆ Sore throat
◆ Dyspnea
◆ Cigarette smoking
◆ Previous pulmonary complications
◆ Hemoptysis

Dyspnea is present when there is demonstrated difficult or labored breathing with shortness of breath. Dyspnea generally increases with the severity of the underlying condition. The presence of dyspnea on presedation evaluation is an ominous sign. Dyspnea occurs when the requirement for oxygen is greater than the patient's ability to physiologically respond to the increased demand. Causes of dyspnea are listed in Box 2-4 on p. 34. **Patients with a history of dyspnea require further presedation pulmonary evaluation. Assessment of dyspnea at rest or at specific levels of exertion is an important indicator of the severity of preexisting pulmonary disease.** It is important to assess the amount and kind of effort that produces dyspnea. Identification of dyspnea at rest, walking (upstairs versus level surface), frequency of rest stops during the climb or walk, and with what other activities of daily life dyspnea occurs are qualitative assessment tools utilized by the healthcare provider assessing the patient before sedation.

Presedation radiographs of the chest are indicated in patients based on the severity of preexisting pulmonary disease. Indications for presedation chest radiographic examination are identified in Box 2-5 on p. 34. Regardless of the presence of preexisting pulmonary disease, the purpose of the presedation pulmonary assessment should focus on identification and treatment of acute infections with appropriate antibiotic therapy. Relief of bronchospastic disease through the use of bronchodilators, implementation of mechanisms

---

BOX 2-3

Antibiotic Prophylaxis Against Endocarditis

Dental, Oral, Nasal, Pharyngeal, Upper Airway, and Esophageal Procedures

Standard
Adults: Amoxicillin, 3 g orally 1 hour before and 1.5 g 6 hours after the procedure, *or* ampicillin, 2 g IV or IM 30 minutes before the procedure
Children: Amoxicillin, 50 mg/kg orally 1 hour before and 25 mg/kg 6 hours after the procedure, *or* ampicillin, 50 mg/kg IV 30 minutes before the procedure

Penicillin Allergy
Adults: Erythromycin, 1 g orally 2 hours before and 500 mg 6 hours afterward *or* azithromycin or clarithromycin, 500 mg orally before, *or* clindamycin, 600 mg orally 2 hours before and 300 mg 6 hours afterward, *or* clindamycin, 600 mg IV 30 minutes before *or* cefazolin, 1 g IV or IM 30 minutes before the procedure*
Children: Erythromycin, 20 mg/kg orally 2 hours before and 10 mg/kg 6 hours afterward *or* clindamycin, 10 mg/kg orally 2 hours before and 5 mg/kg 6 hours afterward *or* clindamycin, 20 mg/kg IV, 30 minutes before and 5 mg/kg 6 hours afterward *or* cefazolin 25 mg/kg IV or IM 30 minutes before and 25 mg/kg 6 hours after procedure*

High Risk (Prosthetic Valve or Prior Endocarditis)
Adults: Ampicillin, 2 g IV or IM, and gentamicin, 1.5 mg/kg (up to 80 mg) IV or IM, 30 minutes before; and amoxicillin, 1.5 g orally 6 hours afterward, or repeat IV regimen 8 hours later
Children: Ampicillin, 50 mg/kg IV or IM, and gentamicin, 2 mg/kg IV or IM, 30 minutes before; and amoxicillin, 50 mg/kg orally 6 hours afterward, or repeat IV regimen 8 hours later

High Risk with Penicillin Allergy
Adults: Vancomycin, 1 g IV, 1 hour before (infuse over 1 hour)
Children: Vancomycin, 20 mg/kg IV, 1 hour before (infuse over 1 hour)

Genitourinary and Gastrointestinal Procedures

Standard
Adults: Ampicillin, 2 g IV or IM, and gentamicin, 1.5 mg/kg (up to 80 mg) IV or IM, 30 minutes before; and amoxicillin, 1.5 g orally 6 hours afterward
Children: Ampicillin, 50 mg/kg IV or IM, and gentamicin, 2 mg/kg IV or IM, 30 minutes before; and amoxicillin, 50 mg/kg orally 6 hours afterward

Penicillin Allergy
Adults: Vancomycin, 1 g IV 1 hour before (infuse over 1 hour), and gentamicin, 1.5 mg/kg (up to 80 mg) IV
Children: Vancomycin, 20 mg/kg IV 1 hour before (infuse over 1 hour), and gentamicin, 2 mg/kg IV

Low Risk
Adults: Amoxicillin, 3 g orally 1 hour before and 1.5 g 6 hours after the procedure
Children: Amoxicillin, 50 mg/kg orally 1 hour before and 25 mg/kg 6 hours after the procedure

*Do not use with a history of immediate hypersensitivity-type allergy to penicillin.
From Morgan, Mikhail, and Murray: *Clinical anesthesiology*, ed 3. Lange Medical Books: McGraw Hill, New York, 2002, pg 409.

---

to improve sputum clearance (postural damage and incentive spirometry), and cessation of cigarette smoking will help to optimize the patient's presedation pulmonary condition.

> Patients presenting for sedation/analgesia should undergo a focused physical examination, including vital signs, auscultation of the heart and lungs, and evaluation of the airway.

Chronic Obstructive Pulmonary Disease

Patients with chronic obstructive pulmonary disease (COPD) frequently have a history of cigarette smoking. Dyspnea, cough, and wheezing may be present. As the disease progresses, barrel chest develops, use of accessory muscles for respiratory excursion, and pursed-lip breathing may ensue. COPD encompasses asthma, chronic obstructive bronchitis (with obstruction of small airways), and emphysema (with enlargement of air spaces and destruction of lung parenchyma, loss of lung elasticity, and closure of small airways).[13]

Asthma

Asthma affects approximately 5% of the adult population and 7% to 10% of children in the United States. Asthma is a chronic condition characterized by airway inflammation and reversible expiratory airway obstruction owing to narrowing of the airway lumen and airway hyperreactivity. Asthma is accompanied by a combination of clinical features, which include the following:

◆ Wheezing
◆ Airway obstruction with reversibility

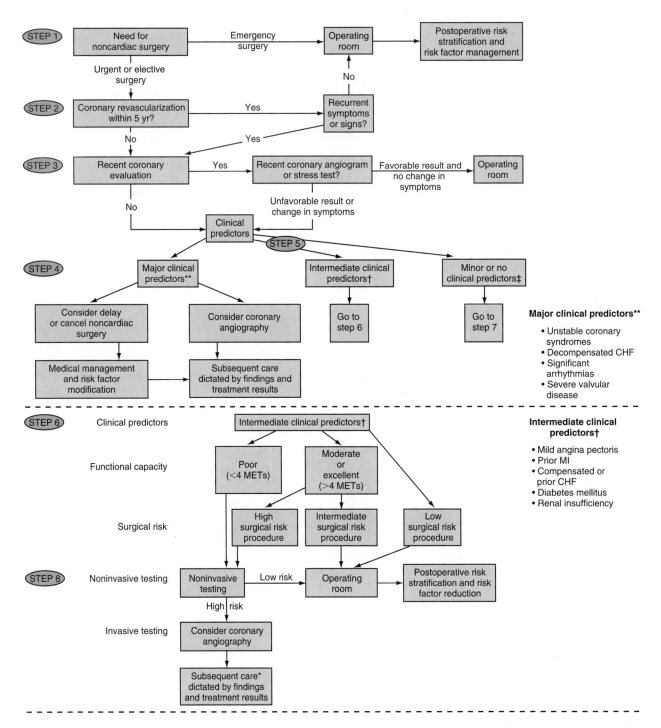

FIGURE 2-1 Guideline update on perioperative cardiovascular evaluation of noncardiac surgery. Stepwise approach to preoperative cardiac assessment. Subsequent care may include cancellation or delay of surgery, coronary revascularization followed by noncardiac surgery, or intensified care. (From American College of Cardiology/American Heart Association Cardiovascular Evaluation Guidelines. ACC/AHA Practice Guidelines, 2002.)

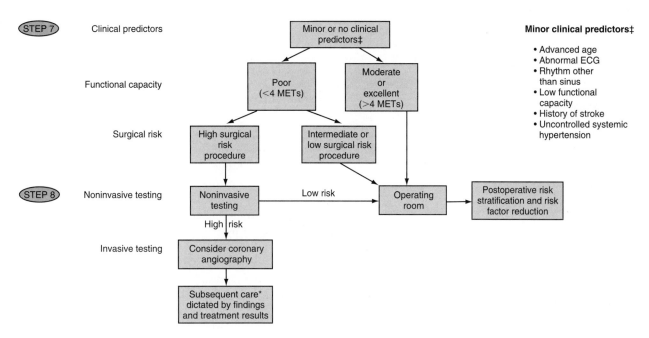

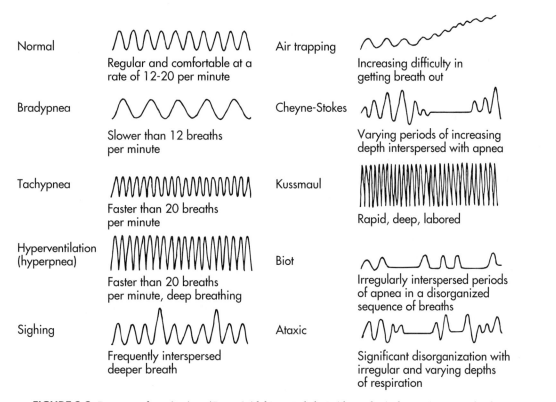

FIGURE 2-1, cont'd

FIGURE 2-2 Patterns of respiration. (From Seidel H. *Mosby's Guide to Physical Examination.* 5th ed. St. Louis: Mosby; 2003:372.)

BOX 2-4

Causes of Dyspnea

- Obstructive pulmonary disease
  - Asthma
  - Bronchitis
  - Emphysema
  - Upper airway obstruction
- Restrictive pulmonary disease
- Cardiomyopathy
- Left ventricular failure
- Obesity
- Anemia
- Neuromuscular disease

- Increased airway responsiveness
- Decreased mucociliary clearance
- Increased mucus production

Before the administration of sedation, the asthmatic patient should exhibit no signs of respiratory infection (fever, productive cough). Eradication of acute and chronic infection with antibiotics is essential. The absence of wheezing, dyspnea, or recent attacks most likely indicates the patient is in a stable phase of the disease. Presedation assessment must include pharmacologic evaluation of the asthmatic patient. Beta agonists (albuterol) are used to produce bronchial dilation. Corticosteroids decrease airway inflammation, and anticholinergic agents (ipratropium bromide) inhibit muscarinic receptors in the lung parenchyma with resultant bronchodilation. Additional presedation assessment includes date of the last asthma attack, severity of the attack, and mechanisms used to relieve symptoms associated with the attack. The patient taking beta agonists should use his or her own metered-dose inhaler (MDI) before the planned procedure. MDIs, oxygen, and breathing treatment equipment should also be available in the procedure room. *Morphine sulfate is relatively contraindicated in the asthmatic patient population because of its histamine-releasing properties.* An estimated 5% of patients with asthma are sensitive to bisulfite and metabisulfite, which are used for preservatives and antioxidants by the food processing industry. These substances are also present in a large number of medications utilized in healthcare today.[14] Fortunately, through identification

---

BOX 2-5

Indications for Presedation Chest Radiograph

- Blood-tinged or colored sputum
- Cigarette smoking greater than 20 pack-years
- Exposure to tuberculosis
- History of congestive heart failure
- Malignancy
- Presence of cardiovascular disease
- Productive cough
- Pulmonary infection
- Sudden change in pulmonary/cardiovascular symptoms

---

of the last attack, its severity, the mechanism of relief, and continuation of the patient's prescribed pharmacologic protocol, many asthmatic patients tolerate the administration of sedation without incident.

Bronchitis

Chronic bronchitis may occur secondary to prolonged exposure of the airways to nonspecific irritants. It is characterized by hypersecretion of mucus and inflammatory changes in the bronchi. Bronchitis is a common cause of COPD and is manifested by permanent or minimally reversible obstruction to air flow during exhalation. Patients with cough, dyspnea, and sputum production may require supplemental oxygenation to avoid hypoxemia and allow the patient the ability to carry out the activities of daily living. **Presedation assessment of the patient with COPD requires a determination of the severity of dyspnea, hypoxia, and infection.** Supplemental oxygen is recommended during the procedure and should remain in place until all residual respiratory depressant effects have dissipated. Depending on the severity of the pathophysiologic disease process, pulmonary function tests, chest radiography, arterial blood gas analysis, bronchodilators, and antibiotic therapy may be ordered by the physician before the planned sedation procedure.

Obstructive Sleep Apnea

A pulmonary disorder of significant concern for the sedation provider is sleep apnea. Sleep apnea occurs when there is cessation of air flow at the mouth for longer than 10 seconds. **Central alveolar hypoventilation syndrome** occurs when there is absence of neural drive to ventilation when voluntary control of breathing is diminished by sleep. **Central sleep apnea** most likely reflects a defect in the function of the medullary ventilatory center. **Obstructive sleep apnea** is due to abnormal relaxation of the genioglossus muscle that normally pulls the tongue forward and relaxation of the pharyngeal muscles. Obstructive sleep apnea may occur secondary to decreased neural input to these muscles from the brainstem.

Regardless of the etiology, sleep apnea is primarily a disorder of the upper airway at the level of the pharynx. Sleep apnea is characterized by episodes of apnea or hypopnea during sleep. Airway obstruction results in snoring and daytime somnolence. The upper airway obstruction leads to fragmented sleep, arterial hypoxemia, hypercarbia, polycythemia, systemic and pulmonary hypertension, and right ventricular failure.

The etiology of obstructive sleep apnea is associated with the dilator muscles responsible for maintaining increased airway tone to prevent collapse and obstruction. Relaxation of the dilator muscles during sleep results in decreased luminar flow with resultant turbulent air flow and snoring. The decreased air flow and partial obstruction leads to sleep disturbances, arterial hypoxemia, and hypercarbia. This pattern ultimately results in arousal from the sleep state.

Diagnosis of sleep apnea is confirmed by polysomnography in a designated sleep laboratory. Polysomnography sleep laboratory technicians monitor the patient for obstructive apneic episodes during sleep. An "episode" is defined as 10 seconds or longer of total cessation of air flow despite continuous inspiratory effort against a partially or completely obstructed airway. Presedation patient assessment includes questioning for signs and symptoms associated with obstructive sleep apnea. These signs and symptoms include:

◆ Morning headache
◆ Hypertension
◆ Stroke
◆ Ischemic heart disease
◆ Loss of initiative
◆ Lassitude
◆ Memory loss
◆ Cognitive dysfunction
◆ Overwhelming somnolence during normal waking hours

Patients presenting for sedation with obstructive sleep apnea should be scheduled as early in the morning as possible. **This patient population is sensitive to the respiratory depressant effects associated with the administration of CNS depressant medications. Clinical management includes careful assessment of the patient's airway before the commencement of the procedure. Titration to clinical effect is required to avoid the development of deep sedative states or general anesthesia.** Institution of the patient's CPAP (continuous positive airway pressure) treatment immediately after the procedure results in a pneumatic splinting effect via positive intraluminal pressure applied to the walls of the upper airway during inspiration. Oxygen therapy is also beneficial during procedural and postprocedural patient care. It is imperative for the sedation provider to realize that patients with obstructive sleep apnea are extremely sensitive to all CNS depressant medications. The administration of these medications increases the potential for increased airway obstruction or the development of apnea with minimal doses of these medications. For this reason, the prudent sedation practitioner should utilize minimal doses of sedation/analgesia medications to avoid unnecessary complications. Dosage of sedative medications must be based on the patients condition and generally are decreased as much as 50% to 70% for this patient population.

> Sleep apneic patients are at high risk for developing arterial hypoxemia during the postprocedure period. The patient should receive written discharge information instructing them not to take any central nervous system depressants or consume any alcohol in the immediate postprocedure period.

Hepatic Assessment

The liver is responsible for the synthesis of proteins and clotting factors and for detoxification of pharmacologic agents and metabolic byproducts. The liver also excretes bodily waste products, stores iron and vitamins, and supplements the body's energy stores. It is the largest organ in the body and receives approximately 29% of the cardiac output.[15] Treatment of patients with impaired hepatic function should attempt to prevent further hepatic deterioration. Patients presenting for sedation services may have acute or chronic liver disease. These patients are predisposed to symptoms associated with hepatic disease, which include:

◆ Ascites
◆ Portal hypertension
◆ Arteriolar vasodilatation
◆ Arterial desaturation
◆ Decreased hematocrit
◆ Encephalopathy
◆ Electrolyte disturbances

Enzyme Induction

An important pharmacologic function of the liver is the breakdown of lipid-soluble medications into water-soluble compounds via the cytochrome P-450 microsomal enzyme system. The degree of metabolism of pharmacologic compounds is dependent on hepatic blood flow and enzyme activity in the endoplasmic reticulum. In some cases, patients with significant liver impairment may exhibit resistance to sedative and analgesic medications because of the accentuated drug metabolism attributed to enzyme induction. Conversely, patients with liver disease may be extremely sensitive to pharmacologic medications because of a decrease in hepatic blood flow and destruction of the hepatocytes, which contain the microsomal enzyme system. **Therefore, with acute or chronic liver failure, careful titration and vigilance are required to assess patient response to the medications administered.**

Hepatitis

Hepatitis is characterized by inflammation of the hepatocytes. Characteristics of hepatitis are listed in Table 2-5. The diagnosis of hepatitis is often confirmed only after presentation with fatigue, anorexia, dark urine, fever, hepatomegaly, ascites, esophageal varices, and peripheral edema. A combination of these symptoms may signify severe hepatic disease. The treatment of hepatitis often focuses on the presenting symptoms. Attention to the nutritional support and hydration status of the patient is imperative. Presedation preparation of the patient with hepatitis should discourage the use of alcohol. Assessment of the coagulation profile, nutritional status, and optimization of presenting symptoms is required before the planned procedure.

Cirrhosis

Cirrhosis is a liver disease that results in scarring and destruction of liver cells. Decreased hepatic blood flow occurs with increased resistance of flow through the portal system.

TABLE 2-5

Characteristic Features of Viral Hepatitis

PARAMETER	TYPE A	TYPE B	TYPE C	TYPE D
Mode of transmission	Fecal-oral Sewage-contaminated shellfish	Percutaneous Sexual	Percutaneous	Percutaneous
Incubation period	20-37 days	60-110 days	35-70 days	60-110 days
Results of serum antigen and antibody tests	IgM early and IgG appears during convalescence	HBsAg and anti-HBc early and persists in carriers	Anti-HVC in 6 weeks to 9 months	Anti-HVD late and may be short-lived
Immunity	Antibodies in 45%	Antibodies in 5%-15%	Unknown	Protected if immune to type B
Course	Does not progress to chronic liver disease	Chronic liver disease develops in 1%-5% of adults and 80%-90% of children	Chronic liver disease develops in 85%	Co-infection with type B
Prevention after exposure	Pooled gamma globulin	Hepatitis B immune globulin Hepatitis B vaccine	Unknown	Unknown
Mortality	<0.2%	0.3%-1.5%	Unknown	Acute icteric hepatitis: 2%-20%

IgM, IgG, Immunoglobulins M and G; HBsAg, hepatitis B surface antigen; HBc, hepatitis B core; HVC, hepatitis virus C; HVD, hepatitis virus D.
From Stoelting R, Dierdorf S. *Anesthesia and Co-Existing Disease.* 4th ed. New York: Churchill Livingstone; 2002:300; adapted from Keefe EB. Acute hepatitis. *Sci Am Med.* 1999;4:1-9.

Cirrhosis and portal hypertension also affect the cardiopulmonary system in the cirrhotic patient. The cardiovascular effects associated with cirrhosis include a hyperdynamic circulation, cardiomyopathy, and portal vein hypertension. **Pulmonary considerations associated with cirrhosis include decreased oxygen affinity for the hemoglobin molecule accompanied by varying degrees of oxygen desaturation. This predisposition to desaturation and hypoxemia requires careful titration with dosage reduction of sedative and analgesic medications.** In cases of advanced liver disease, ascites secondary to portal hypertension, hypoalbuminemia, and edema also predispose cirrhotic patients to hypoxemia. Patients presenting with hepatic disease require careful assessment to ascertain the magnitude of the disease. Predisposition to hypoxemia and decreased drug metabolism require attentive monitoring and careful titration and dosage reduction of all medications.

Renal Assessment

Presedation assessment of the renal system is required to assess for the presence of renal pathology before the scheduled sedation procedure. Functions of the kidney include:

◆ Regulation and maintenance of fluid status
◆ Acid-base maintenance system
◆ Excretion of waste products and electrolyte balance
◆ Detoxification of pharmacologic agents

The kidneys perform these tasks through filtration, reabsorption, and secretion. Presedation evaluation of renal function consists of assessment of the patient for a history of renal surgery or any degree of renal impairment. A history of minor urologic or renal impairment may include cystitis, incontinence, and benign prostatic disease. There are distinct groups of patients with renal impairment who require additional presedation evaluation.

Renal Insufficiency

For patients with renal insufficiency presenting for sedation services, optimization of hydration status is a priority. The goal of the provider is to preserve normal renal function throughout the procedure and in the immediate postprocedure period. Depending on the state of hypovolemia or hypervolemia, many authors advocate titration of saline solution, mannitol, furosemide, or low doses of dopamine.[16-22] Although it is not practical to measure urine output during short diagnostic procedures, urine output should be measured and documented both before and after the procedure. Attention to volume status is ensured through adequate presedation assessment of skin turgor, weight, blood pressure, and heart rate. Patients who appear hyper-volemic may also require diuretic therapy before the planned procedure.

Dialysis

For patients with little or no existing renal function, presedation assessment and planning should focus on preservation of the remaining organ systems in the body. The vascular cannulation site used for dialysis must be carefully guarded against insult. Blood pressure measurement must not be done on the side of the vascular access site. Infection is a leading cause of morbidity and death in patients with compromised renal function. Strict adherence to aseptic or sterile technique must be used for all invasive procedures and intravenous cannula insertion. Anephric patients may be anemic as a result of decreased erythropoietin secretion. Erythropoietin secreted by the kidney is required for the synthesis of hemoglobin molecules. This anemia predisposes the patient to the development of hypoxia. However, issues of anemia can be controlled by the injection of Epogen to supplement lack of erythropoietin secretion improving laboratory values in some renal patients. Presedation laboratory work may reveal hyperkalemia; increased blood urea nitrogen, calcium, and creatinine levels; and acidosis requiring dialysis. Dialysis before the procedure is beneficial for many patients. However, hypovolemia associated with dialysis performed within several hours of the planned procedure may predispose the patient to the development of procedural hypotension. Careful titration of sedative and analgesic medications is required to avoid hypotension and hypoxemia in this specific patient population.

Characteristics associated with chronic renal failure include anemia, metabolic acidosis, pruritus, hypertension, altered fluid and electrolyte status, and susceptibility to infection. During presedation assessment, the clinician must ascertain:

◆ Degree of renal insufficiency
◆ Presence of chronic or acute insufficiency
◆ The last dialysis treatment noted on the chart

Once assessment is completed, presedation treatment of renal disease must address presenting symptoms and focus on:

◆ Fluid volume
◆ Homeostasis
◆ Electrolyte balance
◆ Renal clearance
◆ Hormonal secretion

Hypertension associated with renal disease is a common finding. Hypertension secondary to renal disease is a result of hypervolemia or alterations in the renin-angiotensin mechanism. Hypertension associated with renal disease is often treated as essential hypertension until end-stage renal failure ensues.

> Renal patients may benefit from dialysis before the scheduled procedure. A focus on euvolemia, normotension, assessment of electrolyte disturbances, and correction of clinically significant anemia should precede any sedation procedure.

Pharmacologic Effects of Renal Disease

The presence of preexisting renal disease decreases protein binding, which results in accentuation of pharmacologic effects for highly protein-bound sedative and analgesic medications. Midazolam is 98% protein bound. In the presence of renal failure and a decrease in protein binding there is an increase in the active pharmacologic component of midazolam. **Therefore, accentuation of benzodiazepine effect may be greatly enhanced in patients with renal disease.** Patients with renal impairment also have a greater risk of adverse drug reaction.[23-25] As outlined earlier, pharmacologic effects are accentuated secondary to increased plasma levels of the drug, decreased protein binding, and drug accumulation. Titration and reduction of drug dose must be combined with careful assessment of the cardiopulmonary response to sedative medications in all settings, particularly in those patients with preexisting renal dysfunction.

Neurologic Assessment

Presedation assessment of the patient with neurologic disease attempts to elicit a history of mental deficiency, cerebral vascular insufficiency, or intrinsic metabolic neurologic disease. The goal of a complete neurologic assessment is to ascertain and document presedation levels of consciousness and to evaluate the presence of preexisting neurologic disease.

Cerebrovascular Insufficiency

Cerebrovascular disease may present as:

◆ Transient ischemic attacks (TIAs) with reversible temporary cerebral dysfunction.
◆ Minor cerebrovascular accident with return to a near-normal physiologic state.
◆ Major stroke with resultant severe cerebral dysfunction or death.

Transient ischemic attacks are temporary, reversible, ischemic attacks with full recovery in periods ranging from minutes to 24 hours. Temporary interruption of cerebral blood flow may result from plaque or debris, with recovery occurring after dissolution of the debris. The finding of TIAs on presedation assessment may indicate impending severe neurologic dysfunction or stroke.

Carotid Artery and Vertebral Basilar Disease

Cerebral ischemia may also result from insufficient blood flow to the circle of Willis. The circle of Willis receives blood flow for cerebral circulation from the internal carotid artery and the vertebral arteries, which converge to form the posterior basilar artery. Collection of arterial plaque in the carotid artery results in decreased cerebral circulation with resultant neurologic symptoms, which include:

◆ Visual loss
◆ Paresis
◆ Numbness and tingling of the contralateral extremities

Patients with TIAs or carotid disease may be treated medically or surgically. Medical management consists of antiplatelet medications and anticoagulant therapy. Surgical treatment is indicated when plaque buildup results in lesions that obstruct 80% of blood flow with repeated TIAs. Surgical excision of the obstructive lesion generally results in improvement of the patient's neurologic status. It is important to assess coagulation status during presedation assessment if the planned procedure may predispose the patient to blood loss. Documentation of the incidence, severity, and time to resolution of the TIA symptoms must be performed. Specific documentation must address existing focal neurologic deficits and any functional neurologic limitations before the procedure. These data are critical if a new neurologic deficit is reported after the procedure.

Stroke

Presedation neurologic assessment may reveal a history of hemorrhagic or ischemic stroke. Hemorrhagic insult associated with stroke results from subarachnoid or intracerebral bleeding. Presedation neurologic symptoms that warrant additional investigation include the following:

◆ Headache
◆ Vomiting
◆ Loss of consciousness
◆ Seizures
◆ Slurred speech
◆ Unsteady gait
◆ Hemiparesis

These presedation neurologic symptoms require documentation and consultation before the administration of sedation.

Convulsive Disorders

Patients with a history of epilepsy or convulsive disorder require a thorough assessment of their disease state. Epileptic seizures result from a discharge of abnormally excitable neurons. This excitation may be triggered by discontinuation of medications, infection, neoplasm, drug or alcohol use, electrolyte disturbance, and hypoxia. Presedation assessment must focus on the underlying cause of the seizure. **Recommendations for antiseizure medications include maintenance of therapeutic plasma levels with continued administration of the patient's antiseizure medication.** Initial assessment of patients with seizures requires differentiation of the specific type of seizure. Grand mal seizures are characterized by

◆ Tonic-clonic convulsions
◆ Unconsciousness
◆ Severe muscle clonus
◆ Incontinence
◆ Postictal state

Petit mal seizures are characterized by

◆ Brief periods of staring
◆ Unresponsiveness

Petit mal or focal seizures generally occur in pediatric patients. Assessment of epileptic patients with a seizure history must ascertain compliance with prescribed medications and treatment protocol. Postponement of the procedure should be considered for noncompliant patients or patients who have not received appropriate evaluation and therapy.

Peripheral Nervous System Assessment

Evaluation of the peripheral nervous system includes assessment of extremity strength, color, temperature, capillary refill, and peripheral pulses. Sensory deficits and decreased reflexes may also signify peripheral sensory impairment. When neurologic assessment reveals a peripheral neuropathy, the degree, change over time, and exact nature of the specific neuropathy must be documented before the procedure or the administration of sedative or analgesic agents.

Endocrine System

Presedation assessment of the endocrine system may reveal primary diseases associated with overproduction or decreased production of hormones or by alterations in the stress response.

Diabetes

Diabetes is a chronic disease that is characterized by disruption of glucose metabolism. This altered glucose metabolism results in excessive plasma glucose levels. Hyperglycemia is a result of impaired synthesis, secretion, or use of endogenous insulin. The diagnosis of diabetes is indicated when fasting blood sugar levels are higher than 110 to 120 mg/dL or a 2-hour postprandial blood glucose level is greater than 140 mg/dL.[26] Diabetes affects more than 18 million people in the United States. Ninety percent of diabetic patients do not require insulin and maintain adequate blood sugar levels through dietary restriction, exercise, and weight control. Some patients may require oral hypoglycemic agents. Oral hypoglycemic agents work in one of two ways; they increase insulin release from the pancreas or increase the peripheral response to insulin.[27] This patient population is classified as having type II or non–insulin-dependent diabetes (NIDDM). Specific characteristics of type II diabetes include a gradual decline in pancreatic function. There is evidence of a genetic link related to non–insulin-dependent diabetes mellitus.

Type I diabetes is called insulin-dependent diabetes mellitus (IDDM) and occurs in the remaining 10% of diabetic patients. Patients with type I diabetes tend to be younger and not predisposed to obesity; their disease is referred to as juvenile-onset diabetes. Clinical characteristics of type I and II diabetes are listed in Table 2-6. Patients with IDDM are predisposed to hyperglycemia, acidosis, and ketosis. Diabetes may result in end-organ impairment, which includes the following:

◆ Hypertension
◆ Coronary artery disease
◆ Nephropathy
◆ Retinopathy
◆ Neuropathy
◆ Peripheral vascular disease

Hypertension and coronary disease associated with diabetes mellitus may increase the incidence of cardiovascular complications (labile blood pressure, ischemic changes on ECG, chest pain) during procedural sedation and analgesia.

TABLE 2-6

Clinical Characteristics of Diabetes

CLASS	PREVALENCE	CLINICAL CHARACTERISTICS	DIAGNOSTIC CRITERIA
Insulin-dependent diabetes mellitus (IDDM, type I)	0.4%	Absolute insulin deficiency Usual onset in youth Ketosis-prone Anti-islet cell antibodies	Hyperglycemia Polyuria Polydipsia Weight loss
Non–insulin-dependent diabetes mellitus (NIDDM, type II)	6.6%	Insulin resistance often in the presence of adequate insulin secretion Usual onset after 40 years of age Ketosis-resistant Obese	Same as IDDM Fasting serum glucose >140 mg/dL Abnormal oral glucose tolerance test
Gestational diabetes mellitus	2%-3% of pregnancies	Glucose intolerance with usual onset at 24-30 weeks' gestation Increased perinatal complications Glucose intolerance corrects after delivery NIDDM develops in 30%-50% within 10 years	Abnormal oral glucose tolerance test
Secondary diabetes		Pancreatic disease Drugs (glucocorticoids) Acromegaly Cushing's disease	Same as IDDM

From Stoelting R, Dierdorf S. *Anesthesia and Co-Existing Disease.* 4th ed. New York: Churchill Livingstone; 2002:396.

Autonomic neuropathy may present as silent myocardial ischemia and postural hypotension. Gastroparesis secondary to autonomic neuropathy increases the risk of aspiration and regurgitation.

Ketoacidosis. Ketoacidosis may be triggered by infection, trauma, poor insulin regimen compliance, or the stress of the proposed procedure itself. Ketoacidosis leads to increased resistance to insulin. Characteristics of ketoacidosis include hyperglycemia, hyperosmolarity, hyperkalemia, hyponatremia, and intracellular dehydration with osmotic diuresis. These characteristics predispose the patient to hypotension and hypovolemia. Symptoms of ketoacidosis include nausea, vomiting, lethargy, and hypovolemia. Correction of ketoacidosis includes administration of regular insulin, volume replacement with intravascular fluids, and correction of electrolyte disturbances.

Insulin. A variety of insulins are used for patients who require this therapy. Pork, beef, and human insulin are currently available in the treatment of diabetes mellitus. The pharmacologic profile of insulin types is presented in Table 2-7.

TABLE 2-7

Insulin Formulations*

INSULIN TYPE	ONSET (hr)	DURATION (hr)	PEAK (hr)	OTHER CHARACTERISTICS
Rapid acting (regular, crystalline zinc insulin [CZI])	0.5-1.0	6-8	2-3	Subcutaneous injection does not produce a sharp peak. CZI must be administered 30-60 minutes before meals.
Very rapid acting (lispro)	0.25-0.50	4-6	1-2	As a recombinant human insulin it is more rapidly absorbed. Administer 10-15 minutes before meals.
Intermediate acting (Lente, NPH)	2-4	10-14	4-8	
Long-acting (Ultralente)	8-14	18-24	10-14	Because of long half-life, a new steady state is not achieved for 3-4 days after a change in dose.

*All available in animal and human formulations except for lispro and Ultralente, which are available only as human (recombinant) preparations.
From Stoelting R, Dierdorf S. *Anesthesia and Co-Existing Disease.* 4th ed. New York: Churchill Livingstone; 2002:400; adapted from Nathan DM. Diabetes mellitus. *Sci Am Med.* 1997;3:1-24.

TABLE 2-8

Drug Therapy for Diabetes Mellitus: Oral Blood Glucose-Lowering Agents

DRUG	DOSAGE AND DURATION	NURSING INTERVENTIONS	RATIONALE
First-Generation Sulfonylura/Agents Acetohexamine (Dymelor, Dimelor)	*Usual:* 0.25-1.5 g/day *Maximum:* 1.5 g/day *Duration:* 12-24 hr	Emphasize need for regular eating habits and patterns. Monitor renal function.	There is a high incidence of hypoglycemia in diabetic clients with renal impairment. Older clients can develop exaggerated hypoglycemia responses.
Chlorpropamide (Diabinese, Novo-propamide)	100-500 mg q24h *Maximum:* 500 mg/day *Duration:* 24-60 hr	Emphasize need for regular eating habits and patterns. Monitor weight and intake and output patterns.	The long half-life of the drug is associated with a high incidence of hypoglycemia. There is an increased potential for severe hyponatremia.
Tolazamide (Tolinase)	100-500 mg q12-24h *Maximum:* 2000 mg/day *Duration:* 12-24 hr	Administer with meals.	Taking with meals helps to avoid gastrointestinal upset.
Tolbutamide (Orinase, Mobenol)	750-1500 mg q12-24h *Maximum:* 3000 mg/day *Duration:* 6-10 hr	Administer 30 min before meals. Monitor weight and intake and output patterns.	Taking 30 min before meals gives the best reduction in postprandial hyperglycemia. Use with caution in patients with renal failure.
Second-Generation Sulfonylurea Agents Glipizide (Glucotrol)	2.5-5 mg q12-24h *Maximum:* 40 mg/day *Duration:* 12-24 hr	Administer 30 min before meals	The long half-life of the drug is associated with a high incidence of hypoglycemia.
Glyburide (DiaBeta)	1.25-20 mg/day *Maximum:* 20 mg/day *Duration:* 24 hr	Administer with first main meal. Emphasize need for regular eating habits and patterns.	Hypoglycemia is more likely to occur with insufficient caloric intake. Administration with food helps reduce gastrointestinal side effects.
Glimepiride (Amaryl)	1-4 mg once daily *Maximum:* 8 mg/day *Duration:* 24 hr	Administer with first main meal. Emphasize need for regular eating habits and patterns.	Individuals with impaired renal function are more sensitive to blood glucose–lowering effects of glimepiride.
Nonsulfonylurea Agents Metformin (Glucophage)	500 mg bid or 850 mg once a day *Maximum:* 2550 mg/day *Duration:* 12 hr	Administer with food. Monitor weight and intake and output patterns.	Primary side effects are nausea, diarrhea, and abdominal discomfort. Use with caution in patients with renal failure. Lactic acidosis occurs with greater frequency in patients with impaired renal function.
Repaglinide (Prandin)	0.5-2 mg *Maximum:* 16 mg/day *Duration:* 2-3 hr	Administer 30 min before meals.	Taking 30 min before meals gives the best reduction in postprandial hyperglycemia.
α-Glucosidase Inhibitors Acarbose (Precose)	Individualized *Maximum:* 100 mg tid *Duration:* 2-4 hr	Instruct client to take with the first bite of each main meal.	Acarbose must be taken at the beginning of a meal to be fully effective.

Continued

TABLE 2-8

Drug Therapy for Diabetes Mellitus: Oral Blood Glucose-Lowering Agents—cont'd

DRUG	DOSAGE AND DURATION	NURSING INTERVENTIONS	RATIONALE
Miglitol (Glyset)	Individualized Usual dose: 50 mg tid *Maximum:* 100 mg tid *Duration:* ≈1 hr	Instruct client to take with the first bite of each main meal. Monitor renal function.	Glyset must be taken at the beginning of a meal to be fully effective. Drug may accumulate in clients with renal dysfunction; not recommended for clients with serum creatinine level greater than 2 mg/dL.
Thiazolidinediones Pioglitazone (Actos)	15-30 mg once a day *Maximum:* 45 mg/day	Emphasize need for liver function tests as recommended. Emphasize need to report symptoms of unexplained nausea, vomiting, abdominal pain, fatigue, anorexia, or dark urine. Advise women of childbearing age to use adequate contraception.	Rare cases of liver failure have occurred with pioglitazone. Liver function tests are measured at start of therapy and at regular times thereafter. Administration of troglitazone with certain oral contraceptives may reduce the plasma concentration of the oral contraceptive.
Rosiglitazone (Advandia)	4 mg/day *Maximum:* 8 mg	Emphasize need for liver function tests as recommended. Instruct client to report signs and symptoms of nausea, vomiting, abdominal pain, fatigue, anorexia, or dark urine. Advise women of childbearing age to use adequate contraception.	Rare cases of liver failure have occurred with rosiglitazone. Liver function tests are measured at start of therapy and at regular times thereafter. Improved insulin sensitivity may allow ovulation to resume, increasing the chance of pregnancy.
D-Phenylalanine Derivatives Nateglinide (Starlix)	*Usual:* 60-120 mg tid before meals *Maximum:* Optimal dose has not been defined. *Duration:* 4 hr	Administer 1-30 min before meals. Instruct client to omit medication when skipping a meal.	Stimulates rapid secretion of insulin to reduce increases in blood glucose levels that occur soon after eating. Reduces the risk of hypoglycemia.

From Ignatevicius D, Workman M. *Medical Surgical Nursing, Critical Thinking for Collaborative Care.* Philadelphia: WB Saunders; 2002.

Oral Hypoglycemic Agents. Oral hypoglycemic agents are used when diet and exercise regimens can no longer control blood glucose levels. Oral hypoglycemic agents are listed in Table 2-8. The prolonged duration of action of oral hypoglycemic agents predisposes the patient to hypoglycemia during the procedure and in the immediate postprocedure period. Oral hypoglycemic agents are typically withheld on the morning of the planned procedure to prevent hypoglycemia in the presence of the morning fast. An exception to this recommendation is metformin. Many clinicians require that metformin be discontinued 2 days or more before elective procedures secondary to the rare possibility of the development of lactic acidosis.[28] Some endocrinologists prefer to hold metformin for 2 days after the procedure, particularly when a dye load is used. Patients should be encouraged to closely monitor their glucose values during this postprocedure period. Some physicians will follow glucose values at this time, whereas others will prescribe another oral hypoglycemic agent and return the patient to their metformin at a later date.

Diabetic Procedural Care. Presedation assessment of the diabetic patient includes identification of the type of diabetes. Compliance with diet, exercise, and medication use must also be documented. A thorough assessment for coronary artery disease, hypertension, autonomic neuropathy, and gastroparesis is required before the administration of sedation. For type I diabetic patients treated with insulin, an attempt should be made to maintain blood sugar levels between 120 and 180 mg/dL. A variety of techniques have been advocated to control blood sugar during surgery.[29-31] No matter which diabetic management protocol is selected, it is important to set clear guidelines (blood sugar ranges) and to monitor and document glucose levels frequently. Procedures should be scheduled as early in the morning as possible. Early scheduling allows time to obtain a presedation blood sugar reading and complete the procedure. When fully recovered, the patient may receive the morning dose of insulin or oral hypoglycemic agent along with supplemental nutrition.

Disorders of the Thyroid Gland

The thyroid gland is responsible for regulation of the thyroid hormone. The thyroid gland responds to the pituitary gland's production of thyroid-stimulating hormone (TSH). Increased TSH results in an increase in thyroxine (T_4), which operates through a negative feedback loop. This negative feedback process decreases the release of TSH from the anterior pituitary gland. It is important to ascertain the status of thyroid function secondary to the thyroid hormone's function of regulating metabolic activity.

Hyperthyroidism. Hyperthyroidism produces an increased basal metabolic rate (BMR) secondary to increased secretion of the thyroid hormone. Symptoms of hyperthyroidism include weight loss, heat intolerance, tachycardia, nervousness, tremors, and warm moist skin. This increase in thyroid hormone production may result from thyroiditis, adenoma, or dysfunction of the pituitary gland. Presedation management must focus on return of the patient to a euthyroid state. Procedures on a hyperthyroid patient should be postponed until the patient becomes euthyroid. It may take 2 to 6 weeks of propylthiouracil therapy to decrease the synthesis and conversion of T_4 sufficiently to create a euthyroid state.[32]

Beta-adrenergic antagonists may be prescribed to control tachycardia and hypertension. Additional treatment modalities for hyperthyroidism include gland removal or radioactive iodine (I^{131}). **Presedation examination must assess the prescribed hyperthyroid treatment protocol, cardiovascular status, and state of patient anxiety.** During presedation assessment it is important to assess the size of the thyroid gland. Visual assessment of gland size is recommended because frequent manual palpation of the gland releases thyroxine into the bloodstream. T_4 produces an increase in basal metabolic rate, heart rate, and blood pressure. Additional considerations related to the enlarged thyroid gland include potential difficult airway management because of increased tissue mass. Because of the increased

basal metabolic rate, the pharmacologic effects of intravenous sedatives and analgesics may be reduced in the presence of hyperthyroidism.

Hypothyroidism. Hypothyroidism results from insufficient circulating thyroid hormone. Symptoms of hypothyroidism include intolerance to cold, bradycardia, cardiomegaly, dry skin, hair loss, fatigue, congestive heart failure, decreased mentation, and periorbital edema. Causes of hypothyroidism include surgical ablation, pituitary or hyperthalamic dysfunction, or decreased hormonal biosynthesis. Diagnosis of hypothyroidism includes decreased T_4 and increased TSH on a presedation thyroid serum panel. Treatment of hypothyroidism consists of supplemental thyroid medication. Exogenous T_4 requires 10 days for physiologic effect, whereas triiodothyronine (T_3) exerts physiologic effects in 6 hours.[33] Levothyroxine is often used as an exogenous replacement because of its long half-life and its ability to produce consistent plasma T_4 levels.

Hypothyroid patients generally have a marked sensitivity to intravenous sedatives, analgesics, and hypnotics. Hypothyroidism also reduces the ventilatory response to $Paco_2$ and Pao_2. This marked sensitivity requires a critical reduction in the dose of sedative and analgesic medications. Careful titration of sedatives, analgesics, and hypnotics is required, because even markedly reduced doses have resulted in profound central nervous system and respiratory depression. Patients with hypothyroidism may also have large tongues. This increase in tissue mass coupled with the marked sensitivity to pharmacologic medications requires careful attention to airway management. Airway obstruction is not well tolerated in this patient population and requires immediate intervention.

Diseases of the Adrenal Cortex

The adrenal cortex produces glucocorticosteroids, mineralocorticosteroids, and androgens. These hormones are under the control of the anterior pituitary gland through the secretion of adrenocorticotropic hormone (ACTH). Adrenal cortical disease may occur from decreased or increased production of these hormones. The following conditions may be encountered on presedation assessment of the patient presenting for sedation services.

Glucocorticoid Overproduction: Cushing's Disease

Glucocorticoid steroids regulate protein, carbohydrate, and nucleic acid metabolism. Under normal conditions, 20 to 30 mg of cortisol is produced each day. Cortisol production is significantly increased in the presence of stress, infection, and anxiety. In the face of surgery or diagnostic procedures, the adrenal gland may produce 75 to 150 mg/dL.[34] During periods of extreme stress, the adrenal gland secretes 200 to 500 mg/dL. Cushing's disease may be caused by increased production of ACTH, malignant tumors, or exogenous steroid administration. Glucocorticoid steroids also antagonize the effects of antidiuretic hormone (ADH). As a result of excess cortisol production, the symptoms of Cushing's disease include:

◆ Hypertension
◆ Hyperglycemia
◆ Polyuria
◆ Osteoporosis
◆ Hypokalemia
◆ Truncal obesity
◆ Moon face
◆ Skin striations
◆ Hypovolemia
◆ Plethora

> Presedation preparation of the patient with Cushing's disease must focus on correction of fluid and electrolyte abnormalities, treatment of hypertension, and regulation of blood sugar before the anticipated procedure.

Decreased Cortisol Production: Addison's Disease

Decreased cortisol production may result from hemorrhagic destruction of the adrenal cortical cells, carcinoma, or adrenal cortical suppression secondary to use of exogenous steroids. Use of exogenous steroids to treat asthma, allergy, or associated inflammatory conditions leads to adrenal cortisol suppression. The administration of exogenous steroids on a short-term basis of a 7- to 10-day treatment protocol decreases cortisol-releasing hormone and ACTH release. This decreased hormone release generally returns to normal within several days after cessation of exogenous steroid therapy. However, long-term exogenous steroid supplementation in the presence of inflammatory bowel disease, asthma, and associated inflammatory conditions of more than 10 days' duration may result in adrenocortical insufficiency. The presenting symptoms of adrenal insufficiency mimic hypovolemic shock. Additional symptoms include hypovolemia, hypoglycemia, nausea, vomiting, hypotension, and hemoconcentration. The use of supplemental exogenous steroids has been advocated to prevent intraoperative adrenal crisis. There are limited numbers of documented cases of acute adrenal crisis in the anesthesia literature. However, because of the significant morbidity and mortality associated with adrenal crisis and the minimal side effects associated with exogenous steroid supplementation, many authors advocate the use of exogenous steroid supplementation to prevent the development of adrenal insufficiency. **Presedation steroid replacement is based on the *degree of stress and the magnitude of the procedure*. Presedation steroid coverage may range from no additional exogenous steroids for minor surgical procedures to 200 to 300 mg/70 kg for major surgical or diagnostic procedures.**

Mineralocorticosteroid Production

Conn's Syndrome. Conn's syndrome results from excess production of mineralocorticosteroids. Mineralocortico-

steroids regulate extracellular fluid volume and potassium balance. Increased mineralocorticosteroid production may result from adenomas or adrenal hyperplasia. Symptoms associated with hyperaldosteronism include hypokalemia, hyponatremia, muscle weakness, hypertension, tetany, and polyuria. Hypokalemia is responsible for the kidney's inability to concentrate urine, polyuria, and muscle weakness associated with Conn's syndrome. Presedation preparation of the patient with Conn's disease includes replacement of potassium, administration of antihypertensive agents, and correction of fluid volume status. Presedation serum electrolytes are also warranted.

Hypoaldosteronism. Hypoaldosteronism results in hyperkalemia, with resultant heart block, cardiac conduction defects, hyponatremia, and hypotension. Causes of decreased aldosterone secretion include diabetes, renal failure, and adrenalectomy. Presedation treatment of decreased aldosterone secretion includes return of the patient to a eukalemic state, liberal fluid and sodium intake, and administration of exogenous mineralocorticosteroids (fludrocortisone).

Pheochromocytoma

Catecholamine-secreting tumors located in the adrenal medulla or chromaffin tissue are termed *pheochromocytomas*. Additional sites of these catecholamine-secreting tumors include the spleen, ovary, bladder, and right atria. Symptoms associated with pheochromocytoma are related to an increase in catecholamine release and include palpitations, headache, weight loss, diaphoresis, hypertension, flushing, and hyperglycemia. The main catecholamine released by pheochromocytoma is norepinephrine (80%). Confirmative diagnosis of pheochromocytoma is made after a 24-hour urine collection reveals excess free norepinephrine levels. The combination of diaphoresis, tachycardia, and headache, particularly in young to middle-aged patients, is highly suggestive of the presence of pheochromocytoma. **The presence of pheochromocytoma requires further consultation concerning surgical excision of the catecholamine-producing tumor before performing diagnostic, therapeutic, or minor surgical procedures.** Before tumor resection, antihypertensive treatment with alpha blockers is required to promote vasodilatation and restore blood volume. Phenoxybenzamine (Dibenzyline), prazosin (Minipress), or phentolamine (Regitine) is used to counteract the alpha effects (peripheral vasoconstriction) associated with the increased release of catecholamines. Cardiac dysrhythmias may be controlled with beta blockers. Correction of hypertension with a return of controlled heart rate facilitates a return of volume status. Seventy-five percent of patients who undergo surgical removal of the tumor return to baseline blood pressure within 10 days.[35] Patients presenting for sedation should be past this window period of hemodynamic stabilization before additional diagnostic procedures commence.

Gastrointestinal Assessment

Gastrointestinal assessment includes evaluation for the following conditions:

◆ Obesity
◆ Nausea
◆ Vomiting
◆ Diarrhea
◆ Gastrointestinal bleeding
◆ Gastric reflux

The presence of persistent nausea, vomiting, or diarrhea predisposes the patient to electrolyte abnormalities. Correction of electrolyte status and fluid volume is required before the administration of sedation is initiated. Dryness of mucous membranes, decreased skin turgor, and a large, swollen tongue may indicate significant hypovolemia. Hematocrit, serum osmolality, blood urea nitrogen level, electrolyte profile, and urine output are indicators to quantify volume deficit. Anemia secondary to diarrhea, nausea, vomiting, or gastrointestinal (GI) bleeding requires careful assessment of hemoglobin and hematocrit. Risks and benefits of transfusion must be examined before the procedure. Severe diarrhea results in the excretion of large amounts of water, sodium, and potassium through the colon. In severe cases, shock and cardiovascular compromise may occur. Emergent colonoscopy or endoscopic examination raises several concerns. Bleeding into the stomach or upper GI tract increases gastric volume and the incidence of regurgitation. Anemia and decreased oxygen-carrying capacity of the hemoglobin molecule also increase the risk of hypoxemia. Presedation assessment of GI bleeding must focus on restoration of blood volume, supplemental oxygenation, and a plan to use minimal sedation.

H_2 Antagonists

Patients with a history of pregnancy, recent opioid ingestion, diabetes, pain, abdominal distention, gastric acid reflux, hiatal hernia, or obesity may benefit from the administration of an H_2 (histamine) blocker such as cimetidine (Tagamet), ranitidine (Zantac), famotidine (Pepcid), or nizatidine (Axid) to increase gastric pH.[36] An H_2 dosage schedule is presented in Table 2-9.

ANESTHESIA AND SURGICAL HISTORY

Presedation assessment of the patient's anesthesia and surgical history must ascertain patient recollection of past anesthetic, surgical procedures, and complications related to these procedures. Because medical records and charts may not be readily available from other institutions or physician offices, it is important to obtain an accurate surgical and anesthesia history. Questions related to anesthetic and surgical history may be stated: "What operations have you had in the past?" "Do you recall what type of anesthesia you had?" This question is generally answered with "I went to sleep" or "They knocked me out." It is important to consider the amnestic effects of the benzodiazepines and sedatives used in the operating room. Many patients are under the impression that they received a general anesthetic when in essence they received a local anesthetic with sedation or a regional anesthetic with sedation and monitoring. For elicitation of information concerning past anesthesia and surgical procedures, a sufficient amount of time must be allotted for the patient to answer the question: "Do you recall any anesthesia complications associated with these procedures?" Additional questioning related to past surgery and anesthesia include: "Has anyone in your family ever had any anesthesia complications?" An initial response to this question may be an immediate, "No." However, with some prompting, patients may recall a negative past anesthetic experience. This prompting includes: "Have you ever had nausea or vomiting after any past surgical or diagnostic procedures or been admitted to the intensive care unit unexpectedly?" Positive responses must be followed up with contact with physician

TABLE 2-9				
H_2 Antagonist and Gastrokinetic Agent Dosing Schedule				
MEDICATION	**DOSAGE**	**HALF-LIFE (hr)**	**ONSET OF ACTION (min)**	**DURATION OF ACTION (hr)**
H_2 Antagonist				
Cimetidine	300 mg PO hs and 75 min before the procedure	2	45-60	3-4
Ranitidine	150 mg PO hs and 1-1.5 hr before the procedure	2.5-3	60-90	8-9
Famotidine	20 mg PO 1-1.5 hr before the procedure	2.5-3.5	60	10-12
Gastrokinetic Agent				
Metoclopramide*	10 mg PO	2-4	30-60	
	0.15 mg/kg IV over 3-5 min	2-4	1-3	1-2

*Action: dopamine antagonist that stimulates upper gastrointestinal motility and gastric emptying and increases gastroesophageal sphincter tone.

offices, hospitals, or surgicenters to ascertain specific complications associated with prior surgical or diagnostic procedures. If previous anesthesia records are secured for review, the following items should be documented:

◆ Response to preoperative sedative medications
◆ Verification of ease of airway management
◆ Vascular access
◆ Intraoperative complications
◆ Drug reactions
◆ Hemodynamic parameters
◆ Documented postoperative complications

MEDICATION EVALUATION

The purpose of the presedation evaluation is to decrease morbidity and optimize the patient's condition before the proposed procedure. After organ system assessment, it is important to identify currently prescribed medications and therapeutic rationale. A medication review during presedation assessment includes asking the patient, "What medications are you currently taking?" This question allows the patient to answer with prescription and over-the-counter medications he or she may be using.

When one is questioning the patient about medications, it is important to evaluate and ascertain drug dosage and last dose administered. Once the medication history is complete, it is important to give the patient accurate presedation instructions related to the current medication regimen. An example of this includes the continuation of antihypertensive medications up to and including the morning of the procedure to promote cardiovascular stability. When indicated, aspirin and nonsteroidal anti-inflammatory drugs may be discontinued secondary to bleeding potential associated with platelet dysfunction. Rarely, a patient may indicate uncertainty regarding which medication he or she is taking or report taking "two little white pills and a red pill." It is important to ascertain the name, dosage, and last ingestion of these medications. This may be accomplished after questioning a family member or a significant other. If the patient or family member cannot identify a medication, it may be necessary to contact the prescribing physician or the physician's office staff for confirmation of the prescribed treatment protocol.

> During the presedation assessment, it is important for the healthcare provider to ascertain prescribed medication protocol, treatment efficacy, and patient compliance.

ALLERGIES

A continuation of presedation medication assessment includes the patient's allergy history. Questions related to an allergy history include "Are you allergic to any medication?" At this point, many patients respond with "No" or with a list of several allergies. Allergies reported may include nausea associated with the use of analgesics or gastrointestinal upset with the use of antibiotics. The side effects associated with the use of pharmacologic agents are separate and distinct from an allergic reaction. Side effects may be classified as unpleasant reactions or adverse reactions to prescribed drugs. True allergies to pharmacologic agents occur with less frequency and are manifested by the following conditions:

◆ Bronchospasm
◆ Circulatory collapse
◆ Edema
◆ Hives
◆ Hypotension
◆ Pruritus
◆ Skin wheals
◆ Wheezing

Fortunately, true allergic reactions are rare and the patient's recollection may be insufficient. Many patients may recall rashes and hives, whereas few may recall the development of cardiovascular collapse. This information may be elicited from patient recollection or review of a previous chart. Close observation of all patients after a medication has been administered is the most prudent course.

Anaphylactic vs. Anaphylactoid

Anaphylaxis refers to a life-threatening drug reaction of a severe magnitude. Anaphylactic drug reactions are mediated via the IgE immunoglobulin within the immune system. Therefore, anaphylactic reactions are life-threatening drug reactions mediated by antibodies. The term **anaphylactoid** is used when there is no antibody involvement in the reaction.[37] **Differentiation of anaphylactic vs. anaphylactoid reaction during the procedure is not important.** What is important is the **identification** of an allergic response. Presenting symptoms of allergic reaction include urticaria, hypotension, oropharyngeal edema, hives, wheezing, bronchoconstriction, and cardiovascular compromise requiring immediate diagnosis and treatment. The treatment protocol of an allergic reaction includes:

◆ Preparation
◆ Discontinue suspected allergen
◆ Airway maintenance
◆ Intravenous volume (Several liters [20 mL/kg] may be required if there is massive vasodilatation.)
◆ Epinephrine (in the presence of cardiovascular collapse)
◆ Diphenhydramine
◆ Terbutaline
◆ Aminophylline
◆ Corticosteroids

Presedation assessment of the patient with multiple allergies or documentation of a true anaphylactic or anaphylactoid reaction requires careful preparation and planning before the administration of sedation. The initial step in the prevention of an allergic reaction includes identification of the allergen. It may be difficult to identify an allergen in the patient's history or previous anesthetic/sedation records. When antibiotics, local anesthetics, sedatives, hypnotics, and analgesics have been combined and administered, it may be extremely difficult to specify which medication precipitated the allergic response. A true IgE-mediated allergy to narcotics is rare. In the case of this rare phenomenon, a nonsteroidal analgesic may offer the clinician an analgesic alternative without the need for narcotic adjuncts.

> At this point in the presedation patient assessment, it is also efficacious to ask the patient if he or she has ever been informed of an allergy to latex. The American Association of Nurse Anesthetists Latex Allergy Protocol is featured in Appendix E.

REVIEW OF LABORATORY DATA

The current state of healthcare reimbursement dictates conscientious, efficient presedation laboratory testing and screening. In the past, laboratory or diagnostic testing was reimbursed on a fee-for-service basis. As reimbursement continues to evolve into a capitated system, the clinician must focus on specific laboratory or diagnostic tests that yield beneficial information about the patient. Achievement of these goals in a cost-effective way is a challenge in a capitated healthcare system. In addition, random laboratory testing in the absence of suspicious clinical features or symptoms is not only expensive, it is time consuming and inconvenient for the patient and may result in patient harm. Therefore, it is imperative to use presedation laboratory assessment tools in an efficacious manner to avoid expensive office, surgicenter, or hospital delays on the day of the procedure. On the whole, there is not much direct benefit from unindicated routine laboratory testing. In the absence of preexisting pathophysiologic disease states these diagnostic tests:

◆ Frequently fail to uncover pathophysiologic conditions
◆ Detect abnormalities, which does not necessarily improve clinical outcome
◆ Are inefficient in screening for asymptomatic diseases
◆ Do not alter procedural management of the patient

After completion of a thorough chart review, history, and physical examination, determining factors for laboratory testing include:

◆ Patient age
◆ Magnitude of planned procedure
◆ Medication history
◆ Positive findings during medical history and physical examination

Laboratory testing guidelines for asymptomatic patients, which have been reported in the literature, are featured in Table 2-10.

As the practice of quality patient care continues to be the provider's goal, the judicious ordering of laboratory and diagnostic testing yields relevant clinical data. These data should be used to anticipate complications, decrease morbidity and mortality, and reduce preprocedural delays. On the basis of the broad variety of surgical, therapeutic, and diagnostic

procedures that may be performed with sedation, the clinician must decide which laboratory testing is required for the specific patient population. A Simplified Strategy for Preprocedure Testing Indications postulated by Roizen, Kaplan, and Blery is featured in Figure 2-3 on p. 50.[38-40] An algorithmic approach that may assist the clinician in ordering presedation laboratory testing is featured in Figure 2-4 on p. 51. These recommendations may prove beneficial for the attending physician ordering presedation laboratory and diagnostic testing.

> To have diagnostic testing yield beneficial information, it is important to conduct a thorough patient history and physical examination before considering if a laboratory test is indicated.

DENTITION

Presedation assessment of dentition includes inquiry and visual examination of the oral cavity. The status of the patient's dentition should be documented for the presence of loose, chipped, cracked, or missing teeth. Thorough documentation is beneficial if postprocedure patient claims of loose or missing teeth arise after specific procedures. Medial or lateral chipping should be documented before the procedure. Additional anomalies should be noted, as well as identification of specific dental sites. Figure 2-5 on p. 54 features an oral cavity evaluation table.

SOCIAL HISTORY

During presedation assessment it is important to obtain a social history from the patient. Components of the social history include inquiry and assessment for cigarette smoking, alcohol intake, illicit drug use, and the possibility of pregnancy. Additionally, patients should be assessed for over-the-counter medication use and/or utilization of herbal preparations. When inquiring into a patient's alcohol, drug, or social history, it is best to obtain this information via a matter-of-fact approach. Any attempts to belittle or pressure the patient will result in patient withdrawal and, most likely, an inaccurate history. A variety of mechanisms may be used to elicit this information in a diplomatic and tactful manner.

Cigarette Smoking

A cigarette smoking history must be quantified in pack-years and documented on the presedation assessment form.

$$\text{Pack-years} = \text{Number of packs smoked} \\ \text{per day} \times \text{number of years smoked}$$

The inhaled components of smoke are associated with the development of coronary artery disease, peripheral vascular disease, cerebrovascular disease, stroke, COPD, peptic ulcer disease, esophageal reflux, and lung cancer.[41-43] Nicotine produces an increase in heart rate, blood pressure, myocardial contraction, myocardial oxygen consumption, and myocardial excitement. These sympathetic nervous system changes are undesirable in a patient presenting for sedation who may already be apprehensive and anxious. Therefore, patients should be counseled to consider cessation of smoking 12 hours before the procedure. Patient education should include instruction that this 12-hour abstinence period reduces the deleterious effects of nicotine and carbon monoxide on cardiopulmonary function.[44] The sedation practitioner caring for the pediatric patient subjected to second hand smoke must be prepared to handle complications associated with children who are exposed to passive smoke.[45-47] These complications include:

◆ Increased reactive airway disease
◆ Abnormal pulmonary function tests
◆ Increased respiratory tract infection
◆ Laryngospasm
◆ Postsedation oxyhemoglobin desaturation

Alcohol Intake

Traditional questions to solicit alcohol intake history have included: "Have you ever had a drinking problem?" or "Have you had any alcohol in the last 24 hours?" Aside from appearing abrupt, these questions are also closed ended. An alternative approach in presedation assessment is the broader, more open-ended question, such as "How much alcohol do you consume in 1 week?" The patient can respond in a variety of ways: "I have wine with dinner every night," "None," "A couple of beers on the weekend," or "Two or three scotches every evening." These comments generally lead to further discussion of alcohol history and intake. The **CAGE** approach in evaluating a patient's alcohol consumption has been reported in the literature.[48] It utilizes the following four questions to solicit information related to alcohol use:

◆ Do you feel you should **C**ut down on your alcohol consumption?
◆ Have people **A**nnoyed you by criticizing your drinking?
◆ Have you felt **G**uilty about your drinking?
◆ Have you ever had a drink first thing in the morning to steady your nerves or get rid of a hangover (**E**ye opener)?

Two or more affirmative responses from the patient signifies a high risk for alcoholism and an increased likelihood for experiencing withdrawal symptoms.[49]

Patients with rare social alcohol use afford minimal concern for multisystemic disease states. However, patients with a history of two or three drinks with lunch or dinner may require additional sedative medication during sedation procedures secondary to increased cytochrome P-450 system activity. Chronic use of alcohol frequently leads to stimulation of the cytochrome P-450 system located in the endoplasmic reticulum of the liver. This stimulation requires increased amounts or doses of sedative and analgesic medications. Chronic ingestion of alcohol is associated with multisystemic symptoms. Box 2-6 on p. 55 features the toxic effects associated with chronic alcohol intake. Patients with a history of chronic alcohol use require presedation preparation aimed at the presenting symptoms. Chronic alcoholism

may lead to cirrhosis, elevated liver enzyme levels, esophageal varices, nutritional disorders, gastritis, psychiatric disorders, cardiac myopathy, electrolyte disturbances, and cerebral atrophy. These symptoms predispose patients to increased risks during the administration of sedation. As opposed to chronic alcohol ingestion, a general rule of thumb when dealing with acute alcoholism is to anticipate a decrease in anesthetic requirements. A full stomach and a lack of patient cooperation are also additional risk factors associated with acute alcohol intoxication. If morning presedation assessment reveals the odor of alcohol on the patient's breath, blood for determination of serum alcohol levels should be drawn immediately with the patient's permission. If the patient refuses or if the level is indicative of recent alcohol ingestion, the procedure should be canceled. Cancellation is warranted because of probable noncompliance with NPO instructions and the risks associated with increased gastric volume.

> Chronic alcohol abuse frequently leads to an increase in the amount of sedation required. This occurs secondary to enhanced cytochrome P-450 system activity in the smooth endoplasmic reticulum in the liver.

Stimulant Medications

Stimulants, weight-reduction medications, and "designer drugs" can be ingested orally, inhaled, or used intravenously. Amphetamines cause central nervous system stimulation and may predispose the patient to cardiac dysrhythmias, including palpitations and tachycardia. Amphetamine abuse increases the release of catecholamines. Amphetamines are often used in patients with weight disorders, narcolepsy, and attention deficit disorder and as recreational substances. Chronic abuse of amphetamines leads to tolerance and psychotic states secondary to depleted body catecholamine stores. Dieting fads that result in significant weight reduction in short periods of time require additional laboratory data review. A 12-lead ECG, SMA chemistry, and a complete blood cell count are required to assess electrolyte and hematologic abnormality and to rule out the presence of cardiac conduction abnormalities before the administration of sedation.

Ecstasy

Addiction and many deaths have been reported as a result of designer drug use. The best known and most widely used designer drug is 3,4-methylenedioxymethamphetamine (MDMA, or Ecstasy).[50] Recreational use of Ecstasy began to emerge in the mid 1980s and was commonly utilized during "raves" (large dance parties numbering in the thousands in abandoned warehouses).[51] The drug chemically resembles a combination of amphetamine and mescaline and can be taken orally, injected, smoked, or snorted. Onset is generally within 20 to 45 minutes and the effect may last up to 6 hours.[52]

Text continued on p. 54.

TABLE 2-10

Recommended Test Guidelines for Asymptomatic Patients

AGE	ROIZEN (1994) (SIMPLIFIED) 1	ROIZEN (1994) 2	ROIZEN (1990) 3 ♂	ROIZEN (1990) 3 ♀	ROIZEN (1986) 4 ♂	ROIZEN (1986) 4 ♀	ROIZEN (1981) 5 ♂	ROIZEN (1981) 5 ♀	EISEMAN (1989) 6	VELANOVICH (1991) 7
<6 mo			None	Hb or Hct	None	Hct or Hb	?SGOT ?BUN ?Gluc	Hb or Hct SCOT ?BUN ?Gluc	CBC Elect BUN/Gluc Urin Protime PTT PLT Cnt CXR ECG FOBT	
6 mo 2 y	Hb or Hct	None (♂)								
6 y		Hb or HCT ?Preg test (♀)								
18 y										
30 y										ECG
40 y	Hct ECG	Hct ECG	BUN/Gluc ECG	Hb or Hct BUN/Gluc ECG	BUN/Gluc ECG	Hct or Hb BUN/Gluc ECG	?SGOT BUN/Gluc ECG	Hb or Hct ?SGOT BUN/Gluc ECG		Hct BUN/Gluc Creat Tot Prot/Alb Lymph Cnt CXR ECG
50 y		Hct ECG								
60 y			Hb or Hct BUN/Gluc CXR ECG		Hb or Hct BUN/Gluc CXR ECG		Hb or Hct BUN/Gluc CXR ECG ?SGOT			
65 y	Hct ECG BUN/Gluc	Hct BUN ECG								
70 y										
75 y and over		Hct BUN/Gluc ECG								

[a]Recommendations of the American College of Surgeons.
[b]Recommendations of the Mayo Clinic, Rochester, Minn.
[c]Personal communication with JV Roth (Albert Einstein Hospital, NY).
[d]Personal communication with SL Kaplan (Westfall Surgery Center, Rochester, NY).
Alb, Albumin; BUN/Gluc, blood urea nitrogen and glucose; CBC, complete blood count; Creat, creatinine; ECG, electrocardiogram; Elect, electrolytes; CXR, chest radiograph; FOBT, fecal occult blood test; Gluc, glucose; Hb, hemoglobin; Hct, hematocrit; Lymph Cnt, lymphocyte count; PLT Cnt, platelet count; Preg test, pregnancy test; Protime, prothrombin time; PTT, partial thromboplastin time; SGOT, serum glutamic-oxaloacetic transaminase; Tot Prot, total protein; Urin, urinalysis.
From Miller R: *Anesthesia*, 5th ed. New York: Churchill Livingstone: 2002;854-855.

LARSON (1992)	BLERY ET AL (1986)		MCKEE AND SCOTT (1987)		NARR ET AL (1991)	MACPHERSON ET AL (1990)		ALBERT EINSTEIN HOSPITAL (1993)	WESTFALL SURGICAL CENTER
8	9		10		11	12		13	14
CBC Urin	Minor surg None	Major surg Hct or Hb	None		None	Minor surg None	Major surg CBC	None	None
								CBC	
CBC Urin Elect BUN Creat Gluc CXR ECG	ECG	Hct or Hb ECG	CBC / CBC ECG		ECG Creat/Gluc	BUN ECG	CBC BUN ECG	CBC ECG	ECG
	BUN/ Creat Elect ECG	Hct BUN/ Creat Elect ECG	Minor surg CBC ECG	Major surg CBC BUN Elect ECG CXR	CBC Creat/Gluc ECG CXR	BUN ECG CXR	CBC BUN ECG CXR	CBC BUN CXR Elect Gluc	

PREOPERATIVE CONDITION[b]	Hb M	Hb F	WBC	PT/PTT	PLT, BT	ELECT	CREAT/BUN	BLOOD GLUCOSE OR Hb A_{1c}	SGOT/ALK PTAse	X-RAY	ECG	PREG TEST	ALBUMIN	T/S
Neonates	X	X												
Physiologic age ≥75 y	X	X					X	X		X	X			X
Procedure type C	X	X					X	X			X		X	
Cardiovascular disease							X			X	X			
Pulmonary disease										X	X			
Malignancy	X	X	†	†						X	X			
Radiation therapy			X											
Hepatic disease				X					X					
Exposure to hepatitis									X					
Renal disease	X	X				X	X							
Bleeding disorder				X	X						X			X
Diabetes						X	X	X						
Smoking ≥20 pack-years	X	X								X				
Possible pregnancy												X		
Use of:														
Diuretics						X	X							
Digoxin						X	X				X			
Steroids						X		X						
Anticoagulants	X	X	X	X			X							
Central nervous system disease	X					X	X	X			X			

aFor minimally invasive procedures (type A, e.g., cataracts, diagnostic arthroscopy), no tests are indicated. For moderately invasive surgery (type B procedures, in which blood loss or hemodynamic changes are rare), clinical judgment is needed when selecting tests.

bNot all diseases and pertinent conditions are included in this table. Therefore, the physician should use judgment regarding patients having diseases and conditions that are not listed.

X, obtain test; †, obtain test for leukemias only; BT, bleeding time; Creat/BUN, creatinine or blood urea nitrogen; ECG, electrocardiogram; Elect, electrolytes (i.e., sodium, potassium, chloride, carbon dioxide, and proteins); Hb, hemoglobin (obtain for male [M] or female [F] patients); Hb A_{1c}, glycosylated hemoglobin; pack-y, pack-years, i.e., the smoking of one pack of cigarettes per day for 1 year; PLT, platelet count; PT, prothrombin time; PTT, partial thromboplastin time; SGOT/Alk PTAse, serum glutamic-oxaloacetic transaminase and alkaline phosphatase; T/S, blood typing and screening for unexpected antibodies; WBC, white blood cell count.

Data from Roizen, Kaplan et al, and Blery et al.

FIGURE 2-3 Simplified strategy for preprocedure testing.a (From Miller R. *Anesthesia.* 5th ed. New York: Churchill Livingstone; 2002:856.)

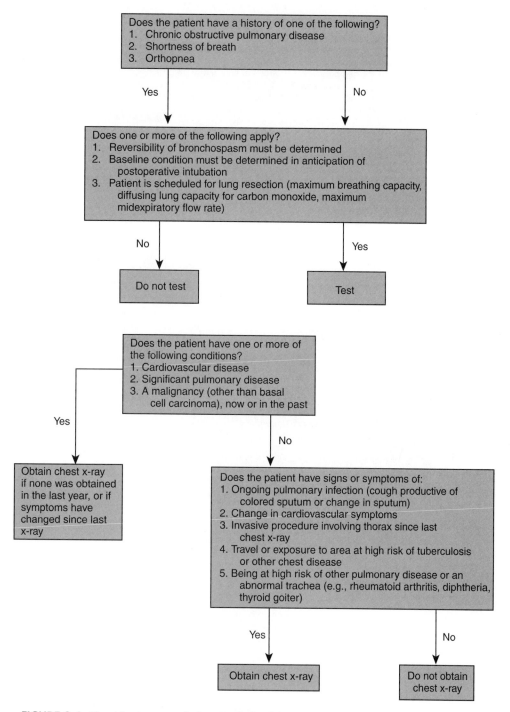

FIGURE 2-4 Algorithmic approach for presedation laboratory testing. (From Miller R. *Anesthesia.* 5th ed. New York: Churchill Livingstone; 2002:858-860.)

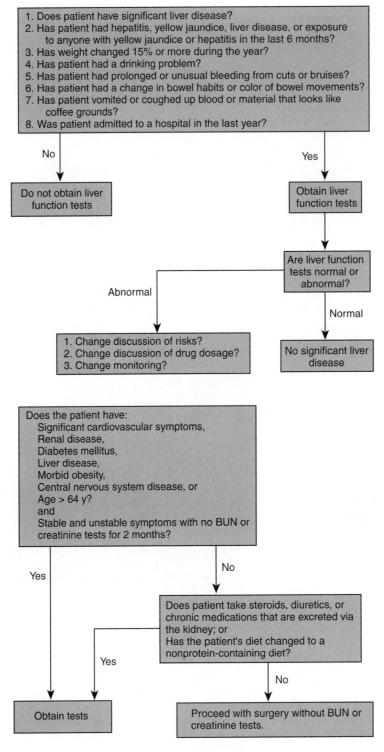

1. Does patient have significant liver disease?
2. Has patient had hepatitis, yellow jaundice, liver disease, or exposure to anyone with yellow jaundice or hepatitis in the last 6 months?
3. Has weight changed 15% or more during the year?
4. Has patient had a drinking problem?
5. Has patient had prolonged or unusual bleeding from cuts or bruises?
6. Has patient had a change in bowel habits or color of bowel movements?
7. Has patient vomited or coughed up blood or material that looks like coffee grounds?
8. Was patient admitted to a hospital in the last year?

No → Do not obtain liver function tests

Yes → Obtain liver function tests

Are liver function tests normal or abnormal?

Abnormal →
1. Change discussion of risks?
2. Change discussion of drug dosage?
3. Change monitoring?

Normal → No significant liver disease

Does the patient have:
  Significant cardiovascular symptoms,
  Renal disease,
  Diabetes mellitus,
  Liver disease,
  Morbid obesity,
  Central nervous system disease, or
  Age > 64 y?
  and
  Stable and unstable symptoms with no BUN or creatinine tests for 2 months?

Yes → Obtain tests

No → Does patient take steroids, diuretics, or chronic medications that are excreted via the kidney; or Has the patient's diet changed to a nonprotein-containing diet?

Yes → Obtain tests

No → Proceed with surgery without BUN or creatinine tests.

FIGURE 2-4, cont'd

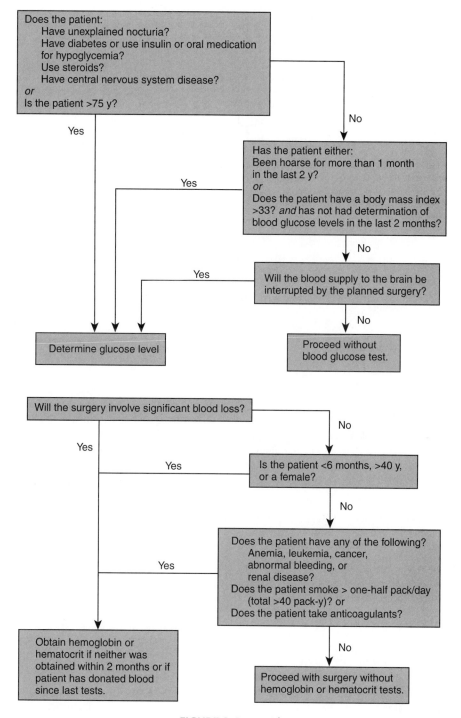

FIGURE 2-4, cont'd

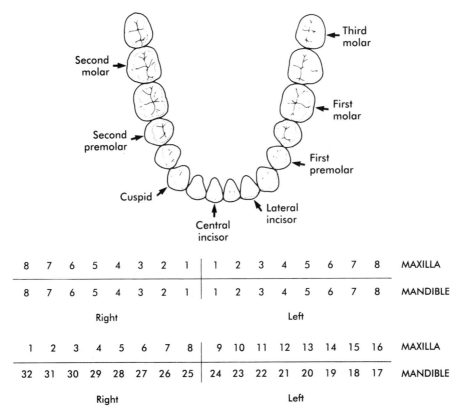

FIGURE 2-5 Oral cavity inspection. (From Longnecker DE, Tinker JK, and Morgan GE: *Principles and Practice of Anesthesiology.* 2nd ed. St. Louis: Mosby; 1998:2452.)

The most common complications associated with its use include hyperthermia and idiosyncratic reactions. Physiologic symptoms associated with the use of Ecstasy include altered mental status, tachycardia, tachypnea, profuse sweating, and hyperthermia.[53] Clinical management is directed at controlling presenting symptomatology. Treatment includes fluids for hypotension, benzodiazepines for agitation and seizures, dopamine or norepinephrine for hypotension unresponsive to fluid challenges, phentolamine or nitroprusside for hypertension, lidocaine for ventricular dysrhythmias, and nitroglycerin for myocardial ischemic pain.[54] A summary of the cardiovascular effects and recommended treatment associated with Ecstasy use is featured in Table 2-11 on p. 56.

Cocaine Abuse

It has been estimated that 30 million Americans have used cocaine and 5 million use it on a regular basis.[55] Cocaine is an ester-based local anesthetic with vasoconstrictive properties. Its alkaloid derivative from the leaves of the *Erythroxylon coca* plant is prepared by dissolving the alkaloid base to form a water-soluble salt (cocaine hydrochloride). It can be sold as crystals, granules, or white powder. Cocaine can be ingested orally (chewing coca leaves), intravenously, intranasally (snorting), or smoked as free base cocaine (crack cocaine). **Cocaine can produce negative inotropic and chronotropic effects on the heart muscle.** In addition, cocaine impairs neural reuptake of dopamine, serotonin, and tryptophan. Illicit use results in a euphoric sensation. Through its vasoconstricting properties, it leads to hypertension, myocardial ischemia, dysrhythmias, myocardial infarction, cerebral hemorrhage, and seizures. ECG evidence of silent ischemia persists for up to 6 weeks in humans after discontinuing cocaine use. In addition, the chronic alteration in cerebral blood flow that cocaine produces in humans does not return to normal after even 30 days of cocaine abstinence. Pulmonary effects include cocaine-induced asthma, hypersensitivity pneumonitis, chronic cough, pulmonary edema, pneumopericardium, and pulmonary hemorrhage. Presedation recommendations for the patient with acute cocaine ingestion include postponement of the procedure for 24 to 48 hours.[56] Patients suspected of cocaine abuse should also be carefully assessed in the following areas before the procedure:

◆ Nasal mucosa for deterioration
◆ Assessment of all extremities for the presence of needle marks
◆ Auscultation of the lungs to exclude asthma
◆ Careful cardiovascular and neurologic examination
◆ Chest radiograph to rule out pulmonary involvement
◆ ECG to identify signs of rhythm disturbance and presence of ischemia/injury/previous myocardial infarction

As noted, complications associated with the procedure secondary to cocaine abuse include cardiac dysrhythmias, tachycardia, and increased myocardial oxygen consumption. **Therefore, ketamine should be avoided or used with extreme caution in this patient population because it can markedly potentiate the cardiovascular toxicity of cocaine.**[57] Additional pharmacologic concerns include using ester-type local anesthetic solutions with caution secondary to their metabolism by plasma cholinesterase. These drugs may compete with cocaine for this metabolic pathway and result in decreased metabolism of both the cocaine and the local anesthetic. Use of naloxone may intensify the actions of cocaine and thus should be used carefully in this patient population.[58] A summary of the cardiovascular effects and recommended treatment associated with cocaine use is featured in Table 2-11.

Opioid Abuse

Opioids are abused via the oral, subcutaneous, or intravenous routes of administration. Opioid ingestion produces a euphoric state with resultant analgesia. Tolerance of the effects of opioids occurs with chronic ingestion. Patients with a history of chronic opioid abuse generally require increased doses of sedative medications during the administration of sedation. It is important to remember that the procedural period is not the time to withdraw an addict from opioid abuse.

Heroin

Heroin was first introduced in the late 1800s as a "less addicting morphine substitute." Chemical alteration of the morphine molecule yields heroin, which is three to four times more potent than morphine. An intense rush is achieved with smoking or injection.[59] Withdrawal symptoms begin 8 to 24 hours after the last use of heroin. Characteristic withdrawal symptoms include:

- Influenza-like syndrome
- Drug craving
- Anxiety
- Sweating
- Tremors
- Rhinorrhea
- Muscle aches
- Sympathetic nervous system discharge

Presenting symptomatology should be controlled through the use of benzodiazepines to control anxiety and agitation and beta blockers for tachycardia and hypertension. Medical problems associated with heroin abuse include malnutrition, chronic anemia, cellulites, bacterial endocarditis (tricuspid valve), pulmonary and systemic septic emboli and infarctions, aspiration pneumonitis, atelectasis, hepatitis, hepatomegaly, and sclerosing glomerulonephritis. **Presedation patient optimization is directed to the organ system affected.** Laboratory testing (blood cell count, liver function tests) is indicated based on the presenting pathophysiology associated with opioid abuse. A baseline ECG is advised secondary to the enhanced automaticity of the heart associated with the heroin-addicted patient. A summary of the cardiovascular effects and recommended treatment associated with opioid abuse is featured in Table 2-11.

Benzodiazepines

Chronic use of benzodiazepines for skeletal muscle relaxation or as antianxiety medication leads to cross-tolerance and addiction. The benzodiazepine-addicted patient will develop a cross-tolerance not only to benzodiazepine medications but to other sedative and analgesic medications as well.

Marijuana

Marijuana is the most common illegal drug used in the United States and approximately one third of all high school seniors have used the drug.[60] The most common means of ingestion of marijuana is smoking. Smoking marijuana increases tetrahydrocannabinol, producing a postinhalation euphoric state in conjunction with sympathetic nervous system stimulation. This increased sympathetic stimulation

TABLE 2-11

Effects of Cardiovascular Complications, Recommended Management of Commonly Misused Drugs

ILLICIT DRUG	EFFECTS	CARDIOVASCULAR COMPLICATIONS	RECOMMENDED MANAGEMENT	
Cocaine	Inhibits reuptake of neuronal catecholamines Class I Na⁺ channel blockade antiarrhythmic effects	Hypertension	Benzodiazepines, nitrates, phentolamine, sodium nitroprusside, or hydralazine	
		Bradyarrhythmias (cocaine)	Atropine (cautiously) temporary transvenous cardiac pacing	
		Supraventricular tachyarrhythmias	Observation (settles with time), adenosine, DCC, beta blocker, alpha blocker in combination	
		Ventricular arrhythmias	DCC, lidocaine, magnesium sulfate	
Amphetamines	Release catecholamines from nerve terminals	Myocardial ischemia and infarction	Aspirin, nitrates, phentolamine, thrombolysis, or coronary intervention	
		Acute heart failure	Diuretics, inotropes, ventilation and intra-aortic balloon pumping may be necessary	
Ecstasy	Releases catecholamines from nerve terminals	NCPO	Ventilation	
		Chronic heart failure	Conventional	
		Endocarditis	Conventional	
LSD, psilocybin ("magic mushrooms")	Serotonergic, dopaminergic, and adrenergic activities	Tachycardia	Observe	
		Supraventricular arrhythmias	Observe, adenosine or verapamil	
		Hypertension	Observe but if severe treat as for cocaine, amphetamine, and ecstasy	
		Myocardial ischemia	As for cocaine, amphetamine, and ecstasy	
Narcotics	Act on the vasomotor center (increase parasympathetic and decrease sympathetic activity)	Bradyarrhythmias	Atropine, temporary transvenous cardiac pacing	May require treatment with an opioid antagonist
		Supraventricular arrhythmias	Adenosine, beta blockers, verapamil, digoxin, DCC	

General measures: ensure adequate airway, breathing, circulation and correct any hypoxic, metabolic, and electrolyte disturbances.
DCC, DC cardioversion; NCPO, noncardiogenic pulmonary edema.
From Kain Z, Barash P. *Anesthetic Implications of Drug Abuse ASA Refresher Course.* Philadelphia: Lippincott, Williams & Wilkins; 2001:29(15):166-167.

Continued

TABLE 2-11

Effects of Cardiovascular Complications, Recommended Management of Commonly Misused Drugs—cont'd

ILLICIT DRUG	EFFECTS	CARDIOVASCULAR COMPLICATIONS	RECOMMENDED MANAGEMENT
	Histamine release from mast cell degranulation	Ventricular arrhythmias	DCC, antiarrhythmic drugs should be used with caution
		Hypotension	IV fluids, vasopressor, inotropic agents
		NCPO	Ventilation
		Endocarditis	Conventional
Volatile substances	Complex multisystem detrimental effects on cardiovascular function	Bradyarrhythmias	Atropine (cautiously), transvenous temporary cardiac pacing
		Supraventricular arrhythmias	Adenosine, beta blockers, digoxin (atrial fibrillation)
		Ventricular arrhythmias	Lidocaine, beta blockers, amiodarone
		Hypotension	IV fluids, calcium gluconate
		Cardiac ischemia	Conventional
		Cardiomyopathy	Conventional
Cannabis (marijuana)	Biphasic dose dependent effect on the autonomic nervous system	Tachycardia with no or slight increase in blood pressure	Support. Significant bradycardia; consider atropine
		Large doses: hypotension, bradycardia	Pronounced hypotension, consider IV fluids: pressor agents rarely needed

increases heart rate and myocardial oxygen consumption and produces orthostatic hypotension in some persons. Patients with a history of chronic marijuana use characteristically present with the following symptoms:

◆ Chronic sinusitis
◆ Tar deposit in the lung
◆ Pulmonary impairment
◆ Conjunctival irritation

The effects of inhaled marijuana last for only several hours. Therefore, it is rare to encounter patients who are acutely intoxicated secondary to marijuana ingestion. **Patients who admit to marijuana ingestion should have resting heart rate and blood pressure documented before initiation of the procedure.** Severe tachycardia should be controlled with beta blockers. To decrease the incidence of pulmonary complications, symptoms of pulmonary impairment should be resolved before the administration of sedation.

Substance Abuse Summary

It is important to approach patients with a history of substance abuse on the basis of the drug abused, the time of last ingestion, and presenting symptoms. Symptoms associated with drug abuse may be life threatening and include the following:

◆ Cellulitis
◆ Abscess of the skin
◆ Cardiomyopathy
◆ Psychotic behavior
◆ Aspiration with overdose
◆ Hepatitis
◆ Acquired immunodeficiency disease
◆ Sepsis
◆ Endocarditis

Counseling and social service support are imperative for this patient population. It is important to approach these patients individually and to realize that they have a disease of addiction, which requires specific treatment and therapy.

Herbal Use

During social and medication history assessment it is important for the clinician to identify patient use of herbal preparations. **The use of herbal preparations has grown in popularity over the past decade.** Annual sales have increased from 3 billion dollars in 1990 to 12 billion dollars in 2000.[61] Sedation patients may utilize herbal preparations for chronic conditions (arthritis, depression, diabetes) or dissatisfaction with traditional medical treatment. Of the Americans utilizing alternative therapies including herbal products, 60% still do not routinely inform their physicians. Among patients who do not discuss use of alternative regimens with their physicians, 55% report that their physicians did not inquire about alternative therapy use.[62] This leaves an estimated 15 million Americans, of whom 3 million are aged 65 and older, at risk for herbal interactions. Although many of these products are recommended or prescribed by conventional medical practitioners, these drugs carry a potential to increase bleeding and can alter the patient's response to sedative, analgesic, and anesthetic agents.

> Healthcare providers need to focus on patient utilization of herbal preparations. It is important for the attending physician to assess for the use of herbal preparations before the procedure.

Ephedra

Ephedra, or ma huang, is a plant derivative that has historically been utilized for its medicinal ingredient ephedrine. North American use of ephedra includes herbal weight loss preparations and central nervous stimulant and ergogenic preparations. Ephedra and its related alkaloids produce sympathetic (adrenergic) nervous system stimulation. Symptoms associated with ephedra use include:

◆ Increased blood pressure
◆ Increased heart rate
◆ Bronchodilation
◆ Peripheral vasoconstriction
◆ Diuresis
◆ Stimulation of smooth muscle contraction

> Careful monitoring to assess for signs of cardiac stimulation is required during the sedation procedure and in the immediate postsedation period.

Feverfew

The principal active ingredient in feverfew is parthenolide, which was historically used to decrease fever. It is also used for its anti-inflammatory effects associated with inhibition of phospholipase. Feverfew inhibits serotonin release from platelets and platelet aggregation. **Long-term users of feverfew should be advised to discontinue use for 7 to 10 days before the planned procedure secondary to feverfew's ability to increase the risk of bleeding.**

Garlic

Garlic is a widely recognized flavoring additive that contains a variety of organosulfur components. Suspected clinical effects associated with garlic use include:

◆ Blood pressure–lowering effects
◆ Decrease in total cholesterol
◆ Decrease in triglyceride levels

Garlic use has been associated with an increase in bleeding potentially through possible antiplatelet effects related to inhibition of thromboxane B_2. **Therefore, sedation patients using garlic should be advised to discontinue use for 7 to 10 days before the planned procedure secondary to garlic's ability to increase the risk of bleeding.**

Ginger

Ginger is a widely recognized spice that has been used medicinally in the Far East for thousands of years. Reported advantages associated with ginger use include antiemesis and symptomatic treatment of migraines and arthritis. Use of ginger results in the inhibition of prostaglandin and leukotriene biosynthesis.[63] **Sedation patients should be counseled to discontinue use for 7 to 10 days secondary to the potential risk associated with bleeding.**

Ginkgo

Ginkgo biloba has been reported to offer beneficial effects for patients with memory loss or cognitive dysfunction. Patients may also take ginkgo for circulatory disorders, tinnitus, sexual dysfunction, asthma, and age-associated macular degeneration. Ginkgo has antioxidant effects, decreases red blood cell aggregation and blood viscosity, and increases blood flow. Side effects associated with ginkgo use include spontaneous bleeding. **Sedation patients should be counseled to discontinue ginkgo use 7 to 10 days before the procedure secondary to the potential increased risk of bleeding.**

Ginseng

Ginseng has been utilized as an adaptogen. Adaptogens allow the body to maintain normal function under times of stress. Adaptogens are believed to enhance mood and cognitive function, relieve stress, increase physical performance, improve cardiovascular function, improve glucose regulation, and enhance hepatic protection. Ginseng decreases platelet aggregation and may produce hypotension through vasodilatory effects. **Sedation patients should be counseled to discontinue use of ginseng for 7 to 10 days before the procedure secondary to its vasodilating properties and potential for bleeding.**

Kava

Kava is an herbal product known for its calming and relaxation effects. Anxiolytic effects may be associated with its effect on GABA receptors. The anxiolytic effects seen with kava may be similar to those associated with benzodiazepine use. Kava has been reported to have dopamine antagonistic effects, monoamine oxidase inhibition, and platelet aggregation inhibition. **Patients should be counseled to discontinue kava use 7 to 10 days before the procedure.**

St. John's Wort

St. John's Wort is used for its antidepressant effects in treating patients with mild to moderate depression. Pharmacologic effects include inhibition of norepinephrine, serotonin, and dopamine uptake at synaptic junctions. Because of its variety of pharmacologic actions, it is not advised to continue St. John's Wort with other antidepressant medications. Additionally, St. John's Wort has the potential to interact with adrenergic stimulants (ephedrine, phenylephrine, and phenylpropanolamine).

A summary of adverse effects and considerations for selected herbs is featured in Table 2-12. Healthcare providers must inquire into a patient's medication history to include use of over-the-counter drugs, herbal products, dietary supplements, vitamins, and minerals. Patients should be asked directly about these products, which can increase bleeding and alter the sympathetic nervous system response.

Pregnancy

Female patients of childbearing age must be questioned regarding the possibility of pregnancy. This question may also be asked in a variety of ways. Some clinicians simply ask, "Is there any possibility that you are pregnant?" A simple "yes" or "no" answer seems to appease some practitioners. However, many providers are more investigative. If a patient is uncertain of her pregnancy status or the healthcare practitioner suspects pregnancy, a presedation pregnancy test should be ordered.[64] Additional issues that must be addressed when deciding whether to order a pregnancy test include:[65]

- Policies of the hospital or health care facility based on medical staff bylaws. The medical facility should have established guidelines that delineate when testing for pregnancy is appropriate.
- The patient should be advised of the fetal risk (e.g., spontaneous abortion) should anesthesia be performed during pregnancy. The incidence of congenital abnormalities is no greater for the pregnant woman undergoing surgery, however, than it is for one with a surgery-free pregnancy.[66] Despite these data, the patient is advised to postpone elective surgery until well after the first trimester, when fetal organogenesis is complete.
- The patient should be privately questioned about the possibility of being pregnant. Female staff should interview the adolescent patient in the absence of family members.

Cardiovascular Effects of Pregnancy

The pregnant patient population presents the clinician with a variety of physiologic changes that may have an impact on the delivery of sedation. These physiologic changes affect multiple organ systems, including cardiovascular, pulmonary, gastrointestinal, and hematologic systems. These effects are mediated through hormonal release associated with the pregnant state. Increased oxygen consumption, decreased vascular resistance, increased cardiac output, and increased blood volume are required to meet the metabolic demands of the mother and the fetus. In the second trimester, compression of the vena cava and aorta by the weight of the gravid uterus is a common finding. Decreased venous return of blood to the heart predisposes the mother to tachycardia, faintness, and ultimately fetal distress. Positioning of the pregnant patient during the second trimester and thereafter requires careful attention to avoid aortocaval compression. Methods to prevent compression of the aorta or vena cava include left uterine displacement. **Placing the patient in the left lateral position or providing left uterine displacement with a towel pack or blanket placed under the right ischial spine takes the weight of the gravid uterus off of the great vessels and helps prevent obstruction of venous return and compression of the aorta.**

Pulmonary Changes Associated With Pregnancy

Edema of the upper airway and mucous membranes occurs as a result of increased extracellular fluid volume and vascular engorgement. **Great care must be taken to maintain a patent airway in this patient population.** Epistaxis is a common complication associated with the insertion of nasal airways secondary to the friability of the mucous membrane. As the fetus develops and the uterus enlarges, functional residual capacity decreases, which predisposes the patient to hypoxemia.

Maternal Gastrointestinal Changes

Gastrointestinal changes associated with pregnancy include decreased gastrointestinal motility, decreased food absorption, increased gastric acidity, and decreased lower esophageal sphincter tone. These changes increase the incidence of gastric acid aspiration. If sedation services are required in the pregnant patient, great vigilance and care are required to avoid the risk of gastric acid aspiration, hypoxemia, or epistaxis in the event of oversedation or airway compromise.

Management of the Parturient

Objectives for the pregnant patient who must receive sedation include:
- Avoidance of teratogenic medications
- Avoidance of fetal hypoxia
- Avoidance of premature labor
- Avoidance of fetal acidosis

> With the numerous physiologic changes associated with pregnancy, pharmacologic implications, and potential airway compromise, it is advised that a member of the anesthesia staff be consulted to care for this specific patient population.

TABLE 2-12

Summary of Adverse Effects for Selected Herbal Preparations

HERB	RELEVANT PHARMACOLOGIC EFFECTS	SEDATION CONCERNS	PRESEDATION DISCONTINUATION
Echinacea	Activation of cell-mediated immunity	Allergic reactions; decreased effectiveness of immunosuppressants; potential for immunosuppression with long-term use	No data
Ephedra	Increased heart rate and blood pressure through direct and indirect sympathomimetic effects	Risk of myocardial ischemia and stroke from tachycardia and hypertension; ventricular arrhythmias with halothane; long-term use depletes endogenous catecholamines and may cause intraoperative hemodynamic instability; life-threatening interaction with monoamine oxidase inhibitors	At least 24 hours before surgery
Garlic	Inhibition of platelet aggregation (may be irreversible); increased fibrinolysis; equivocal antihypertensive activity	Potential to increase risk of bleeding, especially when combined with other medications that inhibit platelet aggregation	At least 7 days before surgery
Ginkgo	Inhibition of platelet-activating factor	Potential to increase risk of bleeding, especially when combined with other medications that inhibit platelet aggregation	At least 36 hours before surgery
Ginseng	Lowers blood glucose; inhibition of platelet aggregation (may be irreversible); increased PT/PTT in animals; many other diverse effects	Hypoglycemia; potential to increase risk of bleeding; potential to decrease anticoagulation effect of warfarin	At least 7 days before surgery
Kava	Sedation, anxiolysis	Potential to increase sedative effect of anesthetics; potential for addiction, tolerance, and withdrawal after abstinence unstudied	At least 24 hours before surgery
St. John's wort	Inhibition of neurotransmitter reuptake, monoamine oxidase inhibition is unlikely	Induction of cytochrome P-450 enzymes, affecting cyclosporine, warfarin, steroids, protease inhibitors, and possibly benzodiazepines, calcium channel blockers, and many other drugs; decreased serum digoxin levels	At least 5 days before surgery
Valerian	Sedation	Potential to increase sedative effect of anesthetics; benzodiazepine-like acute withdrawal; potential to increase anesthetic requirements with long-term use	No data

PT/PTT, prothrombin time/partial thromboplastin time.
Adapted from *JAMA,* July 10, 286(2): p. 213.

NPO STATUS

Aspiration of gastric contents may result in the development of Mendelson's syndrome, which was first described by Mendelson in 1946. This syndrome occurs in the presence of aspiration of gastric contents greater than 25 mL (0.4 mL/kg) with a pH less than 2.5. Sequelae associated with aspiration of gastric contents depend on the character and volume of the aspirate. Aspiration of solid particulate matter results in an anatomic, mechanical obstruction to gas flow. Aspiration of acidic gastric fluid results in chemical burning of the alveoli with severe ventilatory perfusion mismatch. **Aspiration may occur during the administration of sedation in patients who enter into a state of deep sedation with resultant loss of protective airway reflexes.** Mechanisms to avoid aspiration include administration of H_2 blockers and gastrokinetic agents, enforcement of NPO guidelines, and the avoidance of a sedative state sufficient to blunt airway reflexes.

NPO Instructions

Nil per os (NPO) is the Latin term for "nothing by mouth." The NPO principle has been used by anesthesia clinicians and surgeons for years to decrease the risk of gastric acid aspiration. Historically, patients have been instructed to have nothing to eat or drink after midnight. The purpose of the cessation of solid and fluid intake was to assure an "empty" stomach with minimal gastric contents. Various studies that have led practitioners to reevaluate NPO guidelines lend support to the idea that clear liquids administered 2 to 3 hours before the scheduled procedures do not alter residual gastric volume when compared with the standard NPO overnight fast.[67-71] Distinct advantages of the NPO policy revision cited by these authors include patient comfort and decreased incidence of hypoglycemia and hypovolemia. Additional studies demonstrate decreased gastric volume and increased pH when compared with standard overnight fasting regimens.[72-73] It should be noted that the majority of these studies used healthy patient control groups who were not identified as being at high risk of aspiration. Patients at risk of aspiration or patients with decreased gastric emptying were not included in many of these studies.

Many practitioners currently allow ingestion of clear liquids up to 2 hours before the planned procedure. The significance and importance of NPO guidelines associated with the administration of sedation/analgesia are based on varied patient response, total dose of drug administered, and the possibility of patients entering a state of deep sedation. Additional factors that decrease gastric emptying or increase the risk of pulmonary aspiration include the following:

- Delayed gastric emptying
- Diabetes
- Esophageal motility disorders
- Fear
- Obesity
- Opioids
- Pain
- Trauma

Methods to reduce gastric volume include fasting, gastric suction, and administration of medications that increase gastrointestinal motility. Gastric suction is an impractical means of decreasing volume in patients presenting for the administration of sedation. Use of the gastrokinetic drug metoclopramide combined with an H_2 antagonist effectively decreases gastric volume while increasing pH. When indicated, H_2 antagonists should be administered 1 to 2 hours before the planned procedure. To summarize, the adaptation and incorporation of specific NPO guidelines must be based on a sound rationale. As listed in Box 2-7, presedation fasting guidelines have been promulgated by experts in the field of anesthesiology.[74-76]

> Patients at risk for gastric acid aspiration should be treated as having a "full" stomach. It is prudent to avoid deep sedation in this patient population.

INFORMED CONSENT

An important risk-management strategy and legal requirement is to obtain informed consent before the administration of sedation. Informed consent requires that the plan, alternatives, and potential complications be explained to the patient in layperson's terms. The basis for informed consent stems from the fundamental principle that the patient has the right to exercise control over his or her body and over the treatment plan. **Lack of properly obtained informed consent may result in charges of**

BOX 2-7

NPO Fasting Guidelines*

Ingested Material	Minimum Fasting Period[†]
Clear liquids[‡]	2 hr
Breast milk	4 hr
Infant formula	6 hr
Nonhuman milk[§]	6 hr
Light meal[‖]	6 hr

From *Anesthesiology*. April 2002;96(4):1007.
*These recommendations apply to healthy patients who are undergoing elective procedures. They are not intended for women in labor. Following the Guidelines does not guarantee a complete gastric emptying has occurred.
[†]The fasting periods apply to all ages.
[‡]Examples of clear liquids include water, fruit juices without pulp, carbonated beverages, clear tea, and black coffee.
[§]Because nonhuman milk is similar to solids in gastric emptying time, the amount ingested must be considered when determining an appropriate fasting period.
[‖]A light meal typically consists of toast and clear liquids. Meals that include fried or fatty foods or meat may prolong gastric emptying time. Both the amount and type of foods or meat ingested must be considered when determining an appropriate fasting period.

assault and battery. *Assault* is defined as the apprehension or anticipation of the application of unauthorized physical force. *Battery* is defined as the unconsented, unprivileged touching of another person.[77] A separate area on the consent form, which addresses the procedural risks, reasonable alternatives, and expected benefits associated with procedural sedation, is advised. A sample informed consent for sedation services is identified in Figure 2-6.

The legal concept of the reasonable person is used in obtaining informed consent. The reasonable person doctrine centers on material risk. Material risk is one that the provider knows or ought to know would be significant to a reasonable person in the patient's position of deciding whether to submit to a particular medication or treatment procedure.[78] However, all conceivable risks do not require disclosure. In summary, informed consent is an understanding between two persons that incorporates an explanation of the proposed sedation plan and an explanation of risks and alternatives in reasonable layperson terms.

ASA PHYSICAL STATUS CLASSIFICATION SYSTEM

Incorporation of a physical classification system is a beneficial addition to the presedation assessment form. This physical status classification system was developed in 1940 by a committee of the American Society of Anesthetists, currently the American Society of Anesthesiologists.[79] This system was developed to standardize physical status and assign a potential-risk classification. This physical classification system also offers the clinician a numerical summary assessment tool based on the findings of the presedation physical assessment. The ASA Physical Status Classification System is listed in Box 2-8.

PRESEDATION PATIENT INSTRUCTION

Presedation patient instruction must provide detailed patient-specific instruction pertinent to the planned procedure. Examples of specific instruction include the following:
- NPO
- Time of arrival
- Estimated procedure time
- Presence of a responsible adult for discharge
- Medication instructions
- Procedure-specific guidelines
  - Bowel preparation
  - Prophylactic antibiotics
  - Dye preparations
  - Loose-fitting clothing

NPO

When instructing patients concerning NPO guidelines, it is important to tell them that they are to have nothing to eat or *drink* after a specific time. A study in *Anaesthesia* reported that only 28% of patients receiving NPO instructions believed that these instructions pertained only to food and not to water.[80] Therefore, when instructing patients regarding NPO status, the clinician must also specify no food, water, juice, coffee, and so on. Presedation oral medications ordered for the morning of the procedure may be taken with a sip of water. It may be necessary to quantify this amount with the patient to avoid ingestion of large amounts of water.

Sample Consent for the Administration of Moderate Sedation/Analgesia

I, _____, acknowledge that my doctor has explained to me that I will have a surgical, diagnostic, or treatment procedure. Procedural risks and potential complications have been explained to me. I understand that sedation/analgesia services are required so that my doctor can perform the surgical, diagnostic, or treatment procedure. I am aware that the specific sedation/analgesia plan is determined by many factors including my medical and physical conditions, the type of procedure, my doctor's preference, as well as my own desire. It has been explained to me that all forms of sedation and anesthesia involve some risks. I understand that no guarantees or promises can be made concerning the results of my procedure or sedation technique administered. Complications with sedation/analgesia can occur and include the possibility of infection, bleeding, drug reactions, injury to blood vessels, loss of sensation, paralysis, stroke, brain damage, heart attack, or death. I hereby consent to the administration of sedation/analgesia services either by or under the direction of Doctor_____.

Risks, alternatives, and expected benefits have been explained to me in layman's terms, and I have had all questions answered.

_____
Patient or Guardian's Signature/Relationship to Patient Signature

_____/_____/_____   _____AM/PM

Date   *Time*

© 2004, Specialty Health Education, Inc.

FIGURE 2-6 Sample consent for the administration of moderate sedation/analgesia. (© 2004, Specialty Health Education, Inc.)

BOX 2-8

American Society of Anesthesiologists (ASA) Classification of Physical Status

I. Normal, healthy patient with no systemic disease.
Example:
- Patient's health: excellent with no systemic disease
- Limitations on activity: none
- Danger of death: none
- Excluded: Persons at extremes of age (very young, very old)

II. Mild to moderate systemic disease.
Example:
- Patient's health: disease of one body system
- Status of underlying disease: well-controlled
- Limitations on activity: well-controlled
- Danger of death: none

III. Severe systemic disease with functional limitation that is not incapacitating.
Example:
- Patient's health: disease of more than one body system or one major system
- Status of underlying disease: controlled
- Limitations on activity: present but not incapacitated
- Danger of death: no immediate danger

IV. Severe systemic disease that is incapacitating and life threatening.
Example:
- Patient's health: poor with at least one severe disease
- Status of underlying disease: poorly controlled or end-stage
- Limitations on activity: incapacitated
- Danger of death: possible

V. A moribund patient not expected to survive 24 hours without surgical intervention.
Example:
- Patient's health: very poor, moribund
- Limitations on activity: incapacitated
- Danger of death: imminent

Time of Arrival

Patients should be instructed to arrive at the office or procedure unit at a mutually agreed-on time. Sufficient time must be allotted to properly register the patient, obtain baseline vital signs, and prepare the patient for the planned diagnostic examination or procedure. When these presedation duties are performed in an unhurried atmosphere, the patient's anxiety is decreased through reassurance and proper preparation.

Responsible Adult

Patients must be instructed to arrange for a competent adult to accompany them home. Early notification of this requirement allows the patient time to make arrangements for transportation and recovery at home. **It is not acceptable to discharge a sedation patient to home by taxi.** A responsible adult who will assume postsedation care and instructions on behalf of the patient must be present.

Procedure-Specific Guidelines

Procedure-specific guidelines (i.e., bowel preparations, prophylactic antibiotics, or dye preparations) must be clearly outlined before the procedure. Written instructions are extremely helpful for many patients and eliminate numerous telephone calls requesting reiteration of presedation instructions. A sample of presedation patient instructions is summarized in Figure 2-7.

SUMMARY

Patients presenting for therapeutic, diagnostic, and minor surgical procedures often have an inherent fear associated with the planned procedure or medications that will be used during the procedure. Common presedation fears include a "bad" diagnosis (carcinoma), confusion, nausea, vomiting, pain, and, in some cases, death. During presedation assessment the clinician must:

- Conduct the interview in an unhurried manner.
- Use an organized interview format.
- Inform and reassure the patient.

Through the mechanisms outlined, the clinician will alleviate patient anxiety and achieve the goals of presedation patient assessment. A sincere interest in the patient's procedure and treatment plan also helps to decrease patient anxiety.[81,82] When conducted appropriately, presedation assessment is a useful tool, building a trusting patient-clinician relationship.

PATIENTS RECEIVING I.V. MODERATE SEDATION

Dr. _____ has referred you for _____
at the Endoscopy Unit located on the 7th floor of the Johns Hopkins Outpatient Center.

Date _____ Time _____ Please arrive at _____

You will be receiving I.V. (intravenous) moderate sedation. You **must** have a companion (family member/friend) to take you home. You are not allowed to drive or leave the Outpatient Center alone. Your ride must pick you up in the Endoscopy Center by 4:00 p.m. The actual procedure lasts approximately 45 minutes, but you MUST remain in the Endoscopy Center until you recover from sedation. On the average, most patients are discharged 3-4 hours after they arrive. Your procedure will be cancelled if your ride cannot be confirmed.

MEDICATIONS

1 **Do not take aspirin or aspirin products**
   (such as Alka-Seltzer, Ibuprofen, Nuprin, Advil, Aleve, or Motrin) for five days prior to the procedure. For any discomfort or headache, you may take Tylenol.

2 If you are taking medication for high blood pressure, seizures, or if you are taking prednisone, you may take these medications the morning of the procedure or at least two hours before the procedure with a sip of water.

3 **Do not take** any water/fluid pills until after the completion of your procedure.

4 Iron pills should not be taken for seven days prior to your procedure.

5 If you are diabetic:
   - If you take a "sugar" pill, **do not take** it on the day of your procedure.
   - If you are taking regular insulin, **do not take** it on the day of your procedure.
   - If you are taking long acting insulin (NPH), you should take half of your prescribed dose on the morning of your procedure.

6 If you are taking coumadin, contact your G.I. doctor for instructions on when to stop taking this medication.

7 If you are having a procedure, you **must not** have anything to eat or drink eight hours prior to your procedure.

If you have any questions or cannot make your appointment, please call the unit.

FIGURE 2-7 Sample presedation patient instructions. (Modified from The Johns Hopkins Medical Institutions Gastroenterology and Hepatology Division, Baltimore, MD; reprinted with permission.)

LEARNER SELF-ASSESSMENT

In order to achieve maximal educational benefit from this chapter, please complete the Learner Self-Assessment below. This self-assessment tool provides the ability to identify areas requiring additional review. Reference material for each question is provided in Appendix F.

1. Healthcare practitioner considerations associated with **JCAHO Standards** related to presedation patient assessment for moderate sedation include

2. **Practice Guidelines for Sedation and Analgesia by Non-Anesthesiologists** promulgated by the ASA Task Force on Sedation **related to presedation patient assessment** include:

3. **Goals** of presedation patient assessment include:
   a.

   b.

   c.

   d.

4. Two **methods utilized to calculate ideal body weight** include:
   a.

   b.

5. The **components of the patient's medical history** and its impact on planned procedural care include:
   a.

   b.

   c.

   d.

   e.

   f.

   g.

6. Specific alterations in the **cardiovascular, pulmonary, hepatic, renal, neurologic, and endocrine systems** identified in the presedation patient assessment and their implications for procedural patient care include:
   a. Cardiovascular

   b. Pulmonary

   c. Hepatic

   d. Renal

   e. Neurologic

   f. Endocrine

7. Implications for the sedation plan of care **based on the patient's past surgical and anesthetic history** include:

8. Treatment protocol for an **allergic reaction** during a sedation procedure include:

9. The sedation patient population, which requires **presedation laboratory testing** includes:

10. Patient care considerations associated with positive findings on the **presedation social history** include:
    a. Tobacco use

    b. Alcohol consumption

    c. Substance abuse

    d. Herbal product use

    e. Pregnancy

11. **Current NPO guidelines** for sedation patients include:
    a. Solids

    b. Liquids

12. The **ASA Physical Classification System** summarizes physiologic status, which includes:
    a. ASA I

    b. ASA II

    c. ASA III

    d. ASA IV

    e. ASA V

POST-TEST QUESTIONS

Please note: If you are applying for CE credit, you must contact Specialty Health Education, Inc. @ 800-694-8041 for a CE Application Packet.

1. Which of the following methods is utilized to determine lean body weight in the presedation patient? _____.
   A. Basal index
   B. Body mass index
   C. Conversion of pounds into kilograms
   D. Measurement of patient in kilocalories

2. To avoid the development of deep sedative states, dosage requirements for sedative medications should be based on _____.
   A. Actual body weight
   B. Body weight only in kilograms
   C. Ideal body weight
   D. Kilometric weight

3. Presedation administration of H_2 blockers and gastrokinetic agents serve to _____.
   A. Increase gastric volume and decrease gastric acidity
   B. Decrease gastric volume and increase gastric acidity
   C. Decrease gastric volume and decrease gastric acidity
   D. Increase gastric volume and increase gastric acidity

4. *Hypertension* is defined by the American Heart Association as a systolic blood pressure greater than _____ and a diastolic blood pressure greater than _____.
   A. 160/99
   B. 160/95
   C. 140/95
   D. 140/90

5. Current recommendations for managing the hypertensive patient presenting for sedation include _____:
   A. Hold all cardiac medications for 24 hours preprocedure.
   B. Hold all cardiac medications for 12 hours preprocedure.
   C. Administer antihypertensive therapy up to and including the morning of the procedure.
   D. Administer antihypertensive therapy only if the patient has a history of malignant hypertension.

6. Newly diagnosed dysrhythmias or dysrhythmias that impair myocardial performance identified during presedation patient assessment require _____.
   A. Further evaluation and consultation
   B. No further consultation
   C. Administration of presedation digoxin
   D. Administration of presedation lidocaine

7. Which of the following conditions occurs when the requirement for oxygen is greater than the patient's ability to physiologically respond to the increased oxygen demand? _____
   A. Diaphoresis
   B. Lethargy
   C. Dyspnea
   D. Hypovolemia

8. The degree of metabolism of pharmacologic compounds is dependent on hepatic blood flow and enzyme activity in the endoplasmic reticulum.
   A. True
   B. False

9. Accentuation of benzodiazepine effect may be greatly enhanced in patients with renal disease secondary to which of the following physiologic effects?
   A. Increased renal blood flow
   B. Decreased renal blood flow
   C. Ionization of the pharmacologic compounds
   D. Decreased protein binding of the medications

10. Diabetic patients frequently present with joint stiffness and limited joint mobility, which may significantly impact on _____.
    A. Inserting the intravenous line
    B. Airway management
    C. Drug metabolism
    D. Blood sugar management

11. To have diagnostic testing yield beneficial information, it is important to _____.
    A. Order an ECG, CBC, and electrolytes on all patients
    B. Order no presedation laboratory testing at any time
    C. Order presedation laboratory and diagnostic testing based on the patient's past medical history and physical examination
    D. Only follow hospital policy with regard to presedation testing

12. A cigarette smoking history should be quantified in _____ and documented on the presedation assessment form.
    A. Carton years
    B. Pack years
    C. Individual cigarette years
    D. Cigarettes per day

13. Chronic use of alcohol leads to stimulation of the _____, which may require increased doses of sedative and analgesic medications.

    A. Cytochrome P-450 system in the liver
    B. Nephrons in the renal tubules
    C. Nephrons in the gray matter
    D. Hepatocytes in the periductal area

14. Current presedation NPO guidelines include _____.

    A. No solids for 3 hours, clear liquids until 1 hour before sedation
    B. No solids for 6 hours, clear liquids until 2 hours before sedation
    C. No solids for 8 hours, clear liquid ingestion until the procedure
    D. No solids or clear liquids for 12 hours before sedation

15. Utilizing the American Society of Anesthesiologists Physical Classification System, a 36-year-old male with a history of hypertension controlled with daily medications and no evidence of end-organ damage would be classified as an ASA _____.

    A. IV
    B. III
    C. II
    D. I

REFERENCES

1. Sixth report of the Joint National Committee on Prevention, Detection, Evaluation, and Treatment of High Blood Pressure (JNC VI). *Arch Intern Med.* 1997;24:13-20.
2. Stoelting R, Dierdorf S. *Anesthesia and Co-Existing Disease.* 4th ed. New York: Churchill-Livingstone; 2002:93.
3. Stoelting R, Dierdorf S. *Anesthesia and Co-Existing Disease.* 4th ed. New York: Churchill-Livingstone; 2002:94.
4. Tarhan S, Moffit EA, Taylor WF, Guilani ER. Myocardial infarction after general anesthesia. *JAMA.* 1972;220:2566.
5. Steen PA, Tinker JH, Tarhan S. Myocardial reinfarction after anesthesia and surgery. *JAMA.* 1978;239:2566.
6. Nagelhout J, Zaglaniczny K. *Nurse Anesthesia.* 2nd ed. Philadelphia: WB Saunders; 2001:325.
7. Stoelting R, Dierdorf S. *Anesthesia and Co-Existing Disease.* 4th ed. New York: Churchill-Livingstone; 2002:11.
8. Rao T, Jacobs E, El-Etr A. Reinfarction following anesthesia in patients with myocardial infarction undergoing non-cardiac operations. *Anesth Analg.* 1991;71:231-235.
9. Shah K, Kleinman B, Sami H, et al. Reevaluation of perioperative myocardial infarction in patients with prior myocardial infarction undergoing noncardiac operations. *Anesth Analg.* 1991;71:231-235.
10. Slogoff S, Keats A. Does perioperative myocardial ischemia lead to postoperative myocardial infarction? *Anesthesiology.* 1985;62:107-114.
11. Faust R. *Anesthesiology Review.* 3rd ed. New York: Churchill-Livingstone; 2002:343.
12. Goldsmith M. Implanted defibrillators slash sudden death rate in study, thousands more may get them in the future. *JAMA.* 1991;266:3400.
13. Stoelting R, Dierdorf S. *Anesthesia and Co-Existing Disease.* 4th ed. New York: Churchill Livingstone; 2002:177.
14. Stoelting R, Dierdorf S. *Anesthesia and Co-Existing Disease.* 4th ed. New York: Churchill Livingstone; 2002:197.
15. Guyton A. *Textbook of Medical Physiology.* 11th ed. Philadelphia: WB Saunders; 2001.
16. Kleinknecht D, Ganeval D, Gonzalez-Duque LA, et al. Furosemide in acute oliguric renal failure: A controlled trial. *Nephron.* 1976;17:51.
17. Siegel DC, Cochin A, Geocaris T, et al. Effects of saline and colloid resuscitation on renal function. *Ann Surg.* 1971;177:51.
18. Hanley MJ, Davidson K. Prior mannitol and furosemide infusion in a mode of ischemic acute renal failure. *Am J Physiol.* 1981;241:556.
19. Davis RF, Lappas DG, Kirklin JK, et al. Acute oliguria after cardiopulmonary bypass: Renal functional improvement with low-dose dopamine infusion. *Crit Care Med.* 1982;10:852.
20. Polson RJ, Park GR, Lindop MJ, et al. The prevention of renal impairment in patients undergoing orthotopic liver grafting by infusion of low dose dopamine. *Anaesthesia.* 1987;42:15.
21. Paul MD, Mazer CD, Byrick RJ, et al. Influence of mannitol and dopamine on renal function during elective infrarenal aortic clamping in man. *Am J Nephrol.* 1986;6:427.
22. Crowley K, Clarkson K, Hannon V, et al. Diuretics after transurethral prostatectomy: A double-blind controlled trial comparing furosemide and mannitol. *Br J Anaesth.* 1990; 65:337.
23. Bennett WM, Aronoff GR, Golper TA, et al. Drug prescribing in renal failure. In *Dosing Guidelines for Adults.* 2nd ed. Philadelphia: American College of Physicians; 1991.
24. *The Medical Letter on Drugs and Therapeutics Handbook on Antimicrobial Therapy.* New Rochelle, NY: The Medical Letter; 1992.
25. Miller R. *Anesthesia.* 5th ed. New York: Churchill Livingstone; 2000, pg 1459.
26. Morgan E, Mikhail M, and Murray M: *Clinical anesthesiology.* 3rd ed. New York: Lange Medical Books: McGraw-Hill, New York 2002, pg. 737.
27. Davidson J, Eckhardt W, Perese D: *Clinical Anesthesia Procedures of the Massachusetts General Hospital.* 6th ed. Philadelphia: Lippincott, Williams & Wilkins; 2002:73.
28. Mercker S, Maier C, Doz P, et al. Lactic acidosis as a serious perioperative complication of antidiabetic biguanide medication with metformin. *Anesthesiology.* 1997;87:1003-1005.
29. McAnulty G, Robertshaw H, Hall G. Anaesthetic management of patients with diabetes mellitus. *Br J Anaesth.* 2000;85:80-90.
30. Hirsch I, Magill J, Cryer E, et al. Perioperative management of surgical patients with diabetes mellitus. *Anesthesiology.* 1991;74:346-359.
31. Nathan D. Long-term complications of diabetes mellitus. *N Engl J Med.* 1993;328:1676-1685.
32. Walts LF, Miller R, Davidson MB, et al. Perioperative management of diabetes mellitus. *Anesthesiology.* 1981;55:104.
33. Morgan E, Mikhail M, and Murray M: *Clinical anesthesiology.* 3rd ed. New York: Lange Medical Books: McGraw-Hill, 2002:742.
34. Duke J, Rosenberg S. *Anesthesia Secrets.* 2nd ed. Philadelphia: Hanley & Belfus; 2000:281.
35. Jovenich J. Anesthesia in adrenal surgery. *Urol Clin North Am.* 1989;16:583.
36. Dubin SA, Silverstein PI, Wakefield ML, et al. Famotidine, a new H_2 receptor antagonist. *Anesth Analg.* 1989;68:321.
37. Watkins J. Anaphylactoid reactions to IV substances. *Br J Anaesth.* 1979;51-55.
38. Roizen M. Preoperative evaluation. In Miller RD (ed). *Anesthesia.* 3rd ed. New York: Churchill Livingstone; 1990:1:743.
39. Kaplan E, Sheiner L, Boeckmann A, et al. The usefulness of preoperative laboratory screening. *JAMA.* 1985;253:357.
40. Blery C, Szatan M, Fourgeaux B, et al. Evaluation of a protocol for selective ordering of preoperative tests. *Lancet.* 1986;1:139.
41. Centers for Disease Control and Prevention. Selected cigarette smoking initiation and quitting behaviors among high school students—United States, 1997. *Morbid Mortal Wkly Rep.* 1998;47;386-389.
42. Burns DM. Tobacco and health. In Wyngaarden JB, Smith IH Jr (eds). *Cecil Textbook of Medicine.* 17th ed. Philadelphia: WB Saunders; 1985:47.
43. McCrea K, et al. Altered cytokine regulation in the lungs of cigarette smokers. *Am J Respir Crit Care Med.* 1994;150: 696-703.
44. Moller A, Pedersen T. The effect of tobacco smoking on risks in connection with anesthesia and surgery: Development of complications and the preventive effect of smoking cessation. *Ugeskr Laeger.* 1999;161:4273-4276.
45. Wright A, et al. Relationship of parental smoking to wheezing and non-wheezing lower respiratory tract illnesses in infancy. *J Pediatr.* 1991;118:207-214.

46. Martinez F, Cline M, Burrows B. Increased incidence of asthma in children of smoking mothers. *Pediatrics*. 1992; 89:21-26.

47. Chilmonczyk BA, et al. Association between exposure to environmental tobacco smoke and exacerbation of asthma in children. *N Engl J Med*. 1993;328:1665-1669.

48. Kitchems J. Does this patient have an alcohol problem? *JAMA*. 1994;272:1782-1787.

49. Lohr R. Treatment of alcohol withdrawal in hospitalized patients. *Mayo Clin Proc*. 1995;70:777-782.

50. Milroy C. Ten years of "ecstasy." *JR Soc Med*. 1999;92:68-71.

51. Boot B, McGregor I, Hall W: MDMA (Ecstasy) neurotoxicity: Assessing and communicating the risks. *Lancet*. 2000;355: 1818-1821.

52. Milroy C. Ten years of "ecstasy." *JR Soc Med*. 1999;92:68-71.

53. Henry J. Metabolic consequences of drug misuse. *Br J Anaesth*. 2000;85:136-142.

54. Kain Z, Barash P. Anesthetic implications of drug abuse. *ASA Refresher Course*. 2001;29:15.

55. Greenblatt J. Year-End Preliminary Estimates from the 1996 Drug Abuse Warning Network. Rockville, MD: Office of Applied Studies, US Department of Health and Human Services; 1997.

56. Bernard C. Personal communication (letter), December 1996.

57. Kain Z, Rimar S, Barash P. Cocaine abuse in the parturient and effects on the fetus and neonate. *Anesth Analg*. 1993;77: 835-845.

58. Byck R, Ruskis A, Ungerer J, et al. Naloxone potentiates cocaine effect in man. *Psychopharmacol Bull*. 1982;18:214-215.

59. Sporer K. Acute heroin overdose: Update. *Ann Intern Med*. 1999;130:584-590.

60. Kain Z, Barash P. Anesthetic Implications of Drug Abuse. *ASA Refresher Course*. 2001;29:15.

61. Levy S. What and who is behind the growth of supplements. *Drug Topics*. 2000;143-77.

62. Assemi M. Herbal preparations: Concerns for operative patients. *Anesth Today*. 2001;10(3):17.

63. Kiuchi F, Iwakami S, Shibuya M, et al. Inhibition of prostaglandin and leukotriene biosynthesis by gingerols and diarylheptanoids. *Chem Pharm Bull*. 1992;40:387-391.

64. Fischer S. Cost-effective preoperative evaluation and testing. *Chest*. 1999;115(Suppl):96S-100S.

65. Malrey R, Kremer M, Alves S. Preoperative evaluation and preparation of the patient. In Nagelhout JJ, and Zaglaniczny KL: *Nurse Anesthesia*, 2nd ed. Philadelphia: WB Saunders; 2001:337.

66. Duncan P, et al. Fetal risk of anesthesia and surgery during pregnancy. *Anesthesiology*. 1986;65:790-794.

67. Sandhar BK, Goresky GV, Maltby JR, Shaffer EA. Effect of oral liquids and ranitidine on gastric fluid volume and pH in children undergoing outpatient surgery. *Anesthesiology*. 1989;71:327.

68. Splinter WM, Schaefer JD, Zunder IH. Clear fluids three hours before surgery do not affect the gastric fluid contents of children. *Can J Anaesth*. 1990;37:498.

69. Meakin G, Dingwall AE, Addison GM. Effects of fasting and oral premedication on the pH and volume of gastric aspirate in children. *Br J Anaesth*. 1987;59:678.

70. Splinter WM, Schaefer JD. Ingestion of clear fluids is safe for adolescents up to 3 h before anaesthesia. *Br J Anaesth*. 1991;66:48.

71. Splinter WM, Steward JA, Muir JG. The effect of preoperative apple juice on gastric contents, thirst and hunger in children. *Can J Anaesth*. 1989;36:55.

72. Meakin G, Dingwall AE, Addison GM. Effects of fasting and oral premedication on the pH and volume of gastric aspirate in children. *Br J Anaesth*. 1987;59:678.

73. Gray J, Santerrel L, Gaudreau HP, et al. Effects of oral cimetidine and ranitidine on gastric pH and residual volume in children. *Anesthesiology*. 1989;71:547.

74. American Society of Anesthesiologists Task Force on Sedation and Analgesia by Non-Anesthesiologists. Practice guidelines for sedation and analgesia by non-anesthesiologists. *Anesthesiology*. 2002;96:1009-1012.

75. Maltby JR. New guidelines for preoperative fasting. *Can J Anaesth*. 1993;40:R113.

76. Stoelting RK. "NPO" and aspiration pneumonitis: Changing perspectives. 40th Annual Refresher Course Lectures and Clinical Update Program, 1995, Lecture No. 432.

77. Scott R. *Legal Aspects of Documenting Patient Care*. Gainesville, MD: Aspen Publications; 1994.

78. Dornette W. *Legal Issues in Anesthesia Practice*. Philadelphia: FA Davis; 1991.

79. Barash P, Cullen B, Stoelting R. *Clinical Anesthesia*. 2nd ed. Philadelphia: JB Lippincott; 1992.

80. Hume MA, Kennedy B, Asbury AJ. Patient knowledge of anaesthesia and perioperative care. *Anaesthesia*. 1994;49:715.

81. Egbert LD, Battit GE, Turndorf H, Beecher HK. The value of the preoperative visit by an anesthetist. *JAMA*. 1963; 185:553.

82. Leigh JM, Walker J, Janaganathan P. Effect of preoperative anaesthetic visit on anxiety. *BMJ*. 1977;2:987.

CHAPTER 3

Pharmacologic Concepts

At the completion of this chapter, the learner shall:

◆ State the clinical considerations in the sedation/analgesia setting for the following pharmacologic terminology:

- Synergism
- Potency
- Tachyphylaxis

◆ Define *pharmacokinetics.*

◆ List the patient care considerations associated with each of the following pharmacokinetic processes:

- Absorption
- Distribution
- Metabolism
- Excretion

◆ State the role of the cytochrome P-450 system in the biotransformation of sedative and analgesia medications.

◆ Define *pharmacodynamics.*

◆ State the role of agonist/antagonist activity at pharmacologic receptor sites.

Joint Commission on Accreditation of Healthcare Organizations Standards for Operative or Other High-Risk Procedures and/or the Administration of Moderate or Deep Sedation or Anesthesia

Standard PC.13.20
Operative or other procedures and/or the administration of moderate or deep sedation or anesthesia are planned.

Rationale for PC.13.20
Because the response to procedures is not always predictable and sedation-to-anesthesia is a continuum, it is not always possible to predict how an individual patient will respond. Therefore, qualified individuals are trained in professional standards and techniques to manage patients in the case of a potentially harmful event.

Elements of Performance for PC.13.20
1. Sufficient numbers of qualified staff are available* to evaluate the patient, perform the procedure, monitor, and recover the patient.

2. *Individuals administering moderate or deep sedation and anesthesia are qualified[†] and have the appropriate credentials to manage patients at whatever level of sedation or anesthesia is achieved, either intentionally or unintentionally.*

3. A registered nurse supervises perioperative nursing care.

4. Appropriate equipment to monitor the patient's physiologic status is available.

5. Appropriate equipment to administer intravenous fluids and drugs, including blood and blood components, is available as needed.

6. Resuscitation capabilities are available.

---

*For hospitals providing obstetric or emergency operative services, this means they can provide anesthesia services as required by law and regulation.

†**Qualified** The individuals providing moderate or deep sedation and anesthesia have at a minimum had competency-based education, training, and experience in the following:

1. Evaluating patients before moderate or deep sedation and anesthesia.

2. Performing the moderate or deep sedation and anesthesia, including rescuing patients who slip into a deeper-than-desired level of sedation or analgesia. This includes the following:

   a. *Moderate* sedation – are qualified to rescue patients from deep sedation and are competent to manage a compromised airway and to provide adequate oxygenation and ventilation.

   b. *Deep* sedation – are qualified to rescue patients from general anesthesia and are competent to manage an unstable cardiovascular system as well as a compromised airway and inadequate oxygenation and ventilation.

© Joint Commission: Standards for Operative or Other High-Risk Procedures and/or the Administration of Moderate or Deep Sedation or Anesthesia, January, 2004. Reprinted with permission.

Practice Guidelines for Sedation and Analgesia by Non-Anesthesiologists

American Society of Anesthesiologists Task Force on Sedation and Analgesia by Non-Anesthesiologists

Recommendations. Individuals responsible for patients receiving sedation/analgesia should understand the pharmacology of the agents that are administered, as well as the role of pharmacologic antagonists for opioids and benzodiazepines. Individuals monitoring patients receiving sedation/analgesia should be able to recognize the associated complications. At least one individual capable of establishing a patent airway and positive-pressure ventilation, as well as a means for summoning additional assistance, should be present whenever sedation/analgesia is administered. It is recommended that an individual with advanced life support skills be immediately available (within 5 minutes) for moderate sedation and within the procedure room for deep sedation.

Recommendations. Combinations of sedative and analgesic agents may be administered as appropriate for the procedure being performed and the condition of the patient. Ideally, each component should be administered individually to achieve the desired effect (e.g., additional analgesic medication to relieve pain; additional sedative medication to decrease awareness or anxiety). The propensity for combinations of sedative and analgesic agents to cause respiratory depression and airway obstruction emphasizes the need to appropriately reduce the dose of each component as well as the need to continually monitor respiratory function.

Recommendations. Intravenous sedative/analgesic drugs should be given in small, incremental doses that are titrated to the desired endpoints of analgesia and sedation. Sufficient time must elapse between doses to allow the effect of each dose to be assessed before subsequent drug administration. When drugs are administered by nonintravenous routes (e.g., oral, rectal, intramuscular, transmucosal), allowance should be made for the time required for drug absorption before supplementation is considered. Because absorption may be unpredictable, administration of repeat doses of oral medications to supplement sedation/analgesia is not recommended.

Recommendations. Even if moderate sedation is intended, patients receiving propofol or methohexital by any route should receive care consistent with that required for deep sedation. Accordingly, practitioners administering these drugs should be qualified to rescue patients from any level of sedation, including general anesthesia. Patients receiving ketamine should be cared for in a manner consistent with the level of sedation that is achieved.

Recommendations. Specific antagonists should be available whenever opioid analgesics or benzodiazepines are administered for sedation/analgesia. Naloxone or flumazenil may be administered to improve spontaneous ventilatory efforts in patients who have received opioids or benzodiazepines, respectively. This may be especially helpful in cases where airway control and positive-pressure ventilation are difficult. Before or concomitantly with pharmacologic reversal, patients who become hypoxemic or apneic during sedation/analgesia should: (1) be encouraged or stimulated to breathe deeply; (2) receive supplemental oxygen; and (3) receive positive-pressure ventilation if spontaneous ventilation is inadequate. After pharmacologic reversal, patients should be observed long enough to ensure that sedation and cardiorespiratory depression does not recur once the effect of the antagonist dissipates. The use of sedation regimens that include routine reversal of sedative or analgesic agents is discouraged.

From American Society of Anesthesiologists Task Force on Sedation and Analgesia by Non-Anesthesiologists. Practice guidelines for sedation and analgesia by non-anesthesiologists. *Anesthesiology.* 2002;96(4):1009-1012. Reprinted with permission.

As healthcare providers prepare patients for the administration of sedation/analgesia, a working knowledge of the pharmacologic agents used to achieve amnesia, analgesia, and hypnosis is required. Basic pharmacologic principles are presented in this chapter, with an overview of pharmacodynamics and pharmacokinetics. Specific properties of pharmacologic agents used for sedation and analgesia are presented in Chapters 4 and 5. It is important for clinicians engaged in the administration of sedation to understand the pharmacologic profile of sedative and analgesic medications to anticipate side effects associated with their administration. Pertinent pharmacologic definitions associated with the administration of intravenous medications are listed in Box 3-1.

PHARMACOKINETICS

Pharmacokinetics is the quantitative study of the absorption, distribution, metabolism, and excretion of injected drugs and their metabolites.[1] **In essence, pharmacokinetics is the study of what the body does to a drug.** The pharmacokinetic profile of a medication considers the following parameters:

◆ Dose of drug administered
◆ Drug concentration at the receptor site
◆ Drug effect
◆ Patient variability

Before the absorption, distribution, metabolism, and excretion of injected medications, transfer of the pharmacologic agent across cell membranes must occur. This transfer is a result of passive diffusion, active transport, or facilitated diffusion.

1. **Passive diffusion.** Passive diffusion requires the presence of a concentration difference on each side of the cell membrane. The degree of pharmacologic transfer is

---

BOX 3-1

Pharmacologic Definitions

Efficacy: The maximum effect that can be produced by a drug.

Hyperreactive: Refers to the patient population that requires **decreased** doses of pharmacologic agents to produce the desired effect.

Hyporeactive: Refers to the patient population that requires **large** doses of pharmacologic agents to produce the expected pharmacologic effect.

Potency: Pharmacologic dosage required to produce an effect similar to another drug.

Synergism: Occurs with use of one medication in conjunction with another, and results in a pharmacologic effect greater than the algebraic summation associated with each of the two individual drugs (1 + 1 = 3).

Tachyphylaxis: Development of an acute tolerance to a drug.

Tolerance: Development of an increased drug requirement to produce a given effect. Results from chronic exposure to medications or toxins, which results in increased dosages of medications required to achieve the desired pharmacologic effect.

---

dependent on the magnitude of the concentration gradient across the cell membrane.

2. **Active transport.** Active transport requires energy to move molecules across cell membranes. Energy is required to facilitate movement of pharmacologic compounds and molecules across cell membranes against a concentration gradient.

3. **Facilitated diffusion.** Facilitated diffusion is a process by which a specific carrier transport mechanism is used. Therefore, facilitated diffusion cannot move compounds and molecules against an electrochemical or concentration gradient.

Pharmacologic Absorption

The absorption of a medication is dependent on the rate at which the pharmacologic compound leaves the site of administration. An important consideration associated with absorption is bioavailability. **Bioavailability is a pharmacologic term used to indicate the extent to which a drug reaches a site of action or the biologic fluid from which the drug gains access to the site.**[2] The mode of absorption is also an important characteristic to determine the duration and intensity of pharmacologic effect. Several factors may alter absorption. These factors include solubility of the medication, drug form, circulation at the site of absorption, and protein binding. Generally, highly lipid-soluble drugs are capable of crossing cell membranes with ease. The suspension or drug form also affects absorption. To reach the site of action and exert a pharmacologic effect, all drugs must dissolve in water. Therefore, pharmacologic adjuncts delivered in an aqueous medium are absorbed faster than those delivered in pill form or suspension. Circulation at the site of absorption also affects bioavailability. An increase in blood flow at the site of absorption increases the rate of absorption. Decreased blood flow at the site of absorption decreases absorption. Factors that decrease blood flow at the site of absorption include hypotension, shock, or utilization of vasoconstrictors.

Protein Binding

Pharmacologic agents bind to plasma proteins in varying degrees. The bound portion of the drug is inactive. The "free" or unbound portion of a drug is required for pharmacologic effect. Plasma protein binding also contributes to clearance of the drug. The unbound fraction of the drug undergoes metabolism by the hepatic cytochrome P-450 system, glomerular filtration and renal filtration, or both. **Patients with nutritional disorders, carcinoma, recent weight loss, renal disease, or decreased plasma protein levels may demonstrate enhanced or exaggerated effects from pharmacologic adjuncts used to achieve a state of sedation/analgesia.** As always, titration of pharmacologic agents is advised in all situations. Careful assessment of patient response is warranted, particularly in patients with altered hepatic or renal function.

> Patients with decreased plasma proteins or physical conditions associated with altered plasma proteins require careful titration of all central nervous system depressant medications. Administration of small incremental doses slowly over several minutes allows the clinician the ability to fully assess the pharmacologic effects of the medication.

Routes of Administration

Oral. Absorption after ingestion of pharmacologic compounds is dependent on the small intestine and the stomach. Absorption from the gastrointestinal tract generally occurs in the small intestine, where the epithelial lining is thin and has a large surface area.

First-Pass Effect. As depicted in Figure 3-1, medications absorbed through the stomach and intestine require passage (first-pass) through the liver before they gain entrance to the systemic circulation. During this process, some of the active pharmacologic compound is inactivated by liver metabolism or biliary excretion, resulting in decreased bioavailability. As a result of this hepatic metabolism or biliary excretion, some oral medications require larger doses than parenteral medications to exert a pharmacologic effect.

Sublingual. Because of the decreased surface area associated with sublingual administration, the sublingual mode of administration is reserved for highly lipid-soluble medications. A common medication given by the sublingual route is nitroglycerin. Because of venous drainage of the sublingual area directly into the superior vena cava there is no first-pass effect associated with sublingual administration.

Rectal. Pharmacologic agents instilled into the rectum are absorbed through the superior hemorrhoidal veins and transported to the liver.[3] Approximately 50% of rectally administered medications undergo a first-pass effect. Depending on the site of rectal absorption (proximal or distal), bioavailability varies greatly. Rectal administration is generally reserved for unconscious, uncooperative, or pediatric patients who cannot tolerate oral medication administration. Rectal administration is not popular because of a wide variation in patient response, rectal mucosal irritation, and diarrhea.

Subcutaneous. Subcutaneous administration is reserved for nonirritating medications. It offers a more rapid and superior absorption than oral administration. The quantity of medication absorbed depends on:
- Surface area
- Local blood flow
- Drug solubility

A sustained effect after subcutaneous administration provided by a constant plasma level can be pharmacologically advantageous with drugs such as insulin.

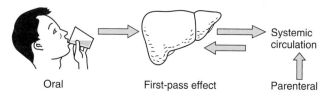

Oral — First-pass effect — Parenteral — Systemic circulation

FIGURE 3-1 First-pass effect. Drugs that are administered orally are absorbed through the gastrointestinal tract and pass through the liver (first-pass effect) before entering the systemic circulation for delivery to tissue receptor sites. Intravenous administration of sedative/analgesic medications allows rapid access to the systemic circulation without undergoing initial metabolism in the liver. This first-pass effect is the physiologic rationale for the large dosage variations in oral and parenteral medications.

Intramuscular. Intramuscular injections afford sustained release and a more rapid pharmacologic effect. An increased bioavailability is directly proportional to blood flow of the muscular bed. Pharmacologic suspensions allow prolonged release. However, organic solvents such as propylene glycol used in the suspension of diazepam often result in erratic intramuscular absorption.

Intravenous. Intravenous administration of medications results in a rapid rise in the blood plasma level. The rapid onset of action is secondary to the direct deposition of pharmacologic agent into the bloodstream. **Although this rapid onset of action is desirable, caution must be exercised during the administration of intravenous medications.** Titration is required, and adequate time should be allowed to assess individual patient response.

Inhalational. Medications may be absorbed through the pulmonary tree (atomized, aerosolized, metered-dose inhaler). The large pulmonary surface area allows pharmacologic agents to be readily absorbed. Alveolar blood flow closely mimics total cardiac output with resultant rapid uptake from the pulmonary epithelium. When used properly, metered-dose inhalers and aerosol delivery are efficacious for the delivery of pharmacologic agents to the systemic circulation.

Topical. Topically administered medications must be lipid soluble, and the quantity absorbed is proportional to the body surface area exposed to the medication. Factors affecting delivery of topical medication to the circulation include the following:

◆ Hydrated skin (more permeable to drug than dry skin)
◆ Occlusive patch (timed-release patch)

Any activity that increases cutaneous blood flow will increase the uptake of topically administered medications. A complete review of the techniques of administration is provided in Table 3-1.

Drug Distribution

Once the absorption process is complete, several phases of pharmacologic distribution occur. The first phase of distribution is a result of cardiac output and regional blood flow. Organs with high blood flow, referred to as vessel-rich organs, receive the majority of the drug during this initial phase. These organs include the heart, brain, liver, lungs, and kidneys. Organ systems that are not considered in the vessel-rich group require minutes to hours to attain equilibrium with pharmacologic agents. These organ systems include muscle, viscera, skin, and fat.

To understand basic pharmacokinetic principles, it is important to envision the body as composed of one or more compartments. Most drugs behave as though they have been distributed within two compartments, one central and the other peripheral. As illustrated in Figure 3-2, an initial drug dose is injected into the central compartment. After introduction into the central compartment, the drug disseminates to the peripheral compartment. The central compartment consists of intravascular fluid and organs in the vessel-rich

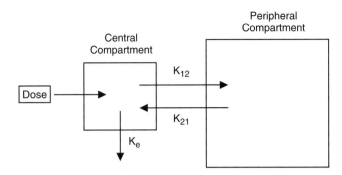

FIGURE 3-2 Two-compartment pharmacokinetic model. K_{12} and K_{21} are rate constants that signify the intercompartmental transfer of drugs. K_e is the elimination rate constant for drug elimination from the body. (From Barash P, Cullen B, Stoelting R. *Clinical Anesthesia.* 4th ed. Philadelphia: JB Lippincott; 2000.)

group. The peripheral compartment consists of all other fluids and tissues of the body. Eventually, drugs return from the peripheral compartment to the central compartment for elimination from the body.

Metabolism

Metabolism and clearance of drugs from the systemic circulation rely on hepatic, biliary, pulmonary, and renal mechanisms. The goal of metabolic degradation is to transform active compounds into water-soluble, pharmacologically inactive substances. In some instances, the process of metabolism yields pharmacologically active metabolites (e.g., desmethyldiazepam during the metabolism of diazepam), which may prolong the drug's duration of action. Metabolic pathways in the liver responsible for biodegradation of pharmacologic compounds include oxidation, reduction, hydrolysis, and conjugation. These complex biochemical processes yield inactive pharmacologic compounds.

Hepatic Microsomal Enzyme System

Sites of drug metabolism include plasma, lungs, kidneys, gastrointestinal tract, and liver. The hepatic microsomal enzyme system lies in the smooth endoplasmic reticulum of the liver. The cytochrome P-450 enzyme system is located on hepatic microsomes. The degree of hepatic microsomal enzyme activity is determined genetically. Aside from genetic predisposition to hepatic microsomal enzyme activity, certain medications may stimulate the cytochrome P-450 system. Prolonged barbiturate, benzodiazepine, or phenytoin use predisposes the patient to an increase in hepatic microsomal enzyme activity. As noted in Chapter 2, it is important to ascertain a thorough patient medication history to assess for the use of enzyme-inducing drugs.

> Enhanced hepatic microsomal enzyme activity generally results in an increased medication requirement for the individual patient.

TABLE 3-1

Techniques of Medication Administration

METHOD	PATTERN OF ABSORPTION	ADVANTAGES	DISADVANTAGES
Oral ingestion	Lower gastrointestinal tract absorption is dependent on local conditions: blood flow, surface area, physical state of the drug.	Safe Convenient Economical	Emesis secondary to gastrointestinal upset Drug destruction secondary to digestive enzymes Ineffective in patients with propulsion disorders Requires patient cooperation Requires intact reflexes First-pass effect
Sublingual	Absorption of highly lipid-soluble, non-ionized pharmacologic preparations; sublingual venous return empties into the superior vena cava.	Convenient Elimination of first-pass effect	Decreased surface area Need for highly soluble and potent agents Requires patient cooperation
Rectal	Proximal absorption via the superior hemorrhoidal veins; distal absorption bypasses hepatic first-pass effect.	Useful in the presence of emesis and nausea	Mucosal irritation Diarrhea First-pass effect Varied absorption
Subcutaneous	Absorption is dependent on the surface area and the absorbing capillary membrane.	May be used for unconscious, uncooperative patients Vasoconstrictors reduce systemic absorption (local anesthetics) Sustained release	Pain, necrosis, tissue sloughing Erratic absorption Suitable for only small volumes of injectate Decreased uptake in the presence of decreased blood pressure
Intramuscular	Rapid absorption of pharmacologic effect is dependent on blood flow to the muscular bed.	May be used in the unconscious, uncooperative patient Sustained release Rapid absorption	Local irritation Erratic absorption May result in increased laboratory results (creatine phosphokinase)
Intravenous	Bypasses absorption processes with resultant immediate blood plasma level of the pharmacologic agent.	Rapid blood plasma level Bypasses limiting factors associated with the absorptive process Utilization of large volumes	Requires vascular access Side effects and complications are immediate Requires careful titration
Inhalational	Pulmonary epithelial absorption Increased alveolar blood flow results in rapid onset of action.	Drug delivery to specific receptor sites of action (i.e., pulmonary: beta agonists) Rapid onset of action	Inability to regulate dose Pulmonary epithelial irritation Improper aerosol delivery
Topical	Highly lipid-soluble medications are absorbed through the epidermis into the systemic circulation.	Slow, timed-release pharmacologic effect Sustained pharmacologic effect Ease of use	Inability to regulate uptake and delivery May require large body surface contact

Excretion

The kidneys are the major organ system for the excretion of drugs and metabolites. Renal excretion of pharmacologic agents or their metabolites depends on:

◆ Glomerular filtration rate
◆ Active tubular secretion
◆ Passive tubular reabsorption

The clearance and excretion of drugs and metabolites require adequate renal function before the administration of sedative medications. Patients with suspected renal disease may require nephrology consultation with baseline testing (e.g., creatinine, blood urea nitrogen). A summary of the pharmacokinetic process is presented in Figure 3-3.

PHARMACODYNAMICS

As pharmacokinetics is the study of what the body does to a drug, **pharmacodynamics is what the drug does to the body.** *Pharmacodynamics* is the study of the effects of pharmacologic agents on the body.[4] It is the study of the effect of pharmacologic agents on target sites, which are typically designated as "receptor sites" or receptors. The pharmacodynamic effects associated with **opioid** use include their clinical and side effects:

Clinical Effect
◆ Suppression of opioid withdrawal
◆ Analgesia
◆ Sedation

Side Effect
◆ Decreased gastrointestinal motility
◆ Dysphoria
◆ Euphoria
◆ Miosis
◆ Nausea

◆ Respiratory depression
◆ Vomiting

The pharmacodynamic effects associated with **benzodiazepine** use include:
◆ Amnesia
◆ Anxiolysis
◆ Muscular relaxation
◆ Anticonvulsant effects

Receptors

Proteins compose one of the most important classes of pharmacologic receptors. Protein macromolecule receptors are present in cell membranes. A signaling process translates information relayed to them by neurotransmitters, hormones, or agonist drugs. Receptors can be "triggered" by conductance or transmembrane signaling. Receptors are identified and classified based on their agonistic or antagonistic clinical effect. Examples of receptor activity include:

◆ Alpha
◆ Beta
◆ Dopamine
◆ Histamine
◆ Mu
◆ Gamma-aminobutyric acid (GABA)

Pharmacologic agents tend to exert their actions on selective receptors to produce a specific drug response. As noted in Figure 3-4, **pharmacologic agents that bind to physiologic receptors to produce a specific effect are termed *agonists*.[5] Pharmacologic *antagonists* are agents that bind to physiologic receptors but have no pharmacologic effect.[5]** Antagonists also inhibit the action of agonists. An example of key agonist and antagonist actions is seen in the autonomic nervous system. Many pharmacologic agents used to control heart rate (e.g., beta blockers) are antagonists. Alpha antagonists phentolamine (Regitine) antagonize

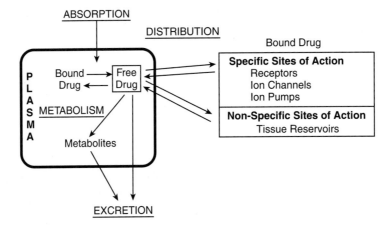

FIGURE 3-3 Overview of pharmacokinetic process. Absorption, distribution, metabolism, and excretion. (From Miller R. *Anesthesia.* 4th ed. New York: Churchill Livingstone; 1994:94.)

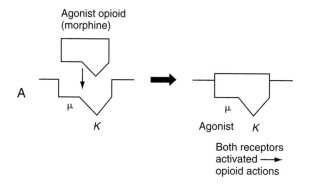

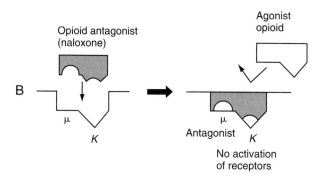

FIGURE 3-4 Pharmacologic agonist/antagonist action. **A,** A pharmacologic agonist stimulates tissue receptor sites resulting in pharmacologic action and effect. **B,** A pharmacologic antagonist occupies the tissue receptor site but does not produce pharmacologic action and effect. Pharmacologic antagonists have no intrinsic activity. (From Miller R. *Anesthesia.* 4th ed. New York: Churchill Livingstone; 1994:277.)

alpha receptors and result in peripheral vasodilatation. Pharmacologic antagonists also include reversal agents for benzodiazepines (flumazenil [Romazicon]) and opioids (naloxone [Narcan]), which competitively bind to their respective receptor sites and reverse the benzodiazepine and opioid effects. Examples of agonist stimulation include beta stimulation (isoproterenol [Isuprel]) to increase heart rate and alpha stimulation (phenylephrine [Neo-Synephrine]) to increase blood pressure.

> Patients who have received flumazenil for the reversal of benzodiazepine effects should be monitored for resedation, respiratory depression, or other residual benzodiazepine effects for an appropriate period (up to 120 minutes) based on the dose and duration of effect of the benzodiazepine employed.[6]

Many of the medications administered during sedation/analgesia act on individual specific receptor sites (opioids and benzodiazepines). **Action on these receptor sites concurrently can result in a synergism that causes analgesia and sedation in excess of either drug alone.** When one is considering pharmacodynamic principles, it is important to consider individual patient response coupled with varied drug dosages required during the administration of sedation and analgesia services.

SUMMARY

It is important for the clinician administering sedation and monitoring the patient to realize that the sedative/analgesic medications selected possess specific pharmacokinetic and pharmacodynamic profiles. Sedation and analgesic medications are generally selected for their pharmacodynamic properties (amnesia, anxiolysis, analgesia, sedation). However, it is equally important for the clinician to understand that a sedative medication may have excellent pharmacodynamic action but a very undesirable pharmacokinetic profile. Prolonged half-lives, unpleasant side effects, poor absorption qualities, and cumulative drug effect must all be considered when selecting a medication for sedation.

LEARNER SELF-ASSESSMENT

In order to achieve maximal educational benefit from this chapter, please complete the Learner Self-Assessment below. This self-assessment tool provides the learner with the ability to identify areas requiring additional review. Reference material for each question is provided in Appendix F.

1. Healthcare practitioner considerations associated with **JCAHO Standards** related to sedation/analgesia medication administration include:

2. **Practice Guidelines for Sedation and Analgesia by Non-Anesthesiologists** promulgated by the ASA Task Force on Sedation **related to sedation/analgesia medication administration** include:

3. What **patient care considerations** arise with regard to the following pharmacologic definitions?
   a. Synergism

   b. Potency

   c. Tachyphylaxis

4. What **patient care considerations are associated with the pharmacokinetic profile** of sedative and analgesic medications?
   a. Absorption

   b. Distribution

   c. Metabolism

   d. Excretion

5. What role does the **cytochrome P-450 system play in the biotransformation** of sedative and analgesic medications?

6. The **pharmacodynamic effects associated** with benzodiazepine and opioid use include:

7. The **clinical pertinence** associated with the utilization of pharmacologic agonists and antagonists in the sedation setting include:

POST-TEST QUESTIONS

Please note: If you are applying for CE credit, you must contact Specialty Health Education, Inc. @ 800-694-8041 for a CE Application Packet.

1. The quantitative study of the absorption, distribution, metabolism, and excretion of injected drugs and their metabolites is defined as _____.
   A. Pharmacodynamics
   B. Synergism
   C. Additive effect
   D. Pharmacokinetics

2. _____ is the maximum effect that can be produced by a drug.
   A. Potency
   B. Efficacy
   C. Tachyphylaxis
   D. Synergism

3. Medications administered via the _____ route must initially undergo a first-pass effect in the liver.
   A. Oral
   B. Intramuscular
   C. Intravenous
   D. Topical

4. The _____ pharmacologic distribution phase is a result of cardiac output and regional blood flow.
   A. First
   B. Final
   C. Delta
   D. Gamma

5. A site of drug metabolism located in the smooth endoplasmic reticulum of the liver is identified as _____.
   A. Golgi apparatus
   B. Hepatic microsomal enzyme system
   C. Mitochondria
   D. Smooth endoplasmic vacuoles

6. Which pharmacokinetic process is dependent on glomerular filtration rate, active tubular secretion, and passive tubular reabsorption? _____
   A. Absorption
   B. Biotransformation
   C. Metabolism
   D. Excretion

7. Which pharmacologic process quantifies the chemical and physical interactions between the pharmacologic agent administered and the effects on target sites and actions of each drug? _____
   A. Pharmacodynamics
   B. Pharmacokinetics
   C. Pharmacologic transfer
   D. Active transfer

8. Which pharmacologic agent binds to physiologic receptors to produce a specific effect? _____
   A. Stereoisomers
   B. Effectors
   C. Agonists
   D. Antagonists

9. Which pharmacologic agents bind to physiologic receptors but have no pharmacologic effect? _____
   A. Stereoisomers
   B. Effectors
   C. Agonists
   D. Antagonists

10. The goal of _____ is to transform active compounds into water-soluble, pharmacologically inactive substances.
    A. Absorption
    B. Metabolic degradation
    C. Distribution
    D. Excretion

REFERENCES

1. Golembiewski J. Pharmacology of neuromuscular blocking drugs and intravenous induction agents. *Anesthesia Today.* 1994;5:2.
2. Barash P, Cullen B, Stoelting R. *Clinical Anesthesia.* 4th ed. Philadelphia: JB Lippincott; 2000:18.
3. Netter F. *Atlas of Human Anatomy.* Summit, NJ; Ciba-Geigy, 1993.
4. Morgan E, Mikhail M, Murray M. *Clinical Anesthesiology.* 3rd ed. New York: McGraw-Hill; 2002:155.
5. Miller R. *Anesthesia.* 5th ed. Philadelphia: Churchill Livingstone; 2000:35.
6. *Physicians' Desk Reference.* 57th ed. Montvale, NJ, Thompson PDR; 2003:2924.

CHAPTER 4

Sedation/Analgesia Medication and Techniques of Administration

CORE COMPETENCIES

At the completion of this chapter, the learner shall:

◆ Identify JCAHO standards related to the administration of sedation/analgesia medications and techniques of administration.

◆ Identify "Practice Guidelines for Sedation and Analgesia by Non-Anesthesiologists" recommendations related to sedation/analgesia medications and techniques of administration.

◆ List the ideal pharmacologic characteristics of sedation and analgesia medications.

◆ State the pharmacokinetic and pharmacodynamic considerations and end-organ effects associated with the following sedation/analgesia medications:

- Benzodiazepines
- Opioids
- Sedative/hypnotics
- Butyrophenones
- Barbiturates
- Dissociative anesthetics
- Local anesthetic solutions

◆ List the advantages, disadvantages, and patient care considerations associated with the following techniques of administration:

- Titration to clinical effect technique
- Bolus technique
- Continuous-infusion technique

Joint Commission on Accreditation of Healthcare Organizations Standards for Operative or Other High-Risk Procedures and/or the Administration of Moderate or Deep Sedation or Anesthesia

Standard PC.13.20

Operative or other procedures and/or the administration of moderate or deep sedation or anesthesia are planned.

Rationale for PC.13.20

Because the response to procedures is not always predictable and sedation-to-anesthesia is a continuum, it is not always possible to predict how an individual patient will respond. Therefore, qualified individuals are trained in professional standards and techniques to manage patients in the case of a potentially harmful event.

Elements of Performance for PC.13.20

1. Sufficient numbers of qualified staff are available* to evaluate the patient, perform the procedure, monitor, and recover the patient.

2. ***Individuals administering moderate or deep sedation and anesthesia are qualified[†] and have the appropriate credentials to manage patients at whatever level of sedation or anesthesia is achieved, either intentionally or unintentionally.***

3. A registered nurse supervises perioperative nursing care.

4. Appropriate equipment to monitor the patient's physiologic status is available.

5. Appropriate equipment to administer intravenous fluids and drugs, including blood and blood components, is available as needed.

6. Resuscitation capabilities are available.

---

*For hospitals providing obstetric or emergency operative services, this means they can provide anesthesia services as required by law and regulation.

[†]**Qualified** The individuals providing moderate or deep sedation and anesthesia have at a minimum had competency-based education, training, and experience in the following:
1. Evaluating patients before moderate or deep sedation and anesthesia.
2. Performing the moderate or deep sedation and anesthesia, including rescuing patients who slip into a deeper-than-desired level of sedation or analgesia. This includes the following:
   a. *Moderate* sedation – are qualified to rescue patients from deep sedation and are competent to manage a compromised airway and to provide adequate oxygenation and ventilation.
   b. *Deep* sedation – are qualified to rescue patients from general anesthesia and are competent to manage an unstable cardiovascular system as well as a compromised airway and inadequate oxygenation and ventilation.

© Joint Commission: Standards for Operative or Other High-Risk Procedures and/or the Administration of Moderate or Deep Sedation or Anesthesia, January, 2004. Reprinted with permission.

Practice Guidelines for Sedation and Analgesia by Non-Anesthesiologists
American Society of Anesthesiologists Task Force on Sedation and Analgesia by Non-Anesthesiologists

Recommendations. Individuals responsible for patients receiving sedation-analgesia should understand the pharmacology of the agents that are administered, as well as the role of pharmacologic antagonists for opioids and benzodiazepines. Individuals monitoring patients receiving sedation/analgesia should be able to recognize the associated complications. At least one individual capable of establishing a patent airway and positive-pressure ventilation, as well as a means for summoning additional assistance, should be present whenever sedation/analgesia is administered. It is recommended that an individual with advanced life support skills be immediately available (within 5 minutes) for moderate sedation and within the procedure room for deep sedation.

Recommendations. Combinations of sedative and analgesic agents may be administered as appropriate for the procedure being performed and the condition of the patient. Ideally, each component should be administered individually to achieve the desired effect (e.g., additional analgesic medication to relieve pain; additional sedative medication to decrease awareness or anxiety). The propensity for combinations of sedative and analgesic agents to cause respiratory depression and airway obstruction emphasizes the need to appropriately reduce the dose of each component as well as the need to continually monitor respiratory function.

Recommendations. Intravenous sedative/analgesic drugs should be given in small, incremental doses that are titrated to the desired endpoints of analgesia and sedation. Sufficient time must elapse between doses to allow the effect of each dose to be assessed before subsequent drug administration. When drugs are administered by nonintravenous routes (e.g., oral, rectal, intramuscular, transmucosal), allowance should be made for the time required for drug absorption before supplementation is considered. Because absorption may be unpredictable, administration of repeat doses of oral medications to supplement sedation/analgesia is not recommended.

Recommendations. Even if moderate sedation is intended, patients receiving propofol or methohexital by any route should receive care consistent with that required for deep sedation.

Accordingly, practitioners administering these drugs should be qualified to rescue patients from any level of sedation, including general anesthesia. Patients receiving ketamine should be cared for in a manner consistent with the level of sedation that is achieved.

Recommendations. Specific antagonists should be available whenever opioid analgesics or benzodiazepines are administered for sedation/analgesia. Naloxone or flumazenil may be administered to improve spontaneous ventilatory efforts in patients who have received opioids or benzodiazepines, respectively. This may be especially helpful in cases where airway control and positive-pressure ventilation are difficult. Before or concomitantly with pharmacologic reversal, patients who become hypoxemic or apneic during sedation/analgesia should: (1) be encouraged or stimulated to breathe deeply; (2) receive supplemental oxygen; and (3) receive positive-pressure ventilation if spontaneous ventilation is inadequate. After pharmacologic reversal, patients should be observed long enough to ensure that sedation and cardiorespiratory depression does not recur once the effect of the antagonist dissipates. The use of sedation regimens that include routine reversal of sedative or analgesic agents is discouraged.

From American Society of Anesthesiologists Task Force on Sedation and Analgesia by Non-Anesthesiologists. Practice guidelines for sedation and analgesia by Non-Anesthesiologists. *Anesthesiology.* 2002;96(4):1009-1012. Reprinted with permission.

The ideal characteristics of injected pharmacologic agents utilized to achieve the desired effects of sedation/analgesia (anxiolysis, amnesia, analgesia, and increased patient cooperation) include the following:

◆ Rapid onset of action
◆ Short duration of action
◆ Lack of cumulative effects
◆ Rapid recovery
◆ Minimal side effects
◆ Rapid metabolism to inactive nontoxic metabolites
◆ Residual analgesia
◆ Optimal patient satisfaction

Unfortunately, there is no single pharmacologic agent or technique that satisfies all of these requirements. In an attempt to produce an amnestic, pain-free, sedated patient, a combination of medications is required. This combination of medications gives the clinician the ability to manipulate the patient's short-term memory and sense of time.[1] Through pharmacologic intervention, the patient's perception of time is altered and patient cooperation is enhanced. To successfully produce a sedate/analgesic state and minimize complications (respiratory distress, cardiovascular depression, and hypoxemia) requires an understanding of the pharmacologic agents used to produce moderate and deep sedation. A complete pharmacologic profile of individual sedative and analgesic medications is provided in Chapter 5, Sedation/Analgesia Pharmacologic Profile. Box 4-1 outlines the advantages and disadvantages of pharmacologic combinations.

PHARMACODYNAMICS AND PHARMACOKINETICS
Benzodiazepines
Pharmacodynamics

Benzodiazepines bind to specific receptor sites in the central nervous system, particularly in the cerebral cortex.

Benzodiazepine receptor binding enhances gamma-aminobutyric acid (GABA) in the brain. Through this GABA interaction (Fig. 4-1), excitatory impulses are inhibited. Pharmacologic effects ranging from anxiolysis to general anesthesia occur depending on the amount of medication administered. Benzodiazepines are used to achieve the following:

◆ Anxiolysis
◆ Sedation
◆ Hypnosis
◆ Anticonvulsive effects
◆ Skeletal muscle relaxation

Pharmacokinetics

Benzodiazepines are generally administered via the following routes of administration:

◆ Orally
◆ Intramuscularly
◆ Intravenously

BOX 4-1

Pharmacologic Combinations

Single pharmacologic agents may produce:
- Adequate sedation in many cases
- Toxicity at increased dosage
- Isolated pharmacologic effect (analgesia, amnesia)
- Cumulative effects

A combination of pharmacologic agents may produce:
- Rapid recovery
- Decreased dosage requirement
- Unpredictable synergistic actions
- Increased likelihood of medication error with multiple injections

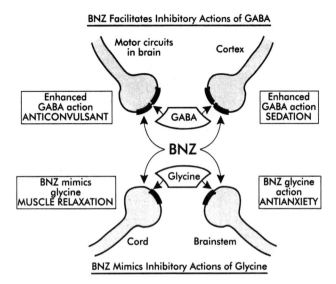

BNZ Facilitates Inhibitory Actions of GABA

Motor circuits in brain

Cortex

Enhanced GABA action ANTICONVULSANT

Enhanced GABA action SEDATION

GABA

BNZ

Glycine

BNZ mimics glycine MUSCLE RELAXATION

BNZ glycine action ANTIANXIETY

Cord

Brainstem

BNZ Mimics Inhibitory Actions of Glycine

FIGURE 4-1 GABA interaction. Through GABA interaction, enhanced inhibition of neurotransmitters occurs, altering normal neuronal function in the central nervous system. (From Richter JJ. Current theories about the mechanisms of benzodiazepines and neuroleptic drugs. *Anesthesiology.* 1981;54:66.)

Benzodiazepines are lipid soluble and readily penetrate the blood-brain barrier. Metabolism of benzodiazepines occurs by means of hepatic metabolism with excretion via the renal system.[2] Initially synthesized in 1959, diazepam (Valium) is the prototype benzodiazepine with which all others are compared. Classified as a long-acting benzodiazepine, intramuscular injections of diazepam are both painful and erratically absorbed.[3] However, diazepam is well absorbed from the gastrointestinal tract, with peak plasma levels achieved in 1 to 2 hours after oral administration and 1 to 2 minutes after intravenous administration. **The initial metabolism of diazepam yields an active metabolite, desmethyldiazepam.** Diazepam has a prolonged half-life (20 to 50 hours) when compared with its short-acting counterpart midazolam (1.7 to 2.6 hours).[4] When compared with midazolam's water-soluble suspension, diazepam's propylene glycol suspension predisposes to venous irritation and phlebitis. The half-life associated with benzodiazepines is secondary to the degree of hepatic extraction and the volume of distribution.

> Geriatric patients may be particularly sensitive to the sedative effects associated with diazepam secondary to the prolonged half-life and active pharmacologic metabolites.

Two new benzodiazepine agonists have been studied in clinical trials.[5,6] Both agonists (RO 48-6791 and RO 48-8684) may offer distinct clinical advantages secondary to their larger volume of distribution, increased clearance, and faster rate of recovery.[7] These benzodiazepine agonists may eventually be introduced into the sedation setting, which is dependent on the results of further clinical trials and ultimately approval by the U.S. Food and Drug Administration.

End-Organ Effects

Cardiovascular System. Arterial blood pressure, cardiac output, and peripheral vascular resistance are slightly decreased with the administration of benzodiazepines. Midazolam reduces blood pressure and vascular resistance more than diazepam. Heart rate variability (increase) with midazolam may occur secondary to decreased vagal tone.[8]

Respiratory System. Benzodiazepines depress the ventilatory response to carbon dioxide. This respiratory effect is generally insignificant unless the benzodiazepine is administered intravenously or in combination with other central nervous system depressant medications. **However, small doses of intravenous benzodiazepines may result in respiratory arrest, especially when given in conjunction with opioids or to patients with pathophysiologic disease processes.** Careful titration and vigilance are required when these medications are administered to avoid respiratory depression and airway obstruction.

Central Nervous System. A reduction in cerebral blood flow, cerebral oxygen consumption, and intracranial pressure occurs with the administration of benzodiazepines. Benzodiazepines are effective in treating seizure disorders and are noted for their centrally mediated muscle relaxant properties. The anterograde amnesia, anxiolysis, and hypnosis provided by benzodiazepines are useful adjuncts during the administration of sedation/analgesia.

Reversal of Pharmacologic Effect. The central nervous system and respiratory depressant effects of benzodiazepines may be reversed with the administration of flumazenil. A complete pharmacologic profile of flumazenil is provided in Chapter 5.

Precautions. To avoid respiratory compromise or cardiovascular depression, caution must be exercised when benzodiazepines are administered to patients with the following conditions:

- Chronic obstructive pulmonary disease
- History of sleep apnea
- Cardiopulmonary depression
- Extremes of age
- Alcohol intoxication
- Morbid obesity
- Potential for difficult airway management
- Presence of pathophysiologic disease processes

Opioids
Pharmacodynamics

The administration of opioids results in binding to specific opiate receptors located within the central nervous system. Opioids occupy mu, kappa, delta, and sigma receptor subtypes.

Mu

- Analgesia
- Respiratory depression
- Miosis
- Decreased gastrointestinal motility
- Euphoria
- Suppression of opiate withdrawal

Kappa

- Analgesia
- Respiratory depression
- Miosis
- Dysphoria

Delta

- Analgesia
- Respiratory depression

Sigma

- Dysphoria
- Hallucinations

The pharmacologic effects of opioids depend on the specific receptor subtypes stimulated. Opioids produce some degree of sedation; however, they are used mainly for their analgesic properties. Increased dosage of narcotics is associated with significant levels of sedation and the potential for severe respiratory depression.

> Potent synergistic effects may occur when combinations of benzodiazepines and opioids are used to produce moderate sedation. Careful titration to clinical effect is required to avoid the development of hypoventilation, airway obstruction, or respiratory insufficiency.

Pharmacokinetics

Intramuscularly, intravenously, and orally administered opioids are readily absorbed to achieve effective plasma levels. Opioid distribution characteristics are presented in Table 4-1. Opioids are metabolized by hepatic biotransformation with pharmacologic end products excreted through the kidneys. Small fractions of opioids are excreted unchanged in the urine.

End-Organ Effects

Cardiovascular System. Meperidine produces tachycardia because of its vagolytic effect. In comparison, morphine sulfate, fentanyl, sufentanil, and alfentanil produce a vagally mediated bradycardia. Blood pressure may decrease secondary to bradycardia, decreased systemic vascular resistance, and alterations in the sympathetic nervous system. Meperidine and morphine sulfate release histamine, which may significantly decrease systemic vascular resistance and produce bronchoconstriction.

Respiratory System. Opioids depress respiratory rate and volume. $Paco_2$ and the apneic threshold for carbon dioxide are increased. **An increase in muscle tone may occur with rapid administration of opioids. This opioid-induced**

TABLE 4-1

Opioid Distribution Characteristics

	MORPHINE	MEPERIDINE (DEMEROL)	FENTANYL
Potency	1	0.1	75-125 × morphine's
Elimination half-life (min)	102-130	220-265	180-220
Protein binding	30%	64%-82%	85%
Heart rate	↓	↑	↓↓
Mean arterial pressure	*	*	↓
Ventilation	↓↓↓	↓↓↓	↓↓↓
Cerebral blood flow	↓	↓	↓
Cerebral metabolic rate of O_2	↓	↓	↓
Intracranial pressure	↓	↓	↓

*Decrease in mean arterial pressure = degree of histamine release.

rigidity results in an increase in muscle tone that may produce chest wall rigidity (wooden chest syndrome) and inability to ventilate the patient. The exact incidence of rigidity varies greatly secondary to patient age, sedation technique utilized, and speed of opioid injection.[9-12] The etiology of opioid-induced muscle rigidity is not clearly understood. Some authors have postulated that it is related to a catatonic state, whereas others have suggested that opioids produce rigidity by altering dopamine concentrations within the striatum of the brain.[13-16] **Treatment protocol for chest wall rigidity includes summoning anesthesia personnel to assist with ventilation, administration of naloxone, and muscle relaxants.**

Central Nervous System. Opioids increase cerebral blood flow and intracranial pressure through respiratory depression and carbon dioxide retention. Additional central nervous system effects include the following:

- Analgesia
- Respiratory depression
- Drowsiness
- Sedation
- Euphoria
- Dysphoria
- Nausea and vomiting

Reversal of Pharmacologic Effect. The central nervous system and respiratory depressant effects of opioids are reversed with the administration of naloxone (Narcan). As identified in Figure 4-2, naloxone is a pure opioid antagonist that competitively binds at the opiate receptors. A complete pharmacologic profile of naloxone is featured in Chapter 5.

Precautions. Because of the potential for respiratory depression, airway obstruction, and respiratory arrest,

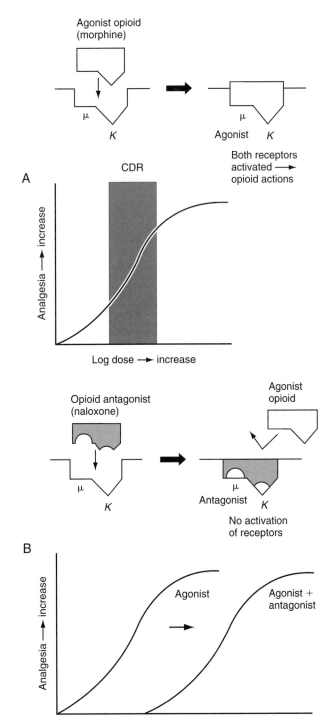

A

B

FIGURE 4-2 Opioid agonist-antagonist action. **A,** An opioid agonist stimulates opioid receptors through a lock and key mechanism to exert pharmacologic effect. **B,** Opioid antagonists reverse the pharmacologic effect of opioids by binding at the opioid receptor but not exerting any pharmacologic response.

extreme caution must be exercised in the following patient populations receiving intravenous opioids:

◆ Chronic obstructive pulmonary disease
◆ History of sleep apnea

◆ Cardiopulmonary depression
◆ Extremes of age
◆ Acute alcohol intoxication
◆ Morbid obesity
◆ Potential for difficult airway management
◆ Presence of pathophysiologic disease processes

Sedative/Hypnotics: Propofol
Pharmacodynamics

Propofol (Diprivan) is a 1% aqueous solution (10 mg/mL) for intravenous use. It consists of an oil in water emulsion containing soybean oil, glycerol, and egg lecithin. As a sedative/hypnotic, propofol produces rapid hypnosis with minimal excitation. It produces nonspecific cortical depression and is characterized by a more complete and rapid awakening than the barbiturate class of induction agents.

It is believed that propofol exerts its pharmacologic effect at the GABA receptor complex. Through an interaction at the GABA receptor complex, opening of the chloride ion channel results in hyperpolarization of cell membranes. Resultant neuroinhibition in the central nervous system is produced (sedation/hypnosis/unconsciousness).

Pharmacokinetics

The high degree of lipid solubility of propofol results in a rapid onset of action with rapid awakening after a general anesthesia induction dose (half-life: 2 to 8 minutes). Plasma clearance of propofol exceeds hepatic blood flow. Inactive water-soluble metabolites are excreted by the kidneys. There is no evidence of drug accumulation in patients, even those with hepatic disease.

End-Organ Effects

Cardiovascular System. Decreased systemic vascular resistance associated with inhibition of sympathetic vasoconstrictor activity, cardiac contractility, and preload occurs. A negative inotropic effect may result from inhibition of intracellular calcium.[17] Changes in heart rate are generally insignificant in the healthy patient; however, cardiac output and contractility manifestations in the elderly patient population may lead to significant hypotension and cardiac dysrhythmias.

Large medication doses, rapid injection, and administration to the elderly or patients with multisystemic disease states results in exacerbation of cardiovascular effects.

Respiratory System. Even small doses of propofol (sedative dosage range) can cause respiratory depression, airway obstruction, and respiratory insufficiency. Propofol inhibits hypoxic ventilatory drive and depresses the normal response to hypercarbia. The ventilatory depression is enhanced with the simultaneous administration of other central nervous system depressant medications. **Therefore, propofol should only be administered by healthcare**

practitioners who demonstrate clinical competency in advanced cardiorespiratory management.

Central Nervous System. Cerebral metabolic rate of oxygen consumption, cerebral blood flow, and intracranial pressure are decreased. Propofol demonstrates significant antipruritic and antiemetic effects. In a small percentage of patients, excitatory phenomenon may be seen (muscle twitching, spontaneous movement, or hiccoughs). The excitatory phenomenon may be secondary to subcortical glycine antagonism.

Pharmacologic Reversal. There is no pharmacologic reversal agent for propofol. In the event of an overdose, cardiovascular and ventilatory support is required.

Precautions. Propofol formulations support bacterial growth. Sterile technique must be utilized when handling. Before drawing propofol into a syringe, the surface of the ampule should be wiped with an alcohol swab before opening. The propofol syringe should be dated/timed and any unused medication should be discarded after 6 hours. Propofol suspension currently utilizes a bacterial retardant but is not antimicrobially preserved. The handling guidelines outlined by the manufacturer must be followed and are outlined in Chapter 5.

Butyrophenones
Pharmacodynamics

Droperidol (Inapsine) structurally resembles and evokes pharmacologic effects similar to the phenothiazines. Butyrophenones decrease anxiety. As a result of their structural similarity to GABA, neuroleptic agents (droperidol) can occupy GABA receptors on the postsynaptic membrane, reducing synaptic transmission and increasing the concentration of dopamine in the intersynaptic cleft. They also inhibit the reuptake of dopamine and norepinephrine into the storage granules at the presynaptic nerve terminals. Thus the normal balance of acetylcholine and dopamine in certain areas of the brain is altered and leads to inhibition of operant behavior and anxiolysis. The antiemetic effect associated with butyrophenones is probably related to their affinity to receptors in the chemoreceptor trigger zone.

Pharmacokinetics

The total body clearance of droperidol is dependent on hepatic blood flow, thus emphasizing the importance of hepatic metabolism in elimination. The short elimination half-life (104 minutes) is not consistent with the prolonged central nervous system effects of droperidol (3 to 6 hours), which may reflect the slow dissociation of the drug from receptors or retention of droperidol in the brain. Droperidol is metabolized in the liver, with maximal excretion of metabolites occurring during the first 24 hours.

End-Organ Effects

Cardiovascular System. Droperidol can decrease systemic blood pressure as a result of actions in the central nervous system and by peripheral alpha-adrenergic blockade (vasodilation). The decrease in blood pressure is usually minimal; however, some patients may experience marked hypotension.

Fatal cardiac arrhythmias have been reported with droperidol (Inapsine) (FDA Alert, 2001).[18] Cases of QT prolongation and/or torsades de pointes have been reported in patients receiving droperidol at or below recommended doses. Cases have occurred in patients with no known risk factors for QT prolongation and some with fatalities. Droperidol is contraindicated in patients with known or suspected QT prolongation, including patients with congenital long QT syndrome. Droperidol should be administered with extreme caution to patients who may be at risk for development of prolonged QT syndrome (congestive heart failure, bradycardia, use of a diuretic, cardiac hypertrophy, hypokalemia, hypomagnesemia, or administration of other drugs known to increase the QT interval). Other risk factors may include age older than 65 years, alcohol abuse, and use of agents such as benzodiazepines, opioids, and volatile anesthetics. Droperidol should be initiated at a low dose and adjusted upward, with caution, as needed to achieve the desired effect.

Respiratory System. Resting ventilation and the ventilatory response to carbon dioxide are not altered by droperidol. Droperidol administered intravenously augments the ventilatory response evoked by arterial hypoxemia, presumably by blocking the action of the inhibitory neurotransmitter dopamine at the carotid body.

Central Nervous System. An outwardly calming effect occurs with droperidol use. Akathisia (most often a feeling of restlessness in the legs) may occur with the administration of droperidol. Droperidol evokes extrapyramidal reactions in approximately 1% of the patient population. Extrapyramidal symptoms occur secondary to droperidol's dopamine antagonistic effects. Butyrophenones occupy GABA receptors on the postsynaptic membrane, reducing synaptic transmission and increasing the concentration of dopamine in the intersynaptic cleft. They also inhibit the reuptake of dopamine and norepinephrine into the storage granules at the presynaptic nerve terminals. Thus, the normal balance of acetylcholine and dopamine in certain areas of the brain is altered and leads to inhibition of operant behavior and anxiolysis. The antiemetic effect associated with the neuroleptic drugs is probably related to their affinity to receptors in the chemoreceptor trigger zone.

Pharmacologic Reversal. Cardiovascular and ventilatory support is required in the event of overdose. There is no pharmacologic reversal agent for the butyrophenone classification of medications.

Precautions. Extreme caution is required in patients with prolonged QT syndrome. Patients with a history of extrapyramidal symptoms (Parkinson's disease), and neuroleptic malignant syndrome should not receive butyrophenones. Droperidol should be administered with caution to hypotensive patients secondary to its alpha-adrenergic (vasodilating) blockade. A complete pharmacologic profile of inapsine is featured in Chapter 5.

Barbiturates
Pharmacodynamics

The use of barbiturates for sedation by non-anesthesia personnel has been reported in the literature.[19] Barbiturates suppress the reticular activating center (sleep-wake center) located in the brain stem and the cerebral cortex on a dose-dependent continuum.[17] They suppress transmission of excitatory neurotransmitters and enhance transmission of the inhibitory neurotransmitter GABA. Barbiturates are used for their sedative, hypnotic, and anticonvulsant properties. Depending on the total dose administered and route of administration, barbiturates are capable of producing effects ranging from sedation to deep coma. **For this reason, the use of barbiturates by non-anesthesia personnel requires clinical skills in advanced airway and cardiovascular management.**

Pharmacokinetics

Barbiturates may be administered intravenously or rectally. Rectal administration is generally reserved for pediatric premedication. Intravenous use includes sedation, induction of general anesthesia, and barbiturate coma. Because of their high lipid solubility, barbiturates reach the brain within 30 seconds. Redistribution from the central compartment (intravascular fluid and highly perfused tissues: lungs, heart, brain, kidneys, liver) to the peripheral compartment (skeletal muscle, fat, bone) is responsible for the duration of action. Repeated doses of barbiturates result in a prolonged duration of action as the peripheral compartment becomes saturated. Metabolism of barbiturates requires hepatic oxidation. Once hepatic oxidation is complete, renal excretion is responsible for eliminating the water-soluble metabolites.

End-Organ Effects

Cardiovascular System. Hypotension, tachycardia, decreased systemic vascular resistance, and decreased venous return may occur with the administration of barbiturates. Cardiovascular changes associated with barbiturate administration are related to decreased cardiac output and reduced systemic vascular resistance. These effects are more pronounced in the hypovolemic patient.

Respiratory System. **The administration of barbiturates for sedation can result in severe respiratory depression and arrest.** Decreased ventilatory response to oxygen and carbon dioxide occurs with the administration of barbiturates. Depression of the medullary respiratory center (hypoventilation and apnea) is associated with increased doses of barbiturates. Smooth muscle constriction may result in bronchospasm. Hiccoughs and tonic-clonic movements occur with the administration of methohexital, particularly after multiple cumulative doses.

Central Nervous System. Barbiturates decrease cerebral metabolic rate, cerebral blood flow, and intracranial pressure by means of cerebral vasoconstriction. Small doses of barbiturates may cause a state of disorientation or excitement. Barbiturates do not have analgesic properties and appear to have an antialgesic effect. Additional central nervous system effects include somnolence, agitation, confusion, nervousness, and anxiety.

Pharmacologic Reversal. There is no pharmacologic reversal agent for barbiturates. Systemic pulmonary and cardiovascular support are required in the event of overdose. For respiratory depression, ventilation is required until recovery from pharmacologic effect.

Precautions. Care should be taken in patients with the following conditions:

- Hepatic dysfunction
- Porphyria
- Cardiopulmonary depression
- Chronic obstructive pulmonary disease
- History of sleep apnea
- Extremes of age
- Acute alcohol intoxication
- Morbid obesity
- Difficult airways
- Pathophysiologic disease process

Dissociative Anesthesia
Pharmacodynamics

Ketamine is a derivative of phencyclidine, which produces a dissociative state. In subanesthetic doses, ketamine provides profound analgesia. Ketamine "dissociates" the thalamus (sensory relay from the reticular activating system to the cerebral cortex) from the limbic system.[20] Characteristic appearance of the dissociative state includes the following:

- Intense analgesia
- Cataleptic state
- Nystagmus
- Open-eyed gaze
- Noncommunicative patient, although the patient gives the appearance of wakefulness
- Skeletal muscle movement

Pharmacokinetics. After intravenous administration, ketamine has a rapid onset and a short duration of action. Distribution half-life is 10 to 15 minutes. Redistribution to the vessel-poor group (fat, skeletal muscle, bone) and biotransformation by the liver results in awakening. Biotransformation results in pharmacologically active metabolites (norketamine), which are excreted in the urine.

End-Organ Effects

Cardiovascular System. Stimulation of the sympathetic nervous system increases heart rate, cardiac output, and arterial blood pressure. Increased myocardial oxygen consumption occurs in conjunction with these changes. Ketamine is contraindicated in patients with coronary artery disease, hypertension, congestive heart failure, or impaired myocardial performance.

Respiratory System. Ketamine produces bronchodilation and minimal reduction of ventilatory drive. Upper airway muscle tone is maintained, and airway reflexes remain intact. Salivary and mucous secretion is enhanced with ketamine administration. These effects may be counteracted with the administration of an antisialagogue (e.g., atropine, glycopyrrolate [Robinul]).

Central Nervous System. Increased cerebral blood flow, cerebral oxygen consumption, and intracranial pressure occur as a result of cerebral vasodilation. Therefore, ketamine use is contraindicated in patients with intracranial disease. **Myoclonic activity is characteristic of ketamine administration. Emergence delirium and undesirable central nervous system side effects include visual and auditory illusions, dreams, and combativeness and may persist for 24 hours.** Emergence delirium generally occurs as the patient is recovering from the pharmacologic effects of ketamine administration. Reassurance and provision of a quiet area in which to recover have been utilized to decrease the incidence of central nervous system excitation.

Pharmacologic Reversal. There is no pharmacologic reversal agent for ketamine. Systemic pulmonary and cardiovascular support are required in the event of overdose. For respiratory depression, ventilation is required until the patient recovers from the pharmacologic effect of ketamine.

Precautions. Extreme caution is required in the presence of increased intracranial pressure, coronary artery disease, and hypertension.

Local Anesthetics

Local anesthetics may be utilized to anesthetize specific anatomic areas (e.g., esophagus, line insertion sites) to complete therapeutic, diagnostic, or minor surgical procedures. It is important for the clinician administering sedation/analgesia to be cognizant of the pharmacodynamics and pharmacokinetics of the local anesthetic utilized.

Pharmacodynamics

Local anesthetics provide temporary loss of motor, sensory, and autonomic nervous system function. Local anesthetic chemical structure generally consists of the following:

◆ A lipophilic group (benzene ring)
◆ A hydrophylic group (tertiary amine)
◆ An intermediate chain (ester or amide linkage)

Local anesthetics are classified as amides or esters. Amide local anesthetics include:

◆ Bupivacaine (Marcaine)
◆ Dibucaine (Nupericaine)
◆ Etidocaine (Duranest)
◆ Lidocaine (Xylocaine)
◆ Mepivacaine (Carbocaine)
◆ Prilocaine (Citanest)
◆ Ropivacaine

Ester local anesthetics include the following:

◆ Chloroprocaine (Nesacaine)
◆ Cocaine
◆ Procaine (Novocaine)
◆ Tetracaine (Pontocaine)

Local anesthetics differ specifically with regard to:

◆ Potency
◆ Time of onset
◆ Duration of pharmacologic effect
◆ Toxicity

Local anesthetics prevent the development of the action potential required for depolarization of nerve cells by blocking sodium channels. For transmission of impulses to occur, movement of sodium and potassium ions through these channels is required. Depolarization occurs when sodium ions move from extracellular fluid to the intracellular space. Repolarization occurs when potassium ions move from the intracellular to the extracellular space. As depicted in Figure 4-3, by preventing development of an action potential, nerve conduction is impaired.

Pharmacokinetics

Local anesthetic absorption is dependent on a variety of factors:

◆ Increased vascularity at the injection site results in increased local anesthetic uptake.
◆ Vasoconstrictors decrease rate of absorption.
◆ Increased protein binding increases duration of action.
◆ Increased lipid solubility increases potency.

Ester local anesthetics are derived from para-aminobenzoic acid (PABA). Ester local anesthetics are metabolized by ester hydrolysis via pseudocholinesterase, which is found in the plasma.[21] Amide local anesthetics are metabolized by dealkylation and hydrolysis in the liver.[21] Local anesthetic potency is determined by lipid solubility. Protein binding determines the duration of effect as the highly bound local anesthetic remains

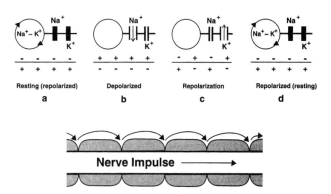

FIGURE 4-3 Local anesthetic agents and nerve conduction. Local anesthetic agents block the conduction of impulses along the nerve fiber. Local anesthetics make changes in the nerve membrane that prevent normal depolarization and repolarization of the nerve cell membrane. (From Chung DC, Lam AM. *Essentials of Anesthesiology.* 3rd ed. Philadelphia: WB Saunders; 1997:81.)

in the lipoprotein of the nerve membrane for a longer duration. Commonly used local anesthetics for therapeutic, diagnostic, and minor surgical procedures are listed in Table 4-2. At times, combinations of local anesthetics are used. This admixture of local anesthetics offers the clinician the beneficial pharmacologic effects of each local anesthetic selected.

Epinephrine may be added to local anesthetics to promote local vasoconstriction. This vasoconstriction limits uptake into the tissue and prolongs local anesthetic effect. The addition of epinephrine to the local anesthetic solution is contraindicated in the following patient populations:

◆ Patients with unstable angina
◆ Patients with cardiac dysrhythmias
◆ Infiltration into areas without adequate collateral blood flow (e.g., fingers, toes)
◆ Hyperthyroid patients
◆ Patients with uteroplacental insufficiency
◆ Patients with increased sympathetic nervous system activity

End-Organ Effects

Cardiovascular System. Intravenous injection of local anesthetics depresses the automaticity of the myocardium.[22] **Myocardial contractility is reduced as local anesthetic concentration is increased. Decreased contractility occurs secondary to cardiac membrane changes and alterations in the response of the autonomic nervous system.** Toxic

TABLE 4-2

Local Anesthetic Solutions

Generic (proprietary)	Ring —	Structure chain	— Amine	Potency and lipid solubility	pK_a	Duration and protein binding	Uses	Maximum dose (mg/kg)
Amides Bupivacaine (Marcaine)	CH₃ / CH₃	—NHCO—	C₄H₉ N	++++	8.1	++++	Epidural, caudal, spinal; infiltration; peripheral nerve block	3
Dibucaine (Nupercaine)	OC₄H₉	—CONHCH₂—	N / C₂H₅ \ C₂H₅	++++	8.8	++++	Spinal; topical	1
Etidocaine (Duranest)	CH₃ / CH₃	—NHCOCH— | C₂H₅	N / C₂H₅ \ C₃H₇	++++	7.7	++++	Epidural, caudal infiltration; peripheral nerve block	4
Lidocaine (Xylocaine)	CH₃ / CH₃	—NHCOCH₂—	N / C₂H₅ \ C₂H₅	++	7.8	++	Epidural, caudal, spinal; infiltration; peripheral nerve block; topical	4.5[1] 7[2]
Mepivacaine (Carbocaine)	CH₃ / CH₃	—NHCO—	CH₃ N	++	7.6	++	Epidural, caudal; infiltration; peripheral nerve block	4.5[1] 7[2]
Prilocaine (Citanest)	CH₃	—NHCOCH— | CH₃	N / H \ C₃H₇	++	7.8	++	Epidural, caudal; infiltration; peripheral nerve block	8
Ropivacaine	CH₃ / CH₃	—NHCO—	C₃H₇ N	++++	8.1	++++	Epidural, caudal, spinal; infiltration; peripheral nerve block	3

Continued

TABLE 4-2

Local Anesthetic Solutions—cont'd

Generic (proprietary)	Ring —	Structure chain —	Amine	Potency and lipid solubility	pK_a	Duration and protein binding	Uses	Maximum dose (mg/kg)
Esters Chloroprocaine (Nesacaine)[3]				+	9.0	+	Epidural, caudal; infiltration; peripheral nerve block	12
Cocaine				++	8.7	++	Topical	3
Procaine				+	8.9	+	Spinal; infiltration; peripheral nerve block	12
Tetracaine (Pontocaine)				++++	8.2	+++	Spinal; topical	3

[1]Maximum dose without epinephrine.

[2]Maximum dose with epinephrine.

[3]Chloroprocaine is metabolized too rapidly to measure lipid solubility or protein binding. It has a rapid onset of action despite a high pK_a.

Redrawn from Morgan G, Mikhail M, Murray M: *Clinical anesthesiology*. 3rd ed. New York: Lange Medical Books/McGraw-Hill; 2002:238.

manifestations associated with local anesthetic overdose include the following:

◆ Bradycardia
◆ Heart block
◆ Hypotension
◆ Cardiac arrest
◆ Circulatory collapse

Treatment of cardiovascular side effects associated with local anesthetic overdose includes:

◆ Administration of oxygen
◆ Airway support
◆ Circulatory support (volume expansion)
◆ Vasopressor and inotropes
◆ Advanced cardiac life support (ACLS) protocol implementation

Respiratory System. Apnea after the administration of local anesthetics may occur following specific nerve paralysis (phrenic, intercostal) or medullary center depression (retrobulbar block). Treatment of local anesthetic–induced respiratory center depression includes administration of oxygen, ventilation, and airway support.

Central Nervous System. Neurologic signs and symptoms of local anesthetic–induced toxicity include the following:

◆ Agitation
◆ Numbness of the tongue and mouth
◆ Dizziness
◆ Visual disturbance
◆ Tinnitus
◆ Restlessness
◆ Slurred speech
◆ Irrational behavior
◆ Muscle twitching
◆ Apnea
◆ Convulsions

> The central nervous system is extremely sensitive to the excitatory effects of local anesthetic solutions.

Central nervous system symptoms may range from mild complaints to life-threatening complications. As symptoms progress, tonic-clonic seizures, respiratory arrest, vomiting with aspiration, and loss of consciousness may ensue. Treatment of neurologic side effects associated with local anesthetic overdose include the following:

◆ Administration of oxygen
◆ Airway support and ventilation
◆ In the presence of seizures, small doses of benzodiazepines (1 to 2 mg midazolam [Versed], or 5 to 10 mg diazepam [Valium]) or barbiturates (50 mg thiopental sodium [Pentothal Sodium]) may be used.

Emergency Resuscitative Medication and Equipment for Local Anesthesia Toxicity Reaction

- Benzodiazepine (midazolam or diazepam) *or* barbiturate (thiopental [Pentothal])
- Advanced Cardiac Life Support protocol medications
- Crash cart
- Oral airways
- Nasal airways
- Laryngoscope
- Endotracheal tubes
- Suction

With proper selection of the local anesthetic combined with sedative/analgesic medications, most therapeutic, diagnostic, and minor surgical procedures are performed uneventfully. As the healthcare provider is cognizant of sedative/analgesic medications and modes of administration, the healthcare provider too must be familiar with local anesthetics used during sedation/analgesic procedures. Preparation for adverse effects associated with the administration of local anesthesia (seizures, cardiovascular depression) is required whenever local anesthetics are administered. Box 4-2 identifies medications and resuscitative equipment required in the event of a toxic reaction to a local anesthetic.

Benzocaine-Induced Methemoglobinemia

Benzocaine is a topical anesthetic that is utilized by a wide variety of sedation practitioners to anesthetize the upper airway before instrumentation (upper endoscopy, transesophageal echocardiography, bronchoscopy).[23] **Physicians and healthcare providers utilizing topical anesthetic solutions (Americaine, Hurricaine, Cetacaine) containing benzocaine should be familiar with the potential complication benzocaine-induced methemoglobinemia.** Prompt recognition of this complication and its prescribed treatment protocol is required by the sedation practitioner to avoid the development of neurologic hypoxia or death.

As of the year 2000, only 58 cases of idiosyncratic benzocaine-induced methemoglobinemia had been reported.[24] **Methemoglobinemia is a condition that is characterized by oxidation of iron within the hemoglobin molecule from the ferrous (Fe^{2+}) form to the ferric (Fe^{3+}) state.** This results in an elevated circulating fraction of methemoglobinemia within the erythrocyte. The result of this oxidation of iron within the hemoglobin molecule includes:

- A significant decrease in the oxygen-carrying capacity of red blood cells
- Central and peripheral cyanosis
- Metabolic acidosis secondary to the cell's inability to carry out aerobic metabolism
- Coma
- Death

Clinical presentation of methemoglobinemia generally would occur after administration of an oxidizing toxin that has been metabolized by the cytochrome P-450 system with resultant free oxygen radicals. The increased levels of methemoglobinemia cause changes in pulse oximetry and oxygen saturation. Oxygen saturation reveals a decreased SpO_2 due to the small difference in light absorption by methemoglobin to hemoglobin. Pulse oximetry yields information based on the differential light absorption of oxyhemoglobin and reduced hemoglobin. Oxyhemoglobin absorbs more light at 940 nm, and reduced hemoglobin absorbs more light at 660 nm. Methemoglobin absorbs light equally at both the wavelengths, with pulse oximetry displaying an SpO_2 of 85%. **The higher the methemoglobin concentration, the closer the SpO_2 value is to 85%.** However, the actual percentage of the arterial oxyhemoglobin concentration can be either underestimated or overestimated in the SpO_2 value.[25,26]

Diagnosis of methemoglobinemia may be difficult. Clinical symptoms generally occur when methemoglobin production exceeds rates of reduction. Patients frequently do not display initial symptoms of respiratory distress. However, as methemoglobin levels begin to rise (normal methemoglobin levels less than 1% to 2% in erythrocytes) the following symptoms may occur:

- Fatigue
- Headache
- Syncope
- Dysrhythmia
- Dyspnea
- Lethargy
- Dizziness
- Metabolic acidosis
- Stupor
- Coma
- Death

The symptoms outlined may occur within 20 to 60 minutes of drug administration. Initial symptoms may occur when methemoglobin concentration exceeds 20% (anxiety, fatigue, dyspnea, dizziness, tachycardia, headache, syncope). As methemoglobin levels increase (> 50%), oxygen delivery decreases and marked dyspnea may occur in conjunction with metabolic acidosis, dysrhythmias, and lethargy. These symptoms may progress to stupor and death. Death has been reported from levels greater than 70% and may be attributed to dysrhythmias, circulatory collapse, or neurologic compromise.[27,28] Elderly, pediatric, and hypoxic patients are also more sensitive to methemoglobin formation.[29,30]

Methemoglobinemia is a medical emergency that requires prompt treatment. Diagnosis should be considered when oxygen saturation levels fall significantly and remain unresponsive to increased oxygen administration.

Treatment protocol includes:

- Identify and discontinue the offending agent immediately.
- Administer supplemental oxygen with high flow rates.

◆ Administer intravenous methylene blue at 1 to 2 mg/kg as a 1% solution over 5 to 10 minutes.

◆ Dose should be repeated within 60 minutes for inadequate response marked by sustained elevation in methemoglobin levels. However, excessive methylene blue can actually promote increased methemoglobin levels.

◆ Monitor arterial blood gases to assess response to therapy.

◆ In severe cases, exchange blood transfusion may be necessary.[23,31]

Benzocaine spray is frequently utilized to produce topical anesthesia for bronchoscopy, upper endoscopy, and transesophageal echocardiography. Chocolate-color cyanosis, which is unresponsive to oxygen therapy coupled with a discrepancy between O_2 saturation and PaO_2 should alert the healthcare provider to confirm the diagnosis with co-oximetry. **Methylene blue should be available in all sedation settings where benzocaine topical spray is administered.**

Although rare, methemoglobinemia is a fatal complication associated with benzocaine topical anesthetic solutions. Initial symptoms mimic other clinical syndromes that may occur during procedural sedation.

TECHNIQUES OF ADMINISTRATION

When administered properly, the use of sedatives and analgesics provides a sedate patient with minimal side effects. The variety of sedative medications and modes of administration offer the clinician a wide range of options to achieve the goals and objectives of sedation/analgesia. Medication selection and administration by a particular technique are dependent on the patient's presedation physical status, the presence of pathophysiologic disease states, age, and the planned procedure. Understanding the technique of administration is equally important to understanding the pharmacokinetics and pharmacodynamics of selected sedative or analgesic medications. Therefore, an explanation of the techniques of medication administration that follow emphasizes clinical approaches designed to avoid the development of deep sedative states or severe respiratory depression.

Titration to Clinical Effect Technique

Medications used for therapeutic, diagnostic, and minor surgical procedures may be administered in a variety of ways. As depicted in Figure 4-4, the titration to clinical effect technique uses individual medications titrated slowly to clinical effect. To establish an analgesic base, opioids are frequently administered before benzodiazepines. Two to 3 minutes before the procedure, intravenous fentanyl, 1 µg/kg (titrated in 25-µg increments), or meperidine, 0.5 mg/kg (titrated in 25-mg increments), or morphine sulfate, 0.05 mg/kg (titrated in 2-mg increments), may be slowly administered to establish analgesia. Some clinicians prefer to administer narcotics by the intramuscular route. For intramuscular injection, the narcotic of choice is administered 45 to 60 minutes before the scheduled procedure. Disadvantages associated with this technique include scheduling conflicts, injection into subcutaneous tissue, poor absorption, and the time required to monitor the patient after an opioid injection.

Combining medications (narcotics and benzodiazepines) reduces total dosage through synergistic action, assists the clinician in the maintenance of the sedate state, and

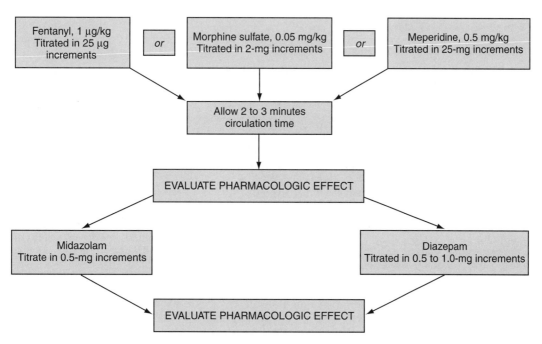

FIGURE 4-4 Titration to clinical effect technique.

promotes rapid patient recovery. **However, respiratory depression is frequently associated with the pharmacologic synergism achieved through concurrent administration of medications.**

Overdose, rapid administration (not allowing adequate circulation time), and failure to appreciate patient pathophysiologic disease processes frequently results in the development of airway obstruction, hypoxia, and respiratory insufficiency.

In conjunction with the preexisting analgesia established with opioids, the addition of benzodiazepines (midazolam in 0.5-mg increments or diazepam in 1-mg increments) titrated to a clinical endpoint of nystagmus or slurred speech provides a sedate patient. To avoid cardiopulmonary depression, it is important to titrate medications slowly to the clinical endpoints outlined earlier. At times, barbiturates or sedative/hypnotics have been advocated in the literature to provide an increase in the depth of sedation. A complete pharmacologic profile for narcotics, benzodiazepines, and sedative/hypnotic agents is outlined in Chapter 5.

Bolus Technique

A popular technique used for procedures of short duration (oral surgery and gastroenterologic procedures) is the bolus technique. Based on a predetermined dosage (mg/kg), the entire dose or a large percentage is administered in a single injection. This technique is particularly popular for administration of benzodiazepines. One advantage of this technique is its ability to provide a rapid medication plasma level immediately before the procedure.

Disadvantages of bolus injection include oversedation leading to respiratory insufficiency, unconsciousness, chest wall rigidity, and cardiovascular depression. The bolus technique eliminates the safety features of slow titration, which assesses for individual patient response and clinical sedation endpoints (nystagmus, slurred speech). Despite the speed with which a desired plasma concentration can be achieved, the risks associated with the bolus technique often outweigh the potential benefits. Small incremental boluses offer the ability to produce therapeutic plasma levels slowly while potentially using less medication to produce the same pharmacologic endpoint.

Continuous-Infusion Techniques

Continuous-infusion techniques permit a constant plasma level through a continuous infusion of medication. **The continuous-infusion technique avoids the fluctuations in plasma levels associated with bolus techniques.** Additional potential benefits include decreased recovery time, less total drug administered, and minimized side effects. Careful titration based on predetermined clinical endpoints (nystagmus, slurred speech, sedation) allows the infusion to be discontinued at the conclusion of the procedure with a rapid return to an alert state. Continuous infusion techniques are popular with propofol administered at a micrograms per kilogram per minute administration rate (Box 4-3). Continuous-infusion techniques require a carrier intravenous solution with the continuous infusion piggybacked into the carrier solution. Extreme care must be exercised to avoid running the carrier solution at a keep-vein-open or slow rate, thereby allowing a buildup of the infusion within the intravenous administration tubing. Once the carrier fluid is opened, the

---

BOX 4-3

Continuous Infusion Technique Sedation Approach

- Initiate intravenous line with carrier solution (e.g., normal saline, lactated Ringer's).
- Establish narcotic medication base:

Fentanyl, 1 µg/kg (titrated in 25-µg increments)

or

Morphine sulfate, 0.05 mg/kg (titrated in 2-mg increments)

or

Meperidine, 0.5 mg/kg (titrated in 25-mg increments)

- Sedation must be initiated slowly with a continuous-infusion technique to achieve the desired level of sedation and to avoid cardiorespiratory depression.
- Begin administration of propofol, 5 µg/kg/min.
- Infusion rate may be increased at 5-µg/kg/min intervals.

Most patients exhibit clinical endpoints associated with sedation/analgesia (nystagmus, slurred speech) at dosage ranges of 5 to 40 µg/kg/min. Dosage and rate of administration must be established slowly. Clinically relevant factors that decrease total dosage of medication administered include presedation patient status, age, presence of pathophysiologic disease, and desired level of sedation.

If a continuous infusion sedation technique with propofol is selected, it is imperative to ensure that the prescribing clinician understands the pharmacokinetics and pharmacodynamics associated with this agent. The prescribing clinician and healthcare provider administering the medication (or monitoring the patient) should possess advanced airway management skills, demonstrate proficiency in managing cardiovascular complications, and recognize that propofol (Diprivan) can induce deep sedative states and/or general anesthesia. Propofol is NOT pharmacologically reversible.

patient then receives a large bolus of medications and may experience a relative overdose and concurrent side effects.

> Regardless of the technique of administration, clinicians must appreciate the pharmacokinetics, pharmacodynamics, and clinical effects associated with sedative and analgesic agents.

Careful titration is warranted in all situations to prevent the development of deep sedation states, respiratory insufficiency, airway obstruction, hypoxia, and cardiovascular depression. Clinician compliance with hospital policy, manufacturer's recommendations, JCAHO standards, professional practice guidelines, and specialty organization position statements is required to provide quality pharmacologic intervention for patients receiving sedation/analgesia.

SUMMARY

When administered properly, the use of sedatives, analgesics, hypnotics, and tranquilizers provides a sedate patient with minimal side effects. The variety of sedative medications and modes of administration offer the prescribing physician and healthcare provider managing the patient with a wide range of options to achieve the goals and objectives of moderate sedation. Selection of any medication or administration by a particular technique is dependent on the patient's presedation physical status, the presence of pathophysiologic disease states, age, and the planned procedure. Table 4-3 identifies specific advantages and disadvantages associated with various techniques of medication administration.

TABLE 4-3

Techniques of Administration

	Advantages	Disadvantages	
Titration to clinical effect technique	1. Allows careful titration of sedative/analgesic medications. 2. Reduces total medication requirement via synergistic action. 3. Provides for a slow, controlled rise in therapeutic plasma level. 4. May provide for more rapid patient recovery.	1. May be time consuming.	**Oversedation** Therapeutic plasma level Small doses of sedation administered Patient awake
Bolus technique	1. Provides a rapid rise in therapeutic plasma level for short procedures. 2. Provides a sedate/analgesic state rapidly based on predetermined mg/kg dosage.	1. Rapid administration of sedative/analgesic medications may result in excess therapeutic plasma level. 2. Respiratory obstruction, ventilatory depression, respiratory insufficiency, hypotension, bracycardia, and cardiovascular instability frequently occurs with excess plasma levels of medication.	**Oversedation** Therapeutic plasma level Small doses of sedation administered Patient awake
Continuous infusion technique	1. Permits constant plasma level through a continuous infusion of medication. 2. Once a therapeutic plasma level is achieved, continuous infusion technique avoids fluctuations in plasma levels. 3. May decrease recovery time secondary to reduction in total dose of medication administered.	1. Difficult for non-anesthesia practitioners to master technique in nonintubated patients. 2. Initial attempts to reach a therapeutic plasma level may result in oversedation. 3. May be difficult to adjust initial continuous infusion rate based on the patient's level of consciousness.	**Oversedation** Therapeutic plasma level Small doses of sedation administered Patient awake

LEARNER SELF-ASSESSMENT

In order to achieve maximal educational benefit from this chapter, please complete the 'Learner Self-Assessment below. This self-assessment tool provides the learner with the ability to identify areas requiring additional review. Reference material for each question is provided in Appendix F.

1. Healthcare practitioner considerations associated with **JCAHO Standards** related to sedation/analgesic medications and techniques of administration include:

2. **Practice Guidelines for Sedation and Analgesia by Non-Anesthesiologists** promulgated by the ASA Task Force on Sedation **related to sedation/analgesic medications and techniques of administration** include:

3. **Healthcare practitioner considerations associated with the pharmacokinetic, pharmacodynamic and end-organ effects** associated with the following sedation/analgesic medications include:
   a. Benzodiazepines

   b. Opioids

   c. Sedative/hypnotics

   d. Butyrophenones

   e. Barbiturates

   f. Dissociative anesthetics

   g. Local anesthetic solutions

4. The **advantages, disadvantages, and patient care considerations** associated with the following techniques of administration include:
   a. Titration to clinical effect technique

   b. Bolus technique

   c. Continuous-infusion technique

POST-TEST QUESTIONS

Please note: If you are applying for CE credit, you must contact Specialty Health Education, Inc. @ 800-694-8041 for a CE Application Packet.

1. Benzodiazepines bind to specific receptors in the central nervous system and enhance the transmission of _____ in the brain.
   A. Norepinephrine
   B. Gamma-aminobutyric acid (GABA)
   C. Dopamine
   D. Epinephrine

2. Which of the following are NOT pharmacodynamic effects associated with the administration of benzodiazepines? _____
   A. Anxiolysis
   B. Sedation
   C. Hypnosis
   D. Analgesia

3. Which of the following sedative medications possesses a long half-life and "yields" an active metabolite?

   _____
   A. Diazepam (Valium)
   B. Midazolam (Versed)
   C. Morphine
   D. Fentanyl

4. Reversal of pharmacologic effect with benzodiazepines can be achieved with which of the following medications? _____
   A. Naloxone (Narcan)
   B. Flumazenil (Romazicon)
   C. Prochlorperazine (Compazine)
   D. Flumazenine

5. Opioids exert pharmacologic action secondary to their pharmacodynamic effects, which include? _____
   A. Occupation of the GABA receptor
   B. Functional dissociation between the reticular activating system and the thalamus
   C. Occupying the mu, kappa, delta, and sigma receptors
   D. Stimulation of dopamine release

6. Chest wall rigidity can occur with which of the following medications? _____
   A. Morphine
   B. Meperidine (Demerol)
   C. Hydromorphone (Dilaudid)
   D. Fentanyl (Sublimaze)

7. Which narcotic analgesic elicits a tachycardia secondary to its vagolytic properties? _____
   A. Morphine
   B. Meperidine (Demerol)

C. Hydromorphone (Dilaudid)
D. Fentanyl (Sublimaze)

8. Which of the following medications must be used with extreme caution in patients with prolonged Q-T syndrome?
   A. Thiopental (Pentothal)
   B. Propofol (Diprivan)
   C. Fentanyl (Sublimaze)
   D. Droperidol (Inapsine)

9. A derivative of phencyclidine that produces a dissociative state and has been used in subanesthetic doses to produce profound analgesia during sedation procedures is identified as _____?
   A. Droperidol (Inapsine)
   B. Lorazepam
   C. Propofol (Diprivan)
   D. Ketamine

10. The incidence of emergence delirium associated with dissociative anesthetics may be decreased with the administration of which of the following medications? _____
    A. Opioids
    B. Phenothiazines
    C. Benzodiazepines
    D. Barbiturates

11. A 77-year-old man presents to the ambulatory care unit with a history of Parkinson's disease. Which of the following medications is contraindicated? _____
    A. Droperidol (Inapsine)
    B. Fentanyl (Sublimaze)
    C. Midazolam (Versed)
    D. Hydromorphone (Dilaudid)

12. Respiratory depression, hypotension, and hypercarbia are frequent complications associated with which of the following techniques of medication administration? _____
    A. Titration technique
    B. Bolus technique
    C. Continuous infusion technique
    D. Liberal flow technique

REFERENCES

1. Spires G. The Big Mac, Conscious vs. Unconscious Sedation. Early Bird Symposium, 63rd AANA National Meeting, August 1996.
2. Stoelting R. *Pharmacology and Physiology in Anesthetic Practice.* 3rd ed. Philadelphia: Lippincott-Raven; 1999:129.
3. Davidson J, Eckhardt W, Perese D. *Clinical Anesthesia Procedures of the Massachusetts General Hospital.* 4th ed. Boston: Little, Brown; 1993:11.
4. Miller R. *Anesthesia.* 5th ed. Philadelphia: Churchill-Livingstone; 2000(1):231.
5. Ihmsen H, Hering W, Albrecht S, et al. Pharmacokinetics of the new benzodiazepines RO48-6791 and RO48-8684 in comparison with midazolam in young and elderly volunteers. *Anesthesiology.* 1996;85:A317.
6. Hering W, Ihmsen H, Albrecht S, et al. CNS effects of the new benzodiazepines RO48-6791 and RO48-8684 compared to midazolam in young and elderly volunteers. *Anesthesiology.* 1996;85:A189.
7. Miller R. *Anesthesia.* 5th ed. Philadelphia: Churchill-Livingstone; 2000(1):237.
8. Morgan G, Mikhail M, Murray M. *Clinical Anesthesiology.* 3rd ed. New York: Lange Medical Books/McGraw-Hill; 2002:161.
9. Bailey PL, Wilbrink J, Zwanikken P, et al. Anesthetic induction with fentanyl. *Anesth Analg.* 1985;64:48.
10. Gergis SD, Hoyt JL, Sokoll MD. Effects of Innovar and Innovar plus nitrous oxide on muscle tone and "H" reflex. *Anesth Analg.* 1971;50:743.
11. Sokoll MD, Hoyt JL, Gergis SD. Studies in muscle rigidity, nitrous oxide, and narcotic analgesic agents. *Anesth Analg.* 1972;51:1620.
12. Freund FG, Martin WE, Wong KC, et al. Abdominal muscle rigidity induced by morphine and nitrous oxide. *Anesthesiology.* 1973;38:358.
13. Mavrojammis M. L'action cataleptique de la morphine chez les rats: Contribution à la théorie toxique de la catalepsie. *CR Soc Biol (Paris).* 1903;55:1092.
14. Jurna I, Ruzdie N, Nell T, et al. The effect of alpha-methyl-p-tyrosine and substantia nigra lesions on spinal motor activity in the rat. *Eur J Pharmacol.* 1972;20:341.
15. Freye E, Kuschinsky K. Effects of fentanyl and droperidol on the dopamine metabolism of the rat striatum. *Pharmacology.* 1976;14:1.
16. Bronson JB, Weinger B, Weinger M. Opiate-induced muscle rigidity is mediated by mu, and not delta or kappa receptors, in the rat. *Anesthesiology.* 1989;71:A599.
17. Stoelting R, Miller R. *Basics of Anesthesia.* 4th ed. New York: Churchill Livingstone; 2000:60.
18. FDA "black box" warning. December 5, 2001. Available at http://www.fda.gov/bbs/topics/answers/2001/ANSO112.html. Accessed February 9, 2003.
19. Glaser C, Stark J, Brown R, et al. Rectal thiopental sodium for sedation of pediatric patients undergoing MR and other imaging studies. *J Neuroradiol.* 1995;16:111.
20. White P. *Intravenous Anesthesia.* Baltimore: Williams & Wilkins; 1997:176.
21. Barash P, Cullen B, Stoelting R. *Clinical Anesthesia.* 4th ed. Philadelphia: Lippincott Williams & Wilkins; 2001:453.
22. Morgan G, Mikhail M, Murray M. *Clinical Anesthesiology.* 3rd ed. New York: Lange Medical Books/McGraw-Hill; 2002:238.
23. Grauer SE, Giraud GD. Toxic methemoglobinemia after topical anesthesia for transesophageal echocardiography. *J Am Soc Echocardiogr.* 1996;9:874-876.
24. Bernstein BM. Cyanosis following use of anesthesia (ethylaminobenzoate). *Gastroenterology.* 1950;17;123-123.
25. Sandza JG Jr, Roberts RW, Shaw RC, et al. Symptomatic methemoglobinemia with a commonly used topical anesthetic, Cetacaine. *Ann Thorac Surg.* 1980;30:187-190.
26. Gupta P, Deepa L, Edward I, et al. Benzocaine-induced methemoglobinemia. *South Med J.* 2000;93:1.
27. Bunn HF. Disorders of hemoglobin. In Wilson JD, Braunwald E, Isselbacher KJ, et al (eds). *Harrison's Principles of Internal Medicine.* 12th ed. New York: McGraw-Hill; 1991: 1543-1552.
28. Douglas WW, Fairbanks VF. Methemoglobinemia induced by a topical anesthetic spray (Cetacaine). *Chest.* 1977;71:587-591.
29. Scott EM, Hoskins DD. Hereditary methemoglobinemia in Alaskan Eskimos and Indians. *Blood.* 1958;13:795-802.
30. Muchmoree EA, Dahl BJ. One blue man with mucositis (letter). *N Engl J Med.* 1992;327:133.
31. Clary B, Skaryak L, Tedder M, et al. Methemoglobinemia complicating topical anesthesia during bronchoscopic procedures. *J Thorac Cardiovasc Surg.* 1997;114:293-295.

Sedation/Analgesia Pharmacologic Profile

CORE COMPETENCIES

At the completion of this chapter, the learner shall:

◆ Identify the pharmacokinetic profile associated with sedative, analgesic, and hypnotic medications utilized in the sedation setting.

◆ Identify the pharmacodynamic profile associated with sedative, analgesic, and hypnotic medications utilized in the sedation setting.

◆ List medications utilized in the sedation setting that are contraindicated in the presence of specific disease states.

◆ Identify the indications, side effects, and clinical pharmacology associated with sedative, hypnotic, and analgesic medications.

◆ State the cardiovascular, respiratory, and central nervous system effects associated with sedative, hypnotic, and analgesic medications utilized for diagnostic, therapeutic, and minor surgical procedures.

Joint Commission on Accreditation of Healthcare Organizations Standards for Operative or Other High-Risk Procedures and/or the Administration of Moderate or Deep Sedation or Anesthesia

Standard PC.13.20
Operative or other procedures and/or the administration of moderate or deep sedation or anesthesia are planned.

Rationale for PC.13.20
Because the response to procedures is not always predictable and sedation-to-anesthesia is a continuum, it is not always possible to predict how an individual patient will respond. Therefore, qualified individuals are trained in professional standards and techniques to manage patients in the case of a potentially harmful event.

Elements of Performance for PC.13.20
1. Sufficient numbers of qualified staff are available* to evaluate the patient, perform the procedure, monitor, and recover the patient.

2. *Individuals administering moderate or deep sedation and anesthesia are qualified†* *and have the appropriate credentials to manage patients at whatever level of sedation or anesthesia is achieved, either intentionally or unintentionally.*

3. A registered nurse supervises perioperative nursing care.

4. Appropriate equipment to monitor the patient's physiologic status is available.

5. Appropriate equipment to administer intravenous fluids and drugs, including blood and blood components, is available as needed.

6. Resuscitation capabilities are available.

*For hospitals providing obstetric or emergency operative services, this means they can provide anesthesia services as required by law and regulation.

†**Qualified** The individuals providing moderate or deep sedation and anesthesia have at a minimum had competency-based education, training, and experience in the following:

1. Evaluating patients before moderate or deep sedation and anesthesia.

2. Performing the moderate or deep sedation and anesthesia, including rescuing patients who slip into a deeper-than-desired level of sedation or analgesia. This includes the following:

   a. *Moderate* sedation – are qualified to rescue patients from deep sedation and are competent to manage a compromised airway and to provide adequate oxygenation and ventilation.

   b. *Deep* sedation – are qualified to rescue patients from general anesthesia and are competent to manage an unstable cardiovascular system as well as a compromised airway and inadequate oxygenation and ventilation.

© Joint Commission: Standards for Operative or Other High-Risk Procedures and/or the Administration of Moderate or Deep Sedation or Anesthesia, January, 2004. Reprinted with permission.

Practice Guidelines for Sedation and Analgesia by Non-Anesthesiologists
American Society of Anesthesiologists Task Force on Sedation and Analgesia by Non-Anesthesiologists

Recommendations. Individuals responsible for patients receiving sedation/analgesia should understand the pharmacology of the agents that are administered, as well as the role of pharmacologic antagonists for opioids and benzodiazepines. Individuals monitoring patients receiving sedation/analgesia should be able to recognize the associated complications. At least one individual capable of establishing a patent airway and positive-pressure ventilation, as well as a means for summoning additional assistance, should be present whenever sedation/analgesia is administered. It is recommended that an individual with advanced life support skills be immediately available (within 5 minutes) for moderate sedation and within the procedure room for deep sedation.

Recommendations. Combinations of sedatives and analgesics may be administered as appropriate for the procedure being performed and the condition of the patient. Ideally, each component should be administered individually to achieve the desired effect (e.g., additional analgesic medication to relieve pain; additional sedative medication to decrease awareness or anxiety). The propensity for combinations of sedative and analgesic agents to cause respiratory depression and airway obstruction emphasizes the need to appropriately reduce the dose of each component as well as the need to continually monitor respiratory function.

Recommendations. Intravenous sedative/analgesic drugs should be given in small, incremental doses that are titrated to the desired endpoints of analgesia and sedation. Sufficient time must elapse between doses to allow the effect of each dose to be assessed before subsequent drug administration. When drugs are administered by nonintravenous routes (e.g., oral, rectal, intramuscular, transmucosal), allowance should be made for the time required for drug absorption before supplementation is considered. Because absorption may be unpredictable, administration of repeat doses of oral medications to supplement sedation/analgesia is not recommended.

Recommendations. Even if moderate sedation is intended, patients receiving propofol or methohexital by any route should receive care consistent with that required for deep sedation. Accordingly, practitioners administering these drugs should be qualified to rescue patients from any level of sedation, including general anesthesia. Patients receiving ketamine should be cared for in a manner consistent with the level of sedation that is achieved.

Recommendations. Specific antagonists should be available whenever opioid analgesics or benzodiazepines are administered for sedation/analgesia. Naloxone or flumazenil may be administered to improve spontaneous ventilatory efforts in patients who have received opioids or benzodiazepines, respectively. This may be especially helpful in cases where airway control and positive-pressure ventilation are difficult. Before or concomitantly with pharmacologic reversal, patients who become hypoxemic or apneic during sedation/analgesia should: (1) be encouraged or stimulated to breathe deeply; (2) receive supplemental oxygen; and (3) receive positive pressure ventilation if spontaneous ventilation is inadequate. After pharmacologic reversal, patients should be observed long enough to ensure that sedation and cardiorespiratory depression does not recur once the effect of the antagonist dissipates. The use of sedation regimens that include routine reversal of sedative or analgesic agents is discouraged.

From American Society of Anesthesiologists Task Force on Sedation and Analgesia by Non-Anesthesiologists. Practice guidelines for sedation and analgesia by non-anesthesiologists. *Anesthesiology.* 2002;96(4):1009–1012. Reprinted with permission.

Title: Endorsement of Position Statement on the Role of the Registered Nurse (RN) in the Management of Patients Receiving IV Conscious Sedation for Short-Term Therapeutic, Diagnostic, or Surgical Procedures

The registered nurse managing the care of patients receiving IV conscious sedation is able to:

- Anticipate and recognize potential complications of IV conscious sedation in relation to the type of medication being administered.
- Possess the requisite knowledge and skills to assess, diagnose, and intervene in the event of complications or undesired outcomes and to institute nursing interventions in compliance with orders (including standing orders) or institutional protocols or guidelines.
- Demonstrate skill in airway management resuscitation.
- Demonstrate knowledge of the legal ramifications of administering IV conscious sedation and/or monitoring patients receiving IV conscious sedation, including the RN's responsibility and liability in the event of an untoward reaction or life-threatening complication.

Excerpt from Endorsement of Position Statement on the Role of the Registered Nurse (RN) in the Management of Patients Receiving IV Conscious Sedation. Washington, DC, American Nurses Association, 1991.

Healthcare practitioners involved with the administration of sedative, analgesic, and hypnotic medications must follow proper monitoring procedures and clinical assessment strategies. It is critical that every licensed independent practitioner prescribing medications and ultimately each healthcare provider administering or monitoring the patient receiving sedation has a clear, definitive understanding of the pharmacodynamics and pharmacokinetics associated with each medication administered. **A failure to appreciate the clinical effects of each medication administered, particularly when combinations are utilized, may result in an increase in patient morbidity and mortality.**

Before the administration of any medication, it is imperative that each healthcare professional be well versed in the pharmacology of the specific medication. A comprehensive understanding of the clinical pharmacology, onset, duration, indications, contraindications, drug interaction, central nervous system and cardiorespiratory effects, metabolism, excretion, and management of an overdose is essential in providing quality patient care.

A detailed summary of the following medications is presented for the sedation provider:

SEDATIVE, ANALGESIC, HYPNOTIC MEDICATIONS
Opioid Agonists

- Alfentanil hydrochloride (Alfenta)
- Meperidine hydrochloride (Demerol)
- Hydromorphone hydrochloride (Dilaudid)
- Morphine sulfate
- Fentanyl citrate (Sublimaze)

Benzodiazepine Agonists

- Diazepam (Valium)
- Midazolam (Versed)

Barbiturates

- Methohexital sodium (Brevital)*
- Thiopental sodium (Pentothal)*

Butyrophenone

- Droperidol (Inapsine)

Hypnotic

◆ Propofol (Diprivan)*

Dissociative Anesthetic

◆ Ketamine hydrochloride*

RESUSCITATIVE MEDICATIONS
Opiate Receptor Antagonist

◆ Naloxone hydrochloride (Narcan)

Benzodiazepine Receptor Antagonist

◆ Flumazenil (Romazicon)

Cardiovascular Stimulants/Antidysrhythmics

◆ Atropine sulfate
◆ Ephedrine
◆ Epinephrine (Adrenalin)
◆ Lidocaine hydrochloride (Xylocaine)

The prescribing clinician and healthcare provider administering the medication (or monitoring the patient) should possess advanced airway management skills, demonstrate proficiency in managing cardiovascular complications, and recognize that each medication can induce deep sedative states and/or general anesthesia. The medications indicated with an asterisk in the previous list are NOT pharmacologically reversible.

Sedation/analgesia is an ever-changing field. The medications listed here are provided as a guide for the sedation clinician. A variety of dosing protocols have been proposed in the literature and are outlined in Tables 5-1 through 5-3. A schedule of controlled substances is featured in Box 5-1 on p. 107. Licensed independent practitioners are advised to check the product information currently provided by the manufacturer of each drug to be administered to verify the recommended dose associated with the specific procedure, patient physiologic status, and level of sedation desired. It is the responsibility of the treating physician relying on experience and knowledge of the patient to determine dosages and the best treatment for the patient. Neither the publisher nor the author assumes any responsibility for any injury and/or damage to persons or property.

---

*It is the author's opinion that these medications should be administered only by anesthesia providers (physician anesthesiologists or certified registered nurse anesthetists), unless extensive didactic and clinical education is completed. Licensed independent clinicians and healthcare professionals who are non-anesthesia providers should not under any circumstance administer these drugs unless they have received comprehensive education and are credentialed appropriately. If these medications are utilized by non-anesthesia providers, it is imperative to assure that the prescribing clinician understands the pharmacokinetics and pharmacodynamics associated with each agent.

Alfentanil Hydrochloride (ALFENTA) (OPIOID AGONIST)	
Schedule:	Alfentanil is subject to Schedule II control under the Controlled Substances Act of 1970.
Clinical Pharmacology:	Alfentanil is an opioid analgesic with rapid onset of action. Alfentanil is one fifth to one tenth as potent as fentanyl and has one third the duration of action of fentanyl. Lower doses provide analgesia whereas higher doses promote hypnosis and attenuate the catecholamine response. Opioids bind to opiate receptors located throughout the CNS. Opioid receptors that have been identified include mu, kappa, delta, and sigma. The pharmacodynamic properties of each opioid are dependent on which specific opioid receptor is occupied.
Onset:	IV = immediate, produces analgesia in 1 minute
Peak Effect:	IV = 1 to 2 minutes
Duration:	IV = 5 to 15 minutes
Indications:	For use as an adjunct in the maintenance of anesthesia, for continuous infusion, as a primary anesthetic agent, and as the analgesic component for monitored anesthesia care.
Contraindications:	Known hypersensitivity to alfentanil, depressed ventilatory function, increased intracranial pressure.
Protein Binding:	92%
Half-Life:	90 to 111 minutes
Considerations:	Individualize dose. Titrate medication to effect. Reduce dosage (30%-50%) in elderly and debilitated patients. Calculate drug dose based on lean body weight in obese patients (more than 20% above ideal body weight). Alfentanil crosses placental barrier and is excreted in breast milk.
Drug Interactions:	Pronounced synergism and respiratory depression occurs when used in conjunction with CNS depressants (barbiturates, benzodiazepines, sedatives, hypnotics).
Respiratory Effects:	Apnea, respiratory depression, hypoxia, bronchospasm as well as diminished respiratory reserve. Extreme caution must be utilized in patients with pulmonary disease, decreased respiratory reserve, or compromised respiratory status. Dose-related muscle rigidity (particularly truncal rigidity) may occur. Facilities must be fully equipped to monitor and treat respiratory depression. Respiratory depressant effects outlast analgesic effects.

Continued on p. 104.

TABLE 5-1

Sedation Dosing Protocols (Sample 1)

AGENT	SUGGESTED DOSING	ONSET AND DURATION	CLINICAL CONSIDERATIONS
Analgesics Morphine sulfate	1-mg increments; peak clinical effects not apparent for up to 20 min	*Onset:* 5-10 min, peak CNS effect delayed up to 20 min *Duration:* 2-4 hr	*Respiratory:* potent respiratory depressant in presence of other sedatives; in absence of pain may produce excessive sedation and dysphoria; respiratory monitoring (pulse oximetry, respiratory rate and depth) essential *Cardiovascular:* hypotension may follow administration to hypovolemic patient *Gastrointestinal:* nausea and vomiting; excessive sedation may lead to aspiration *Genitourinary:* urinary retention
Meperidine (Demerol) 1/10 as potent as morphine (8-10 mg equivalent to 1 mg morphine)	Dilute and titrate 5- to 10-mg increments, evaluating patient response within onset time	*Onset:* 3-5 min *Duration:* 1-3 hr	In equal analgesic doses produces same sedation, respiratory depression, and incidence of nausea and vomiting as morphine
Fentanyl (Sublimaze) 100 times more potent than morphine	50 µg/mL; titrate 0.5 to 1 mL (25-50 µg) to patient response	*Onset analgesia:* 3-5 min *Duration analgesia:* 30-60 min period of respiratory depression longer than analgesic duration (3.5 hr) *Onset sedation:* 103 min dependent on concomitant drug administration *Duration sedation:* highly variable but generally 15-90 min	*Respiratory:* potent respiratory depressant alone and when combined with benzodiazepines; skeletal muscle (chest wall) rigidity with rapid administration; rigidity may be so pronounced that ventilation is difficult or impossible *Cardiovascular:* vagotonic producing bradycardia; hypotension in hypovolemic patient
Benzodiazepines Diazepam (Valium)	Titrated in 2-mg increments; large interpatient variability in response to titrated doses	*Onset:* 1-2 min *Duration:* in hours equal to the patient age (20-yr old = 20 hr; 70-yr old = 70 hr)	*Respiratory:* minimal respiratory depression unless large doses or concomitant opioid administration *Cardiovascular:* minimal depressant effects, although the occasional patient may experience hypotension *Other:* Pain on injection may cause phlebitis, local irritation, and venous thrombosis

Continued

TABLE 5-1

Sedation Dosing Protocols—cont'd

AGENT	SUGGESTED DOSING	ONSET AND DURATION	CLINICAL CONSIDERATIONS
Midazolam (Versed) Four times as potent as Diazepam	Titrate 0.5- to 1-mg doses and never exceed 2.5 mg; most rapid-acting benzodiazepine; allow a minimum of 2 min between doses to assess patient effect; like diazepam, large interpatient variability to titrated doses; following established sedation, decrease subsequent doses 20-40%	*Onset:* 3-5 min *Duration:* 1-5 hr in healthy patient; duration doubled in elderly and obese patients	*Respiratory:* central respiratory depressant and may produce apnea with rapid administration; effects are pronounced with concomitant opioid administration; observant respiratory monitoring critical to avert potential problems *Cardiovascular:* hypotension in hypovolemic patient; incidence of hypotension increased with concomitant opioid administration
Antagonist Agents Naloxone (Narcan)	0.1-mg increments titrated to obtain respiratory rate of 12 breaths per minute	*Onset:* 1-2 min *Duration:* 30-45 min; opioid may outlast expected opioid duration; repeat doses are often necessary	Opioid antagonist; titrate to achieve an acceptable respiratory rate; continued evaluation of respiratory function essential; will reverse previously established analgesia following painful procedure
Flumazenil (Romazicon)	0.2 mg administered over 10-15 sec; additional 0.2 mg after 45 sec, repeating at 60-sec intervals up to 1 mg; no more than 3 mg is recommended in any 1-hr period	*Onset:* 1-2 min *Duration:* 30-60 min	Specific benzodiazepine antagonist; titrated to reverse respiratory depression and sedation; duration of benzodiazepines exceed duration of flumazenil; continued ventilatory assessment required

From Biddle C, Aker J. Conscious sedation: Between Scylla and Charybdis. *Quality of Life: A Nursing Challenge.* 1995;4(4):107.

Alfentanil Hydrochloride *cont'd*

CV Effects: Dysrhythmias, bradycardia, tachycardia, hypotension. Bradycardia may be treated with atropine. Use with caution in patients with bradyarrhythmias.

CNS Effects: The magnitude and duration of CNS effects is enhanced when alfentanil is used with other CNS depressant drugs. Dosages of alfentanil and other CNS depressant drugs should be reduced when used in combination. Caution should be exercised in patients with increased intracranial pressure or head injury. Increased intracranial pressure is associated with the development of hypercapnia and the respiratory depressant effects associated with opioid use. Additional neurologic effects include confusion or euphoria.

Metabolism: Alfentanil is metabolized to inactive metabolites via hepatic mechanisms. Erythromycin can inhibit alfentanil metabolism.

Elimination: Excretion via urine.

Overdose: Signs and symptoms of narcotic overdose include decreased respiratory rate and volume, extreme somnolence, cold clammy skin, bradycardia, and hypotension. In the event of an overdose, maintenance of a patent airway coupled with cardiac and respiratory support is required. Ventilation and oxygenation must be maintained until the respiratory depressant effects have dissipated.

Narcan (naloxone), a narcotic antagonist, will reverse the respiratory and cardiovascular depressant

TABLE 5-2

Sedation Dosing Protocols (Sample 2)

MEDICATION	SIDE EFFECTS	ROUTE	TOTAL DOSE*	ONSET	DURATION
Barbiturates					
Methohexital	Respiratory depression, hypotension	IV PR	0.75-1 mg/kg 20-30 mg/kg	45 sec 8-10 min	5-10 min 45-60 min
Pentobarbital	Respiratory depression, hypotension	IV IM PO/PR	2.5 mg/kg 2.5 mg/kg 2-6 mg/kg	45 sec 10-15 min 15-60 min	15 min NA 1-4 hr
Benzodiazepines					
Midazolam	Respiratory depression	IV IM PO PR Nasal	0.02-0.1 mg/kg 0.05-0.15 mg/kg 0.5-0.75 mg/kg 0.7-1 mg/kg 0.2-0.4 mg/kg	2-3 min 2-5 min 15-20 min 10-15 min 10-15 min	30 min 30-40 min 45-60 min 45 min 45 min
Opioids					
Fentanyl	Respiratory depression	IV	2 µg/kg	1-2 min	20-30 min
Morphine	Respiratory depression, hypotension, nausea and vomiting	IV IM/SQ	0.1-0.2 mg/kg 0.1-0.2 mg/kg	1-5 min 30 min	3-4 hr 4-5 hr
Other Sedative Agents					
Chloral hydrate	Prolonged sedation	PO/PR	50-75 mg/kg	30-60 min	1-8 hr
Ketamine	Postemergence delirium	IV IM PO PR Nasal	0.5-1 mg/kg 4 mg/kg 5-10 mg/kg 5-10 mg/kg 3-6 mg/kg	1 min 5 min 30-40 min 5-10 min 5-10 min	15 min 15-30 min 2-4 hr 15-30 min 15-30 min
Propofol	Respiratory depression, hypotension	IV IV bolus	0.05-0.1 mg/kg/min 1 mg/kg	30 sec 30 sec	8-10 min
Reversal Agents					
Flumazenil	Withdrawal symptoms (agitation)	IV	0.2 mg 0.01 mg/kg (pediatrics)	1-3 min	30-45 min
Naloxone	Withdrawal symptoms (agitation)	IV/IM/SQ	0.1-0.2 mg	1-2 min (IV)	15-45 min

IM, Intramuscular; *IV,* intravenous; *NA,* not available; *PO,* oral; *PR,* rectal; *SQ,* subcutaneous.
*Doses should be administered in fractional boluses (e.g., one fourth to one half) and titrated to effect.
From Spitalnic S, Blazes C, Anderson A. Conscious sedation: A primer for outpatient procedures. *Hosp Phys.* 2000(May):25.

effects associated with alfentanil overdose. Naloxone may also reverse additional side effects associated with narcotic administration. These side effects include urinary retention, pruritus, respiratory depression, nausea, and vomiting. Careful titration is required to avoid full reversal of analgesia.

Patients treated with naloxone must remain adequately monitored and reassessed post sedation for a minimum of 120 minutes to avoid the development of re-narcotization and respiratory depression.

Dosage: 3 to 8 µg/kg based on lean body weight titrated in 12-µg increments. Dosage should be individualized and reduced in the elderly, debilitated, patient with renal/hepatic disease, or patient with hypothyroidism. Titration to individual patient response is required. If utilized for sedation/analgesia, slow IV injection is required.

Supplied: 500 µg/mL

| TABLE 5-3 |

Sedation Dosing Protocols (Sample 3)

DRUG	ONSET OF ACTION	USUAL DOSAGE	DURATION
Benzodiazepines			
Midazolam	1-5 min	0.5-2.0 mg IV over 2 min; may repeat at 5-min intervals with 0.5 mg to a maximum of 5 mg	60-90 min
Diazepam	3-10 min IV 15-30 min PO	2-5 mg IV over 5 min; may repeat at 5-min intervals with 2 mg to a maximum of 10 mg	2-8 hr
Lorazepam	5-10 min	0.5-2.0 mg IV slow to a maximum of 4 mg	4-6 hr
Opioids			
Morphine	2-5 min	2-5 mg IV over 5 min; may repeat at 5-min intervals in increments of 2-5 mg to a maximum of 20 mg	2-7 hr
Meperidine	1-3 min	25-50 mg IV over 2 min; may repeat at 5-min intervals in increments of 10-15 mg to a maximum of 150 mg (use with caution in patients with renal disease)	2-4 hr
Fentanyl	1-2 min	25-50 μg IV over 2 min; may repeat at 5-min intervals in increments of 25 μg to a maximum of 500 μg/4 hr	30-60 min
Reversal Agents			
Flumazenil (for benzodiazepines)	1-2 min	0.2 mg IV over 15 sec; may repeat in 1-min intervals to a maximum of 1 mg	1-2 hr
Naloxone (for opioids)	1-2 min	0.02-0.04 mg IV over 30 sec; may repeat at 1-min intervals to a maximum of 10 mg (dilute 0.4 mg naloxone in 10 mL to make 0.04 mg/mL)	1-4 hr

From Messinger J, Hoffman L, O'Donnell J, Dunworth B. Getting conscious sedation right. *Am J Nurs.* 1999;99(12):47.

Meperidine Hydrochloride (DEMEROL)
(OPIOID AGONIST)

Schedule: Meperidine is subject to Schedule II control under the Controlled Substances Act of 1970.

Clinical Pharmacology: Meperidine is a synthetic opioid analgesic similar to morphine sulfate but less potent. Meperidine is one tenth as potent as morphine (8 to 10 mg equivalent to 1 mg morphine). Its principal therapeutic actions are analgesia and sedation. Pain threshold is elevated, and the CNS is depressed. Meperidine may cause less spasm of smooth muscle, constipation, and suppression of the cough reflex than morphine. Opioids bind to opioid receptors located throughout the CNS. Opioid receptors that have been identified include mu, kappa, and delta. The pharmacodynamic properties of each opioid are dependent on which specific opioid receptor is occupied.

Onset: IV = 1 to 5 minutes; IM = 10 to 15 minutes; PO = 15 to 45 minutes

Peak: IV = 5 to 7 minutes; IM = 30 to 50 minutes; PO = 60 to 90 minutes

Duration: 2 to 4 hours

Indications: Meperidine is indicated for the short-term relief of moderate to severe pain.

Contraindications: Known hypersensitivity to meperidine, depressed ventilatory function, acute asthma, increased intracranial pressure. It has been reported that patients receiving monoamine oxidase (MAO) inhibitors have had fatal reactions when treated with meperidine, although the exact mechanism is unclear. Reactions include severe respiratory depression, cyanosis, hypotension, hyperexcitability, convulsions, tachycardia, and hypertension. When narcotics are required in this patient population, meperidine is contraindicated. Monitoring and follow-up is required if narcotics are utilized in the presence of MAO inhibitors.

Protein Binding: 60% to 80%

BOX 5-1

Schedule of Controlled Substances

Drugs that come under the jurisdiction of the Controlled Substances Act are divided into five schedules. Adherence to Federal and State guidelines regarding administration, dispensing, distribution, and accountability is imperative. Copies of the Controlled Substances Act may be obtained from the Superintendent of Documents, U.S. Government Printing Office, Washington, D.C. 20402.

Schedule I
The substances in this schedule are those that have no accepted medical use in the United States but have a high abuse potential. Some examples are heroin, LSD, peyote, and methaqualone.

Schedule II
The substances in this schedule have a high abuse potential with severe psychic or physical dependence. Schedule II substances consist of specific narcotics, stimulants, and depressant medications. Examples include opium, morphine, codeine, fentanyl, sufentanil, hydromorphone, meperidine, and oxycodone. Additional Schedule II medications are amphetamines, methylphenidate (Ritalin), pentobarbital, and secobarbital.

Schedule III
Schedule III substances have an abuse potential less than those in Schedules I and II and include compounds containing limited quantities of certain narcotic and non-narcotic medications. Examples of Schedule III drugs include derivatives of barbituric acid (except those identified in earlier schedules), phentermine, paregoric, and any compound, mixture, preparation or suppository dosage form containing amobarbital, secobarbital, or pentobarbital.

Schedule IV
The substances in this schedule have an abuse potential less than those listed in Schedules I, II, and III. Examples of Schedule IV medications include chloral hydrate, meprobamate, paraldehyde, methohexital, diazepam, midazolam, lorazepam, and pentazocine.

Schedule V
The substances in this schedule have an abuse potential less than those listed in Schedules I, II, III, and IV. These substances consist primarily of medications containing limited quantities of narcotics and stimulant drugs utilized for their antitussive, antidiarrheal, and analgesic effects. Examples include buprenorphine and propylhexedrine.

Half-Life:	3 to 5 hours
Considerations:	The administration of intravenous meperidine must be titrated to effect and injected slowly. Rapid injection increases the incidence of adverse reactions, which include severe respiratory depression, apnea, hypotension, circulatory collapse, and cardiac arrest. Pharmacologic breakdown results in a toxic metabolite (normeperidine); therefore, long-term use is not recommended in the elderly.
Drug Interactions:	Dry mouth, constipation, spasm of the sphincter of Oddi (biliary spasm), flushing, urinary retention, pruritus, urticaria, rash, skin wheals, local irritation at the injection site, and antidiuretic effect. Drug effects are potentiated by antacids, anticholinergics, cimetidine, tricyclic antidepressants, oral contraceptives, phenothiazines, and CNS depressant medications.
Respiratory Effects:	Severe respiratory depression and arrest may occur with the IV administration of meperidine. Extreme caution should be exercised in patients with asthma, chronic obstructive pulmonary disease, cor pulmonale, decreased respiratory reserve, hypoxia, or hypercapnia. Facilities must be fully equipped to monitor and treat respiratory depression.
CV Effects:	Tachycardia, bradycardia, shock, cardiac arrest, palpitations, syncope, orthostatic hypotension. Hypotension may be severe in hypovolemic, critically ill patients.
CNS Effects:	Euphoria, dysphoria, weakness, headache, sedation, convulsions, agitation, tremor, uncoordinated muscle movements, transient hallucinations, disorientation, and visual disturbances. Extreme caution should be exercised with utilization of any narcotic in patients with increased intracranial pressure or head injury. Increased intracranial pressure is associated with the development of hypercapnia and the respiratory depressant effects of opioids.
Metabolism:	Meperidine undergoes extensive metabolism in the liver to normeperidine. Normeperidine's extended half-life of 15 to 30 hours may lead to cumulative effects.
Excretion:	Urinary excretion is pH dependent. Meperidine is secreted in breast milk.
Overdose:	Signs and symptoms of overdose include decreased respiratory rate and volume, extreme somnolence, cold clammy skin, bradycardia, and hypotension. In the event of an overdose, maintenance of a patent airway coupled with cardiac and respiratory support is required. Ventilation and oxygenation must be maintained until the respiratory depressant effects have dissipated.
Reversal:	Narcan (naloxone), an opioid receptor antagonist will reverse the respiratory and cardiovascular depressant effects associated with meperidine overdose. Naloxone may also reverse additional side effects associated with opioid administration. These side effects include urinary retention, pruritus, respiratory depression, nausea, and vomiting.

Careful titration is required to avoid full reversal of analgesia.

Patients treated with naloxone must remain adequately monitored and reassessed post sedation for a minimum of 120 minutes to avoid the development of re-narcotization and respiratory depression.

Dosage: Should be individualized and reduced in the elderly, debilitated, patient with renal/hepatic disease, or patient with hypothyroidism. Titration to individual patient response is required. If utilized intravenously for sedation/analgesia, slow IV injection is required.

IV: 0.25 to 1 mg/kg slowly in 5- to 10-mg increments titrated to patient effect.

Supplied: Ampules = 50 mg/mL, 100 mg/mL; vials = 50 mg/mL, 100 mg/mL; Carpojects and Tubex dispensers also available.

Hydromorphone Hydrochloride (DILAUDID)
(OPIOID AGONIST)

Schedule: Hydromorphone is subject to Schedule II control under the Controlled Substances Act of 1970.

Clinical Pharmacology: Hydromorphone is a semisynthetic opioid agonist (derivative of morphine). It is six times as potent as morphine with a shorter duration of action and a more rapid onset. It produces potent analgesia, more sedation, and less euphoria than morphine.

Onset: IV = 1 minute

Peak: IV = 15 to 30 minutes

Duration: IV = 2 to 3 hours

Indications: Analgesic agonist for the relief of moderate to severe pain.

Contraindications: Known hypersensitivity to hydromorphone; patients who are not already receiving increased doses of parenteral narcotics and patients with increased intracranial pressure, depressed ventilatory function, or acute asthma.

Protein Binding: Less than 30%

Half-Life: 2 to 3 hours

Considerations: Respiratory depression is dose related. Hydromorphone must be given slowly when utilized for IV administration (over 3 minutes). Rapid administration of hydromorphone increases narcotic-related side effects.

Drug Interactions: Hypotension, bradycardia, urinary retention, dysphoria, constipation, nausea, pruritus, and urticaria. Patients taking other CNS depressants may have synergistic effects when hydromorphone is utilized. Decreased doses of hydromorphone are required when utilized in the presence of other CNS depressant drugs.

Respiratory Effects: Respiratory depression and decreased respiratory rate and tidal volume with resultant cyanosis and hypoxemia. Facilities must be fully equipped to monitor and treat respiratory depression.

CV Effects: Orthostatic hypotension, syncope, circulatory depression, bradycardia, hypotension.

CNS Effects: Sedation, drowsiness, lethargy, mental/physical impairment, anxiety, fear, dysphoria, dizziness, mood alterations, psychological dependence.

Metabolism: Conjugation in the liver.

Excretion: Excreted as glucuronidated conjugate via the kidney. Hydromorphone may be excreted in breast milk.

Overdose: Narcan (naloxone), a narcotic antagonist, will reverse the respiratory and cardiovascular depressant effects associated with hydromorphone overdose. Naloxone may also reverse additional side effects associated with narcotic administration. These side effects include urinary retention, pruritus, respiratory depression, nausea, and vomiting. Careful titration is required to avoid full reversal of analgesia.

Patients treated with naloxone must remain adequately monitored and reassessed post sedation for a minimum of 120 minutes to avoid the development of re-narcotization and respiratory depression.

Dosage: Slow IV administration 0.5-mg increments titrated to patient response. Should be individualized and reduced (30%-50%) in the elderly or debilitated, in the presence of renal/hepatic disease, or in patients with hypothyroidism. Titration to individual patient response is required.

Supplied: Injection: 1 mg/mL, 2 mg/mL, 3 mg/mL, 4 mg/mL

Morphine Sulfate
(OPIOID AGONIST)

Schedule: Morphine sulfate is subject to Schedule II control under the Controlled Substances Act of 1970.

Clinical Pharmacology: Morphine is an alkaloid derivative of opium that produces analgesia, sedation, euphoria, and dose-related respiratory depression. Hypotension and decreased systemic vascular resistance is related to the degree of histamine release.

Nausea and vomiting associated with morphine sulfate administration is associated with stimulation of the chemoreceptor trigger zone. Morphine induces sleep and inhibits perception of pain by binding to opiate receptors, decreasing sodium permeability, and inhibiting transmission of pain impulses. Opioids bind to opiate receptors located throughout the CNS. Opioid receptors that have been identified include mu, kappa, and delta. The pharmacodynamic profile of each opioid is dependent on which specific opioid receptor is occupied.

Onset: IM = 10 to 30 minutes; IV = 5 to 10 minutes; CNS effect delayed up to 20 minutes.

Peak: IM = 30 to 60 minutes; IV = 20 minutes

Duration: IM = 4 to 5 hours; IV = 4 to 5 hours

Indications: Morphine is a systemic opioid receptor agonist that may be administered through a variety of routes, which include oral, intramuscular, and intravenous. Morphine may be utilized as a narcotic analgesic for the relief to moderate to severe pain. It is the analgesic of choice associated with myocardial infarction. It is used to treat acute pulmonary edema associated with left ventricular failure.

Contraindications: Known hypersensitivity to morphine or natural opioids, bronchial asthma, decreased respiratory reserve, and increased intracranial pressure.

Protein Binding: 33%

Half-Life: 2 to 4 hours

Considerations: As with all opioid adjuncts, individualized dosing is required with titration to patient effect.

Drug Interactions: Histamine release (urticaria, skin wheals, local tissue irritation), constipation, headache, anxiety, depression, convulsions, bradycardia, dysphoria, pruritus, nausea, vomiting, urinary retention, and biliary colic as well as interference with thermal regulation.

Respiratory Effects: Caution must be utilized in patients with decreased respiratory reserve and increased intracranial pressure. Acute respiratory failure and bronchospasm may occur in patients with chronic obstructive pulmonary disease, acute asthma, or signs of respiratory embarrassment. The degree of bronchoconstriction is dependent on the magnitude of histamine release associated with the administration of morphine sulfate. Facilities must be fully equipped to monitor and treat respiratory depression.

CV Effects: Hypotension, bradycardia, and chest wall rigidity. Extreme caution must be exercised in patients with decreased circulating blood volume or impaired myocardial function. Hypotension may occur after IV injection secondary to histamine-mediated vasodilation.

CNS Effects: Euphoria, somnolence. The utilization of CNS depressant drugs, sedatives, and hypnotics potentiates morphine sulfate's CNS depressant effects.

Metabolism: The principal site of metabolism is the liver.

Excretion: Ninety percent of urinary excretion occurs within 24 hours, and 7% to 10% of morphine is excreted in the feces.

Overdose: Signs and symptoms of opioid overdose include decreased respiratory rate and volume, extreme somnolence, cold clammy skin, bradycardia, and hypotension. In the event of an overdose, maintenance of a patent airway coupled with cardiac and respiratory support is required. Ventilation and oxygenation must be maintained until the respiratory depressant effects have dissipated.

Narcan (naloxone), an opioid antagonist, will reverse the respiratory and cardiovascular depressant effects associated with morphine overdose. Naloxone may also reverse additional side effects associated with narcotic administration. These side effects include urinary retention, pruritus, respiratory depression, nausea, and vomiting. Careful titration is required to avoid full reversal of analgesia.

Patients treated with naloxone must remain adequately monitored and reassessed post sedation for a minimum of 120 minutes to avoid the development of re-narcotization and respiratory depression.

Dosage: 0.03 to 0.1 mg/kg in 1-mg increments titrated to patient response. Dosage should be individualized and reduced in the elderly, debilitated, patients with hypothyroidism, or those with renal/hepatic disease.

Supplied: Injection: = 1 mg/mL; 2 mg/mL; 4 mg/mL; 8 mg/mL; 20 mg/mL; 15 mg/mL

Fentanyl Citrate (SUBLIMAZE)
(OPIOID AGONIST)

Schedule: Fentanyl is subject to Schedule II control under the Controlled Substances Act of 1970.

Clinical Pharmacology: Fentanyl is a phenylpiperidine derivative that is a potent opioid agonist and descending CNS depressant. The analgesic activity of 100 μg (2 mL) of fentanyl is equivalent to 10 mg of morphine or 75 mg of meperidine. It is 75 to 125 times more potent than morphine milligram for milligram. It has a rapid onset and relatively short duration of action. Its use is associated with little hypnotic activity, and histamine release rarely occurs. Opioids bind to opiate receptors located throughout the CNS. Opioid receptors that have been identified include mu, kappa, delta, and sigma. The pharmacodynamic properties of each opioid are dependent on which specific opioid receptor is occupied. Fentanyl's principle actions are analgesia and sedation.

Onset: IV = 3 to 5 minutes; transmucosal = 5 to 15 minutes

Peak Effect: IV = 5 to 15 minutes; transmucosal = 1 to 2 hours

Duration: IV = 30 to 60 minutes; transmucosal: 1 to 2 hours

Indications: Analgesic action of short duration during anesthetic periods, premedication, induction, and maintenance of anesthesia. Fentanyl is a narcotic analgesic supplement in general or regional anesthesia. It is useful in short-duration minor surgery in outpatients and in diagnostic procedures or treatments that require the patient to be awake or lightly sedated.

Contraindications: Known hypersensitivity to fentanyl. Depressed ventilatory function, presence of airway obstruction, acute or severe bronchial asthma, increased intracranial pressure. Fentanyl is contraindicated in patients taking monoamine oxidase inhibitors.

Protein Binding: 80% protein bound

Half-Life: 1.5 to 6 hours

Considerations: Titration to effect is required. Dosage reduction and extreme caution must be utilized when administering to elderly or debilitated patients and patients susceptible to respiratory depression. When administered in large doses or injected rapidly, chest wall rigidity may result in inability to ventilate the patient. Chest wall rigidity may be treated with narcotic antagonist, paralysis by muscle relaxant, and positive pressure ventilation.

Drug Interactions: Circulatory and respiratory depression. Profound synergism occurs when utilized with sedatives and CNS depressants. Concurrent use with diazepam (Valium) with higher doses of fentanyl may produce vasodilation and prolonged hypotension and result in delayed recovery.

Respiratory Effects: Duration of respiratory depression may last longer than analgesic effects. As the dose of narcotic is increased, the degree of pulmonary exchange is decreased. Apnea, respiratory depression, and chest wall rigidity may occur. Extreme caution must be exercised when administering to patients with chronic obstructive pulmonary disease, decreased respiratory reserve, and compromised respiratory status. Facilities must be fully equipped to monitor and treat respiratory depression. In healthy individuals, respiratory rate returns to normal more quickly than with other opiates.

CV Effects: Vagally mediated bradycardia, shock, cardiac arrest, palpitations, syncope, hypotension.

CNS Effects: Euphoria, dysphoria, weakness, sedation, agitation, tremor. Extreme caution should be exercised with patients with intracranial hypertension. Addition of CNS depressant drugs produces a synergistic effect and potentiates the effects of CNS depressant drugs.

Metabolism: Hepatic biotransformation

Elimination: Renal excretion. Caution should be exercised in elderly patients owing to decreased clearance rates and those with liver and kidney disease. Fentanyl is excreted in breast milk.

Overdose: Signs and symptoms of narcotic overdose include decreased respiratory rate and volume, extreme somnolence, cold clammy skin, bradycardia, and hypotension. In the event of an overdose, maintenance of a patent airway coupled with cardiac and respiratory support is required. Ventilation and oxygenation must be maintained until the respiratory depressant effects have dissipated.

Narcan (naloxone), a narcotic antagonist, will reverse the respiratory and cardiovascular depressant effects associated with fentanyl overdose. Naloxone may also reverse additional side effects associated with narcotic administration. These side effects include urinary retention, pruritus, respiratory depression, nausea, and vomiting. Careful titration is required to avoid full reversal of analgesia.

Patients treated with naloxone must remain adequately monitored and reassessed post sedation for a minimum of 120 minutes to avoid the development of re-narcotization and respiratory depression.

Dosage: 0.5 to 2 μg/kg or 25 to 100 μg titrated in 25-μg increments to patient response. Dosage should be individualized and reduced in the elderly or debilitated, patients with renal/hepatic disease, or patients with hypothyroidism. Titration to individual patient response is required. If utilized for sedation/analgesia, slow IV (over 3 to 5 minutes) injection is required.

Supplied: 50 μg/mL

Diazepam (VALIUM)
(BENZODIAZEPINE AGONIST, SEDATIVE-HYPNOTIC, ANXIOLYTIC, ANTICONVULSANT, AMNESTIC)

Schedule: Diazepam is subject to Schedule IV control under the Controlled Substances Act of 1970.

Clinical Pharmacology: Diazepam is a benzodiazepine that depresses the central, autonomic, and peripheral nervous systems to produce amnesia, anxiolysis, muscle relaxation, and a calming effect. The pharmacologic effects of benzodiazepines are primarily exerted via facilitated action of the inhibitory neurotransmitter gamma-aminobutyric acid (GABA). This GABA interaction enhances the inhibitory effects of various neurotransmitters. Benzodiazepines affect the limbic system, thalamus, and hypothalamus, producing a calm, sedate state. The effects of diazepam on the CNS are based on:

- ◆ Dose administered
- ◆ Route of administration
- ◆ Presence of other premedicants
- ◆ Concurrent medications administered (opioids)

Diazepam is the benzodiazepine to which all other benzodiazepines are compared. It possesses a long half-life, active metabolites, and a propylene glycol suspension that causes pain on injection.

Onset: IV = 2 to 5 minutes; PO = 30-90 min

Peak: IV = 3 to 5 minutes

Duration: IV = 15 to 60 minutes; PO = 3 to 8 hours

Indications: Anxiety, acute alcohol withdrawal, skeletal muscle spasm, sedation, sedation/analgesia procedures, preoperative sedation, status epilepticus, severe recurrent seizures.

Contraindications: Known hypersensitivity to diazepam. Avoid in patients with acute narrow-angle glaucoma, untreated open-angle glaucoma, shock, coma, and acute alcohol intoxication and in children younger than 6 months of age.

Protein Binding: 98%

Half-Life: 30 to 50 hours or equal to the patient's age in hours (20-year old = 20 hours, 70-year old = 70 hours)

Considerations: When utilized intravenously, diazepam must be injected slowly. A large vein must be used to prevent venous irritation and possible thrombophlebitis. Utilization of hand and wrist veins may result in increased incidence of venous irritation. Extreme caution must be utilized to avoid extravasation or intra-arterial administration. Hypoalbuminemia may increase the incidence of side effects. A new formulation as a lipid emulsion has decreased the incidence of pain on injection.

Drug Interactions: Drug effect is accentuated (synergism) by concomitant use of sedatives, hypnotics, or narcotic analgesics. Drug dosage should be decreased based on the type, amount, and time adjunct medications are administered.

Complications associated with IV diazepam include venous thrombosis, phlebitis, local irritation, swelling, and vascular impairment. It is recommended not to mix or dilute the medication once it is withdrawn into the syringe.

Respiratory Effects: Intravenous diazepam may cause respiratory depression and apnea. Respiratory depression is generally minimal unless large doses were used or there was concomitant opioid administration. Extreme caution should be used in patients with decreased respiratory reserve. Coughing and laryngospasm have been reported with the administration of diazepam during endoscopic procedures.

CV Effects: Decreased systemic vascular resistance and cardiac output. Vagotonic action may lead to bradycardia and hypotension particularly in hypovolemic and debilitated patients. Extreme caution should be utilized in critically ill or hypovolemic patients.

CNS Effects: Drowsiness, confusion, depression, dysarthria, headache, hypoactivity, slurred speech, syncope, vertigo, tremor, ataxia, restlessness, anterograde amnesia, venous irritation, blurred vision, diplopia, rash, urticaria, and hiccoughs. Diazepam may also cause increased CNS depression with concomitant administration of other CNS depressant medications. Physical and psychological dependence has been reported as well as acute withdrawal after sudden discontinuation in addicted patients.

Metabolism: Hepatic metabolism yields metabolite (desmethyldiazepam) with active pharmacologic effect.

Excretion: Urine

Overdose: In the event of an overdose (respiratory depression, apnea, cardiovascular collapse) maintenance of a patent airway and respiratory and cardiovascular support are required. Reversal with flumazenil, which is a specific benzodiazepine antagonist, generally restores the patient to a clear-headed state. **Patients who have responded to flumazenil should be carefully monitored (up to 120 minutes) for signs of re-sedation.**

Patients must be continuously monitored post sedation to assess for:

◆ Re-sedation
◆ Respiratory depression
◆ Residual depressant effects of benzodiazepines

Dosage: 0.05 to 0.15 mg/kg titrated in 1- to 2-mg increments; there is a large interpatient variability in response to titrated doses. Before the planned procedure, 1 to 2 mg of intravenous diazepam titrated over 2 minutes may be administered. Additional 1-mg increments administered over several minutes provide sedation for the planned procedure. Additional time must be allowed to evaluate pharmacologic effect in geriatric or debilitated patients or patients with decreased cardiac output. Do not administer by rapid or single bolus injection. Titration to effect includes administration of drug until somnolence, slurring of speech, or nystagmus occurs. Extreme care must be exercised when administering diazepam in the presence of concurrent opioid administration.

Supplied: Injection: 5 mg/mL; emulsion: 5 mg/mL; tablets: 2 mg, 5 mg, 10 mg; extended release capsules: 15 mg; PO solution: 5 mg/5 mL or 5 mg/mL

Midazolam (VERSED)
(BENZODIAZEPINE AGONIST, SEDATIVE-HYPNOTIC, ANESTHETIC ADJUNCT, AMNESTIC)

Schedule: Midazolam is subject to Schedule IV control under the Controlled Substances Act of 1970. It was approved by the U.S. Food and Drug Administration in 1986.

Clinical Pharmacology: Midazolam is a water-soluble benzodiazepine. It is classified as a short-acting benzodiazepine CNS depressant with potent amnestic activity. It is three to four times more potent than diazepam. Depressant effects are dependent on dose, route of administration, and the presence or absence of other CNS depressant drugs. The pharmacologic effect of benzodiazepines is primarily exerted via facilitated action of the inhibitory neurotransmitter gamma-aminobutyric acid (GABA). This GABA interaction enhances the inhibitory effects of various neurotransmitters. Benzodiazepines affect the limbic system, thalamus, and hypothalamus, producing a calm, sedate state. The effects of midazolam on the CNS are based on:

◆ Dose administered
◆ Route of administration
◆ Presence of other premedicants

◆ Concurrent medications administered (opioids)

Specific advantages of midazolam use include a short half-life, superior sedation, amnesia, and anxiolysis when compared with other benzodiazepines. Midazolam is a water-soluble benzodiazepine. Diazepam and lorazepam utilize a propylene glycol suspension that causes pain on injection, venous irritation, and phlebitis.

Onset: IV = 1 to 5 minutes; IM = 5 to 15 minutes; intranasal = less than 5 minutes

Peak: IV = Immediate; IM = 15 to 60 minutes; intranasal = 10 minutes

Duration: 2 to 6 hours

Indications: Preoperative medication, sedation, anxiolysis, and intravenous induction agent for general anesthesia.

Contraindications: Known hypersensitivity to midazolam, acute narrow-angle glaucoma, dosage reduction in debilitated patients, shock, coma, or acute alcohol intoxication.

Protein Binding: 97%

Half-Life: 1 to 4 hours

Considerations: Individualized dosage. Reduce dose in elderly patients. Titrate medication to effect. Midazolam must never be used without individualization of dose. Bolus administration is not recommended for sedation/analgesia procedures.

Drug Interactions: Drug effect is accentuated (synergism) by concomitant use of sedatives, hypnotics, or narcotic analgesics. Drug dosage should be decreased based on the type, amount, and time that adjunct medications are administered. Patients receiving erythromycin and cimetidine may have a decrease in the plasma clearance of midazolam.

Respiratory Effects: Potent respiratory depressant. Midazolam may cause a decrease in respiratory rate and tidal volume. Apnea, respiratory depression, and cardiac arrest can occur. The drug can depress the ventilatory response to carbon dioxide stimulation. It may produce apnea with rapid administration; effects are pronounced with concomitant opioid administration. Patients with chronic obstructive pulmonary disease are extremely sensitive to the respiratory depressant effects associated with midazolam.

CV Effects: Mean arterial pressure, cardiac output, stroke volume, and systemic vascular resistance may be slightly decreased. Hypotension and brady-cardia occur more frequently in patients premedicated with a narcotic. Patients with congestive heart failure eliminate midazolam more slowly.

CNS Effects: Anxiolytic, hypnotic, sedative effects. Agitation, involuntary movement, hyperactivity, and combativeness may occur and may be due to:

◆ Excessive dosing
◆ Inadequate dosing
◆ Hypoxia
◆ Use of other CNS depressant medications accentuates the respiratory depressant effects of midazolam.

Metabolism: Midazolam undergoes hepatic microsomal metabolism (hydroxymidazolam). There are no active metabolites. Hepatic clearance may be decreased with use of enzyme-inhibiting drugs.

Elimination: Metabolites are excreted in the urine.

Overdose: In the event of an overdose (respiratory depression, apnea, cardiovascular collapse) maintenance of a patent airway and respiratory and cardiovascular support are required. Reversal with flumazenil, which is a specific benzodiazepine antagonist, generally restores the patient to a clear-headed state. Patients must be continuously monitored post sedation to assess for:

Re-sedation

Respiratory depression

Residual depressant effects of benzodiazepines

Dosage: **WARNINGS: VERSED must never be used without individualization of dosage particularly when used with other medications capable of producing CNS depression. Before the intravenous administration of VERSED in any dose, the immediate availability of oxygen, resuscitative drugs, age- and size-appropriate equipment for bag/valve/mask ventilation and intubation, and skilled personnel for the maintenance of a patent airway and support of ventilation should be ensured. Patients should be continuously monitored with some means of detection for early signs of hypoventilation, airway obstruction, or apnea, that is, pulse oximetry. Hypoventilation, airway obstruction, and apnea can lead to hypoxia and/or cardiac arrest unless effective countermeasures are taken immediately.**

Sedation: 0.025 to 0.1 mg/kg titrated to clinical effect. Do not administer by rapid or single bolus injection. Titration to effect includes administration of drug until somnolence, nystagmus, or slurring of speech occur.

Healthy Adults Younger than the Age of 60: Titrate slowly to the desired effect (e.g., the initiation of slurred speech). Some patients may respond to as little as 1 mg. No more than 2.5 mg should be given over a period of at least 2 minutes. Wait an additional 2 or more minutes to fully evaluate the sedative effect. If further titration is necessary, continue to titrate, using small increments, to the appropriate level of sedation. Wait an additional 2 or more minutes after each increment to fully evaluate the sedative effect. A total dose greater than 5 mg is not usually necessary to reach the desired endpoint. If narcotic premedication or other CNS depressants are used, patients will require approximately 30% less midazolam than unpremedicated patients.

Patients Age 60 or Older and Debilitated or Chronically Ill Patients: Because the danger of hypoventilation, airway obstruction, or apnea is greater in elderly patients and those with chronic disease states or decreased pulmonary reserve, and because the peak effect may take longer in these patients, increments should be smaller and the rate of injection slower. Titrate slowly to the desired effect (e.g., the initiation of slurred speech). Some patients may respond to as little as 1 mg. No more than 1.5 mg should be given over a period of no less than 2 minutes. Wait an additional 2 or more minutes to fully evaluate the sedative effect. If additional titration is necessary, it should be given at a rate of no more than 1 mg over a period of 2 minutes, waiting an additional 2 or more minutes each time to fully evaluate the sedative effect. Total doses greater than 3.5 mg are not usually necessary. If concomitant CNS depressant premedications are used in these patients, they will require at least 50% less midazolam than healthy young unpremedicated patients.

Methohexital Sodium (BREVITAL)
(BARBITURATE, GENERAL ANESTHETIC)

Schedule: Methohexital sodium is subject to Schedule IV control under the Controlled Substances Act of 1970.

Clinical Pharmacology: Methohexital sodium is an ultra-short-acting barbiturate and is twice as potent as thiopental. The duration of action is approximately 50% shorter than thiopental with less cumulative effect. Its primary mechanism of action is through its effect on the reticular activating center and interaction with the gamma-aminobutyric acid receptor complex. Methohexital is a methylated barbiturate that depresses the sensory cortex, decreases motor activity, and produces dose-dependent degrees of drowsiness, hypnosis, and sedation. It is not an analgesic agent.

Onset: IV = 30 seconds; rectal = less than 5 minutes

Peak Effect: IV = 45 seconds; rectal = 5 to 10 minutes

Duration: IV = 5 to 10 minutes; rectal = 30 to 90 minutes

Indications: Induction of general anesthesia. Methohexital is used as an adjunct to inhalational anesthesia during short procedures. Some clinicians utilize methohexital as an IV anesthetic adjunct for diagnostic and minor surgical procedures.

Contraindications: Known hypersensitivity to barbiturates. Dosage reduction is required in the presence of shock, coma, porphyria, or acute alcohol intoxication. Caution must be exerted when administering this drug to a patient with concomitant disease states.

Half-Life: 6 to 8 hours

Considerations: **Methohexital sodium should be administered by qualified personnel specially trained in the administration of anesthesia and in the management of the airway and cardiovascular system.**

In the presence of extravascular or intra-arterial injection, necrosis and gangrene may occur. Utilization of local or intra-arterial injection with an alpha blocker (phentolamine, 2.5 to 5 mg in 10 mL) produces vasodilation in the affected extremity.

Respiratory Effects: Respiratory depression, hypoxia, laryngospasm, apnea, hiccoughs, cardiorespiratory arrest, bronchospasm, dyspnea.

CV Effects: Circulatory depression, thrombophlebitis, vascular collapse, hypotension, cardiorespiratory arrest, tachycardia, and local irritation and pain at the injection site.

CNS Effects: May have additive effects with other CNS depressants. Tonic/clonic movements, seizures, nerve injury near the injection site, restlessness, anxiety, and emergence delirium may occur.

Metabolism: Methohexital is extensively metabolized by the liver.

Elimination: Renal

Overdose: In the event of an overdose, maintenance of a patent airway and respiratory and cardiovascular support are required.

Dosage: Individualization and titration of dosage is required. Decrease dose by 30% to 50% in elderly and debilitated patients. Methohexital should not be administered intravenously in a concentration form greater than 1% (10 mg/mL).

For sedation procedures: Increments of 10 mg have been utilized to augment the effects of benzodiazepines and opioids. To avoid deep sedation states or general anesthesia, extreme caution must be utilized when administering supplemental methohexital. Incremental doses must be given slowly over several minutes and adequate circulation time allowed to assess the pharmacologic effect.

Pediatric dosage: 25 to 30 mg/kg rectally has been administered to achieve deep levels of sedation by healthcare practitioners trained in the administration of anesthetic agents.

If methohexital is utilized by non-anesthesia providers, it is imperative to assure that the prescribing clinician understands the pharmacokinetics and pharmacodynamics associated with this agent. In addition, the clinician should also possess advanced airway management skills, demonstrate proficiency in managing cardiovascular complications, and recognize that methohexital can induce deep sedative states and/or general anesthesia. Methohexital is NOT pharmacologically reversible.

Supplied: In powder form for injection: 500 mg, 2.5 g, 5.0 g, with diluent.

Thiopental Sodium (PENTOTHAL)
(BARBITURATE, GENERAL ANESTHETIC, ANTICONVULSANT)

Schedule: Thiopental is subject to Schedule III control under the Controlled Substances Act of 1970.

Clinical Pharmacology: Thiopental is an ultra-short-acting barbiturate that causes CNS depression, a hypnotic state, and anesthesia. Its primary mechanism of action is via its effect on the reticular activating center and interaction with the gamma-aminobutyric acid (GABA) receptor complex. It is not an analgesic agent. Repeated doses lead to accumulation of the drug secondary to its increased lipid solubility and prolonged elimination phase.

Onset: IV = 10 to 20 seconds

Peak: IV = 30 to 40 seconds

Duration: IV = 5 to 15 minutes

Indications: For the induction of general anesthesia and as an adjunct for supplementary regional anesthesia and monitored anesthesia care procedures. Thiopental is used as an anticonvulsant and induction agent for barbiturate coma (to decrease cerebral metabolic rate and intracranial pressure).

Contraindications: Porphyria, known hypersensitivity to barbiturates, status asthmaticus, shock, severe heart disease.

Protein Binding: 80%

Half-Life: 3 to 8 hours

Considerations: **Thiopental should be administered by qualified personnel specially trained in the administration of anesthesia and in the management of the airway and cardiovascular system.** Due to its high pH (10 to 12), signs and symptoms of extravascular (necrosis, pain) or intra-arterial injection (gangrene, spasm, or thrombosis of vessel) require immediate intervention. Treatment includes infiltration of the area with 5 to 10 mg of phentolamine diluted in 10 mL of normal saline. Intra-arterial injection of papaverine (40 to 80 mg) may decrease the incidence of smooth muscle spasm.

Respiratory Effects: Decreased tidal volume and rate secondary to depression of the medullary breathing centers. Apnea, laryngospasm, histamine release, bronchospasm, sneezing, and coughing.

CV Effects: Venous dilation, decreased cardiac output, hypotension, decreased systemic vascular resistance, and coronary perfusion pressure.

CNS Effects: Potentiates CNS, sedative, narcotic, and hypnotic medications. Headache, prolonged recovery, somnolence, emergence delirium. Thiopental decreases cerebral blood flow, intracranial pressure, and cerebral metabolic rate. Depresses electroencephalographic and evoked potentials.

Metabolism: Primary mechanism of metabolism is the liver.

Excretion: Inactive metabolites are excreted via the kidneys.

Overdose: In the event of overdose, maintenance of a patent airway and respiratory and cardiovascular support are required.

Dosage: *Sedation procedures:* Ten- to 20-mg increments have been utilized to augment the effects of benzodiazepines and opioids. To avoid deep sedation states or general anesthesia, extreme caution must be utilized when administering supplemental doses of thiopental sodium. Incremental doses must be given slowly and adequate circulation time allowed to assess the pharmacologic effect.

If thiopental is utilized by non-anesthesia providers, it is imperative to assure that the prescribing clinician understands the pharmacokinetics and pharmacodynamics associated with this agent. In addition, the clinician should also possess advanced airway management skills, demonstrate proficiency in managing cardiovascular complications, and recognize that thiopental can induce deep sedative states and/or general anesthesia.

Supplied: Injection (syringes) 250 mg, 400 mg, 500 mg; vials with diluent: 500 mg, 1000 mg; kits: 1 g, 2.5 g, and 5 g

---

Droperidol (INAPSINE)
(NEUROLEPTIC/ANTIPSYCHOTIC)

Schedule: Inapsine is not a controlled substance.

Clinical Pharmacology: Droperidol is a neuroleptic tranquilizing agent that produces marked tranquilization and sedation. It allays apprehension and provides a state of mental detachment and indifference. In addition, it is also a potent antiemetic agent.

Onset: 3 to 5 minutes

Peak: 30 minutes

Duration: 2 to 4 hours; may be extended up to 12 hours

Indications: Sedation, tranquilization, emesis

Contraindications: Known hypersensitivity to droperidol and hypotension secondary to alpha-blocking effects. In the presence of other CNS depressants, the addition of droperidol results in synergistic effects.

Half Life: 2 to 3 hours

Drug Interactions: Extrapyramidal symptoms (1% of patients treated), dysphoria, drowsiness, restlessness, hyperexcitatory phenomenon, anxiety.

Respiratory Effects: Resting ventilation and the ventilatory response to carbon dioxide are not altered by droperidol. Droperidol administered IV augments the ventilatory response evoked by arterial hypoxemia, presumably by blocking the action of the inhibitory neurotransmitter dopamine at the carotid body.

CV Effects: Droperidol can decrease systemic blood pressure as a result of actions in the CNS and by peripheral alpha-adrenergic blockade (vasodilation). The decrease in blood pressure is usually minimal, however a patient may experience marked hypotension.

Extreme caution is required in patients with prolonged QT syndrome. Fatal cardiac arrhythmias have been reported with droperidol (FDA Alert, 2001). Cases of QT prolongation and/or torsades de pointes have been reported in patients receiving droperidol at doses at or below recommended doses. Some cases have occurred in patients with no known risk factors for QT prolongation, and some cases have been fatal. Droperidol is contraindicated in patients with known or suspected QT prolongation, including patients with congenital long QT syndrome. Droperidol should be administered with extreme caution to patients who may be at risk for development of prolonged QT syndrome (congestive heart failure, bradycardia, use of a diuretic, cardiac hypertrophy, hypokalemia, hypomagnesemia, or administration of other drugs known to increase the QT interval). Other risk factors may include age older than 65 years, alcohol abuse, and use of agents such as benzodiazepines, opioids, and volatile anesthetics. Droperidol should be initiated at a low dose and adjusted upward, with caution, as needed to achieve the desired effect. Patients with a history of extrapyramidal symptoms (Parkinson's disease) and neuroleptic malignant syndrome should not receive butyrophenones. Droperidol should be administered with caution to hypotensive patients secondary to its alpha-adrenergic blockade.

CNS Effects: An outwardly calming effect occurs with droperidol use. Akathisia (most often a feeling of restlessness in the legs) may occur with the administration of droperidol. Droperidol evokes extrapyramidal reactions in approximately 1% of the patient population. Extrapyramidal symptoms occur secondary to droperidol's dopamine antagonistic effects. Butyrophenones occupy GABA receptors on the postsynaptic membrane, reducing synaptic transmission and increasing the concentration of dopamine in the intersynaptic cleft. They also inhibit the reuptake of dopamine and norepinephrine into the storage granules at the presynaptic nerve terminals. Thus the normal balance of acetylcholine and dopamine in certain areas of the brain is altered and leads to inhibition of operant behavior and anxiolysis. The antiemetic effect associated with the neuroleptic drugs is probably related to their affinity to the GABA receptors in the chemoreceptor trigger zone.

Metabolism: Primary mechanism of metabolism is hepatic.

Overdose: Cardiovascular support is required in the event of overdose. There is no pharmacologic reversal agent for the butyrophenone classification of medications.

Dosage: Antiemetic doses of 0.625 to 1.25 mg and sedative doses of approximately 2.5 mg have been reported in the literature.

Precautions: **Extreme caution is required in patients with prolonged QT syndrome. Patients with a history of extrapyramidal symptoms (Parkinson's disease) and neuroleptic malignant syndrome should not receive butyrophenones. Droperidol should be administered with caution to hypotensive patients secondary to its alpha-adrenergic blockade.**

Propofol (DIPRIVAN)
(SEDATIVE/HYPNOTIC)

Schedule: Not currently a controlled substance.

Clinical Pharmacology: Propofol is a sedative/hypnotic for intravenous use. It produces rapid hypnosis with minimal excitation. It produces nonspecific cortical depression and a more complete and rapid awakening than thiopental or methohexital. Rapid awakening is associated with extensive redistribution from the CNS to other tissues and high metabolic clearance. It possesses intrinsic antiemetic effects and has no analgesic properties. Action is dose and rate dependent.

Onset: 40 seconds

Peak Effect: 1 minute

Duration: 5 to 10 minutes

Indications: For the induction and maintenance of general anesthesia, sedation, and analgesia.

Contraindications: Known hypersensitivity to propofol or its components (soybean oil, glycerol, egg lecithin, sodium hydroxide).

Protein Binding: 97% to 99%

Considerations: Individualize dose and titrate to effect. Reduce dose in elderly, hypovolemic, and high-risk patients. Potentiation occurs when combined with narcotic analgesics and CNS depressants. Pain on injection has been reported. **Propofol should be administered by qualified personnel specially trained in the administration of anesthesia and in the management of the airway and cardiovascular system.**

Special Handling Procedures: Propofol is available as an oil in water emulsion (intralipid) that contains soybean oil, glycerol, and egg lecithin. A history of egg allergy is not a definitive contraindication to its use. Patients with egg allergies generally have a reaction to egg whites (albumin), whereas egg lecithin is extracted from egg yolk. When originally released from production, propofol contained no antimicrobial preservatives. Sepsis and death have been reported by the Centers for Disease Control and Prevention related to contaminated propofol solution. Propofol now contains 0.005% disodium edetate. Disodium edetate retards the rate of growth of microorganisms in the event of contamination. For this point, the manufacturer requires strict aseptic technique must be maintained in its handling.

WARNING: **Strict aseptic techniques must always be maintained during handling. Propofol injectable emulsion is a single-use parenteral product that contains 0.005% disodium edetate to retard the rate of growth of microorganisms in the event of accidental extrinsic contamination. However, propofol injectable emulsion can still support the growth of microorganisms because it is not an antimicrobially preserved product under USP standards. Accordingly, strict aseptic technique must still be adhered to. Do not use if contamination is suspected. Discard unused portions as directed within the time limits. There have been reports in which failure to use aseptic technique when handling propofol injectable emulsion was associated with microbial contamination of the product and with fever, infection/sepsis, other life-threatening illness, and/or death.**

Manufacturer Handling Instructions: Propofol (Diprivan) injection should be prepared just before initiation of each individual anesthetic/sedative procedure. The vial/prefilled syringe rubber stopper should be disinfected using 70% isopropyl alcohol. Diprivan Injectable Emulsion should be drawn into sterile syringes immediately after vials are opened. When withdrawing Diprivan Injectable Emulsion from vials, a sterile vent spike should be used. The syringe(s) should be labeled with appropriate information, including the date and time the vial was opened. Administration should commence promptly and be completed within 6 hours after the vial was opened. Diprivan Injectable Emulsion should be prepared for single-patient use only. Any unused portions of Diprivan Injectable Emulsion, reservoirs, dedicated administration tubing, and/or solution containing Diprivan Injectable Emulsion must be discarded at the end of the anesthetic procedure or at 6 hours, whichever occurs sooner.

The IV line should be flushed every 6 hours and at the end of the anesthetic procedure to remove residual Diprivan Injectable Emulsion.

Respiratory Effects: Dose-dependent respiratory depression, apnea, hiccoughs, laryngospasm, bronchospasm, wheezing, and coughing.

CV Effects: Hypotension associated with a decrease in cardiac output, cardiac contractility and preload, arrhythmias, tachycardia, bradycardia, and decreased cardiac output.

CNS Effects: Headache, dizziness, confusion, euphoria, myoclonic/clonic movement, seizures, sexual illusions, and possible additive effect with other CNS drugs, sedatives, and opioids.

Metabolism: Hepatic conjugation to inactive metabolites.

Elimination: Inactive metabolites are eliminated via urine.

Overdose: In the event of an overdose, maintenance of a patent airway and respiratory and cardiovascular support are required. There is no pharmacologic reversal agent for overdose.

Dosage: *For sedation procedures:* Increments of 10 mg have been utilized to augment the effects of benzodiazepines and opioids. To avoid deep sedation states or general anesthesia, extreme caution must be utilized when administering supplemental propofol. Incremental doses must be given slowly over several minutes and adequate circulation time allowed to assess full pharmacologic effect.

Continuous infusion techniques: Utilized for sedation, particularly in critical care unit settings. Dosage (25 to 75 μg/kg/min) varies according to patient physiologic status, presence of pathophysiologic disease states, age, diagnosis, and level of sedation required. This technique is generally reserved for intubated patients.

If propofol is utilized by non-anesthesia providers, it is imperative to assure that the prescribing clinician understands the pharmacokinetics and pharmacodynamics associated with this agent. In addition, the clinician should also possess advanced airway management skills, demonstrate proficiency in managing cardiovascular complications, and recognize that propofol can induce deep sedative states and/or general anesthesia. Propofol is NOT pharmacologically reversible.

Supplied: 10 mg/mL (20 mL ampule, 50 mL vial, 100 mL infusion vial);10 mg/mL (prefilled syringe)

Ketamine
(DISSOCIATIVE ANESTHETIC)

Clinical Pharmacology:	A phencyclidine derivative that produces rapid dissociative anesthesia, which causes the patient to appear conscious (eyes open, swallowing, enhanced laryngeal-pharyngeal reflexes, muscle contractures, respiratory stimulation). However, the patient loses the ability to process or respond to sensory input. Ketamine has been demonstrated to be an N-methyl-D-aspartate receptor (a subtype of the glutamate receptor) antagonist. Through selective disorganization of nonspecific pathways in the midbrain and thalamic areas, it produces analgesia, amnesia, and unconsciousness. Central sympathetic stimulation occurs with systemic, pulmonary arterial pressure, heart rate, and cardiac output increases. Ketamine also produces significant bronchodilation.
Onset:	IV = less than 60 seconds; IM = 3 to 8 minutes
Peak:	IV = 5 to 10 minutes; IM = 5 to 20 minutes
Duration:	IV = 5 to15 minutes; IM= 12 to 25 minutes
Indications:	IV and IM anesthetic induction agent. Ketamine is utilized as a sedation/analgesia agent for therapeutic, diagnostic, and therapeutic procedures.
Contraindications:	Patients with increased intracranial pressure, open eye injury, or patients with psychiatric illness. Caution must be exercised in patients with ischemic heart disease, hypertension, and dysrhythmias. It is contraindicated for procedures of the pharynx, larynx, and bronchus secondary to increased secretions.
Protein Binding:	12%
Half-Life:	3 hours
Considerations:	Due to ketamine's ability to produce hypertension and tachycardia, increased myocardial oxygen consumption occurs. Psychologic reactions (illusions, dreams, fear, anxiety, excitement, and out of body experiences) termed "emergence delirium" occur in approximately 40% of patients. Emergence reactions generally manifest within the first several hours of recovery and are diminished with the administration of small doses of benzodiazepines.
	Ketamine should be administered by qualified personnel specially trained in the administration of anesthesia and in the management of the airway and cardiovascular system.
Drug Interactions:	A combination of theophylline and ketamine may produce seizures. Diazepam and lithium prolong the elimination half life of ketamine.
Respiratory Effects:	Minimal decrease in ventilatory drive. It is a potent bronchodilator. Increased upper airway secretions are exhibited particularly in children.
CV Effects:	Hypertension, tachycardia, increased cardiac output.
CNS Effects:	Euphoria, unconsciousness, disassociation and production of a cataleptic state. There may be an increase in intracranial pressure, cerebral oxygen consumption, and cerebral blood flow.
Metabolism:	Biotransformation to active and inactive metabolites.
Elimination:	Excretion via the kidney.
Overdose:	In the event of overdose, maintenance of a patient airway and respiratory and cardiovascular support are required.
Dosage:	Sedation and analgesia: IV = 0.2 to 1 mg/kg; IM = 1 to 2.5 mg/kg
	If ketamine is utilized by non-anesthesia providers, it is imperative to assure that the prescribing clinician understands the pharmacokinetics and pharmacodynamics associated with this agent. In addition, the clinician should also possess advanced airway management skills, demonstrate proficiency in managing cardiovascular complications, and recognize that ketamine can induce deep sedative states and/or general anesthesia. Ketamine is NOT pharmacologically reversible.
Supplied:	10 mg/mL (20, 25, 50 mL vials); 50 mg/mL (10 mL vials); 100 mg/mL (5 mL vials)

Naloxone Hydrochloride (NARCAN)
(OPIOID RECEPTOR ANTAGONIST)

Clinical Pharmacology:	Naloxone hydrochloride is a pure opioid antagonist with no agonist activity. Through competitive inhibition at the opiate receptors, reversal of respiratory depression, hypotension, hypercapnia, sedation, and euphoria associated with the administration of narcotics is reversed. Naloxone has not been shown to produce tolerance or physical or psychological dependence. In the presence of physical dependence, naloxone will produce withdrawal symptoms. Requirement for repeat doses is dependent on amount, type, and route of opioid administration.
Onset:	IV = 2 minutes
Peak Effect:	5 to 15 minutes

Duration:	30 to 45 minutes, dependent on dose and route of naloxone administration.
Indications:	Complete or partial reversal of opioid depression (respiratory depression, sedation and hypotension) induced by the administration of opioids. Additional indications include diagnosis of suspected acute opioid overdosage. Unlabeled uses include reversal of alcoholic coma and improvement of circulation in refractory shock.
Contraindications:	Known hypersensitivity to naloxone. Caution must be utilized when administering to patients with preexisting cardiac disease or patients with known or suspected physical dependence on opioids.
Half-Life:	30 to 60 minutes
Considerations:	Titrate slowly to the desired effect. Excessive reversal with naloxone may result in total reversal of analgesia with additional side effects (e.g., hypertension, excitation). The short duration of action is presumed to be due to its rapid removal from the brain. **Therefore, the duration of action of some opioids may exceed that of naloxone and patients must be carefully monitored post sedation for signs of respiratory depression/arrest. Repeated doses of naloxone may be administered as required.**
Respiratory Effects:	Reversal of respiratory depression. Rapid intravenous administration may induce pulmonary edema.
CV Effects:	Hypotension, hypertension, ventricular tachycardia/fibrillation.
CNS Effects:	Excitement, tremors, seizures
Metabolism:	Hepatic conjugation
Excretion:	Renal
Overdose:	Larger than necessary dosages of naloxone may result in significant reversal of analgesic effects (e.g., hypertension, tachycardia).
Dosage:	1 to 4 µg/kg titrated in 0.1-mg increments promptly reverses opioid-induced analgesia and depression of ventilation.
Supplied:	0.4 mg/mL; 1 mg/mL; 0.02 mg/mL

Flumazenil (ROMAZICON)
(BENZODIAZEPINE RECEPTOR ANTAGONIST)

Class:	A benzodiazepine receptor antagonist.
Clinical Pharmacology:	Flumazenil is utilized for complete or partial reversal of benzodiazepine sedation. It competitively inhibits the activity of the benzodiazepine receptor sites on the GABA/benzodiazepine receptor complex. Flumazenil has been shown to antagonize sedation and psychomotor impairment. The duration and degree of reversal of benzodiazepine effects are related to total dose administered and plasma benzodiazepine concentrations. Duration and degree of reversal are dose and plasma content related (both for amount of benzodiazepine and amount of flumazenil).
Onset:	IV = 1 to 2 minutes. An 80% response will be achieved within 3 minutes of administration.
Peak:	6 to 10 minutes
Duration:	45 to 90 minutes. Duration of effect is dependent on the total benzodiazepine plasma concentration.
Indications:	Complete or partial reversal of the sedative effects of benzodiazepines. Flumazenil is used in the management of benzodiazepine overdose.
Contraindications:	Known hypersensitivity to flumazenil or benzodiazepines. Patients on long-term benzodiazepine therapy for control of life-threatening disorders (status epilepticus) or in patients who show signs of serious cyclic antidepressant overdose.
Half-Life:	41 to 79 minutes.
Considerations:	Individualized dosage is required. Safety and effectiveness for reversal of sedation/analgesia induced with benzodiazepines have been established in patients 1 to 17 years of age. Re-sedation may occur, especially in children 1 to 5 years of age. Safety and effectiveness of repeated flumazenil doses in children experiencing re-sedation have not been established. Serious adverse effects of flumazenil are related to the reversal of benzodiazepine effects. Utilization of more than the minimally effective doses is tolerated by most patients but may complicate the management of patients who are physically dependent on benzodiazepines. Flumazenil has been associated with seizures. Flumazenil-induced seizures have been reported in patients treated with benzodiazepines to control seizures or chronic physical dependence on benzodiazepines. **Patients who have responded to flumazenil should be carefully monitored (up to 120 minutes) for signs of re-sedation.** To avoid pain and inflammation at the site of injection, administration of flumazenil via a large vein is recommended.

Drug Interactions:	Flumazenil is not recommended in cases of tricyclic antidepressant overdosage.
Respiratory Effects:	Respiratory depression is related to the duration of effect of the benzodiazepine administered that has exceeded the therapeutic effects of flumazenil.
CV Effects:	Cutaneous vasodilation, sweating, and flushing. Arrhythmias (atrial, nodal, ventricular extrasystole, bradycardia, tachycardia) and hypertension may occur.
CNS Effects:	Dizziness, headache, insomnia, abnormal or blurred vision, confusion and benzodiazepine withdrawal–induced seizures.
Additional Adverse Reactions:	Fatigue, pain at the injection site, thrombophlebitis, or rash.
Metabolism:	Hepatic metabolism is dependent on hepatic blood flow.
Excretion:	Inactive metabolites excreted via the urine
Overdose:	In the presence of benzodiazepine agonists, excessive doses of flumazenil result in anxiety, agitation, increased muscle tone, and possibly benzodiazepine-induced seizure activity.
Dosage:	Individualized dosage is required based on patient response:
Adult reversal of sedation:	Slow IV bolus, 0.2 mg over 15 seconds. If desired level of consciousness is not obtained after waiting an additional 45 seconds, a further dose of 0.2 mg can be injected and repeated at 60-second intervals where necessary (up to a maximum of 4 additional times) to a maximum total dose of 1 mg. No more than 3 mg is recommended in any 1-hour period.
Pediatric reversal of sedation:	Recommended initial dose is 0.01 mg/kg (up to 0.2 mg) administered IV over 15 seconds. If the desired level of consciousness is not obtained after an additional 45 seconds, further injections of 0.01 mg/kg (up to 0.2 mg) can be administered and repeated at 60-second intervals where necessary (up to a maximum of 4 additional times) to a maximum dose of 0.05 mg/kg or 1 mg, whichever is lower.
Supplied:	0.1 mg/mL in 5 mL vials; 0.1 mg/mL in 10 mL vials

Atropine Sulfate
(ANTICHOLINERGIC)

Class:	Anticholinergic
Clinical Pharmacology:	Atropine is a white crystalline alkaloid. Atropine antagonizes the action of

acetylcholine at the muscarinic receptor producing local, central, and peripheral effects. Atropine decreases salivary, respiratory, and gastrointestinal secretions. Bronchial and lower esophageal sphincter muscle tone is relaxed. As a parasympatholytic medication, atropine increases sinus node automaticity and atrioventricular conduction through a direct vagolytic mechanism of action.

Onset:	IV = 45 to 60 seconds; IM = 5 to 40 minutes; Intratracheal = 10 to 20 seconds; PO = 30 minutes to 2 hours; Inhalation = 3 to 5 minutes
Peak:	IV = 2 minutes; Inhalation = 1 to 2 hours
Duration:	IV/IM (vagal blockade) = 1 to 2 hours
Indications:	To decrease salivary, bronchial, and gastric secretions. Treatment of sinus bradycardia, vagal episodes, and incorporation within the ACLS algorithm.
Contraindications:	Extreme care must be used in patients with tachyarrhythmias, congestive heart failure, acute myocardial infarction, and myocardial ischemia. Use with caution in patients with atrioventricular block at the His-Purkinje level (type II atrioventricular block and new third-degree blocks with wide QRS complexes).
Considerations:	Large doses may produce mental disturbances, confusion, delirium, flushed hot skin, and blurred vision. Exercise caution in obstructive uropathy and obstructive diseases of the gastrointestinal tract. Transient decreases in heart rate have been associated with the administration of low dosages (<0.5 mg) due to weak peripheral muscarinic effects.
Respiratory Effects:	Respiratory depression in excessively large doses may be due to paralysis of the medullary center. Smooth muscle relaxation and suppression of secretions may occur.
CV Effects:	Tachycardia is associated with high dosages, and bradycardia is associated with low dosages and palpitations.
CNS Effects:	Confusion, hallucinations, drowsiness, excitement and agitation, blurred vision, dilation of pupils, and psychosis.
Metabolism:	Enzymatic hydrolysis
Elimination:	Thirteen to 50 percent of the drug is excreted unchanged in the urine.
Overdose:	If marked excitement is present, a short-acting barbiturate or benzodiazepine may be utilized for sedation. Physostigmine salicylate (Antilirium) reverses most cardiovascular and CNS effects; however, it may cause severe bradycardia, seizures, or asystole. Ice bags

and alcohol sponges help to reduce fever in the presence of hot flushed skin or febrile states, particularly in children.

Dosage: *Bradyarrhythmias:* 0.4- to 1-mg bolus repeated every 3 to 5 minutes up to a total dose of 2 mg can be used to achieve a desired pulse rate above 60 beats per minute. American Heart Association guidelines recommend a total dose not to exceed 0.04 mg/kg and the use of shorter dosing intervals (3 minutes) and higher maximum dose range (0.04 mg/kg) in severe clinical conditions. Subsequent doses of 0.5 to 1 mg may be given at 4- to 6-hour intervals. Doses under 0.5 mg may cause paradoxical slowing of heart rate. *Smooth muscle relaxation and suppression of secretions:* 0.4 to 0.6 mg every 4 to 6 hours.

Supplied: 0.4 mg to 1 mg/1 mL; 0.4 mg/0.5 mL

Ephedrine
(INDIRECT-ACTING, SYNTHETIC, NONCATECHOLAMINE, SYMPATHOMIMETIC)

Clinical Pharmacology: Ephedrine causes endogenous catecholamine release via indirect mechanism of action and stimulation of adrenergic receptors via a direct effect. A sympathomimetic drug, it is less potent than epinephrine. Through positive inotropic action, increased strength of myocardial contraction occurs. Through these combined effects (alpha and beta stimulation) blood pressure, heart rate, contractility, and cardiac output increase. Ephedrine is also a bronchodilator via stimulation of $beta_2$ stimulation. CNS stimulation occurs, and metabolic and respiratory rate is increased.

Onset: IV = 30 to 45 seconds (immediate); IM = less than 5 minutes

Peak: IV = 2 to 5 minutes; IM = less than 10 minutes

Duration: 10 to 60 minutes

Indications: Treatment of procedural hypotension and emergency treatment of hypotension of unknown origin. Ephedrine may be used to treat bronchospasm, bradycardia, and allergic disorders.

Contraindications: Cautious utilization in patients with hypertension, tachycardia, or unstable cardiovascular profile. Ephedrine is contraindicated in patients with narrow-angle glaucoma. Do not use to treat overdosage of phenothiazines: a further drop in blood pressure and irreversible shock may occur.

Considerations: Tachyphylaxis occurs with repeated doses; however, temporary cessation of the drug restores its original effectiveness.

Drug Interactions: Decreased responsiveness has been observed in patients treated with beta blockers. Unpredictable effects occur in patients with depleted catecholamine stores. Hypertensive crisis may occur in patients treated with monoamine oxidase inhibitors or tricyclic antidepressants.

Respiratory Effects: Pulmonary edema, bronchodilation

CV Effects: Hypertension, tachycardia, dysrhythmias

CNS Effects: Agitation, anxiety, insomnia, tremors

Metabolism: Hepatic

Elimination: Renal

Overdose: Signs and symptoms associated with an overdose (tachycardia, dysrhythmias, hypertension, agitation) generally dissipate within several minutes. Symptoms associated with an exaggerated pharmacologic response may be treated with alpha or beta blockade.

Dosage: *Adults:* IV = 2.5- to 10-mg increments titrated to effect. IM = 25 to 50 mg. Supplemental doses may be increased to prevent the development of tachyphylaxis. *Children:* 0.1 mg/kg titrated to effect.

Supplied: 50 mg/1 mL ampule

Epinephrine Hydrochloride (ADRENALIN)
(DIRECT-ACTING, NONSYNTHETIC CATECHOLAMINE)

Class: Sympathomimetic

Clinical Pharmacology: Epinephrine is a naturally occurring catecholamine that is secreted from the adrenal medulla. It possesses both alpha (peripheral vasoconstriction) and beta (increase in heart rate, bronchodilation) activity. However, its most prominent actions are on the beta receptors of the heart, vascular, and other smooth muscle. When given intravenously it produces a rapid rise in blood pressure and direct stimulation of cardiac muscle (positive chronotropic and inotropic effects), which increases the strength of ventricular contraction and cardiac output.

Onset: IV = 30 to 60 seconds; Subcutaneous = 6 to 15 minutes; Inhalation = 3 to 5 minutes; Intratracheal = 5 to 15 seconds

Peak: 2 to 3 minutes

Duration of Action: IV = 5 to 10 minutes; Intratracheal = 15 to 25 minutes; Inhalational/Subcutaneous = 1 to 3 hours

Indications:	Treatment of cardiac arrest, ventricular fibrillation, and asystole. Epinephrine is useful in conditions that require increased inotropy, for bronchodilation, in treatment of allergic reactions, and for prolongation of local anesthetic activity.
Contraindications:	Cardiac dilation, coronary insufficiency, cardiovascular disorders, thyroid toxicosis, diabetes mellitus, and organic brain damage
Considerations:	Caution in patients with hypertension, cardiovascular disease, diabetes, and hyperthyroidism. Epinephrine is contraindicated for intravenous regional anesthesia and local anesthesia supplement to end organs (digits, ears, nose).
Drug Interactions:	The cardiovascular effects of epinephrine may be potentiated by tricyclic antidepressants and antihistamines (diphenhydramine). Use in caution in patients taking monoamine oxidase inhibitors. Vasodilators (alpha-blocking agents) may counteract the pressor effects of epinephrine.
Respiratory Effects:	Pulmonary edema, bronchodilation, dyspnea.
CV Effects:	Hypertension, tachycardia, chest pain.
CNS Effects:	Anxiety, headache, hemorrhage.
Metabolism:	Enzymatic degradation (hepatic, renal, and gastrointestinal tract)
Elimination:	Renal
Overdose:	Excessive doses of epinephrine may result in precordial distress, vomiting, headache, dyspnea, and hypertension. Alpha or beta blockers may be required to counteract excessive dosage of epinephrine.
Dosage:	*Cardiac arrest:* AHA guidelines recommend 1 mg (10 mL of a 1:10,000 concentration IV; may repeat every 3 to 5 minutes. Follow each dose with a 20-mL flush to ensure delivery to systemic circulation. *Endotracheal:* A diluted solution may be given through the endotracheal tube before an IV is established. American Heart Association guidelines recommend 2 to 2.5 mg diluted in 10-mL of normal saline. *Vasopressor:* 1 to 10 μg/min titrated to desired response. *Hypersensitivity:* 0.1 to 0.25 mg (1 to 2.5 mL of a 1:10,000 concentration). Start with a small dose, giving only as much as required to alleviate undesirable symptoms, and repeat as necessary (usually every 20 to 30 minutes).
Supplied:	0.01 mg/mL 10 μg/mL; 0.1 mg/mL 100 μg/mL; 0.5 mg/mL 500 μg/mL; 1 mg/mL 1000 μg/mL

Lidocaine Hydrochloride (XYLOCAINE)
(ANTIARRHYTHMIC)

Class:	Antiarrhythmic
Clinical Pharmacology:	Lidocaine is a local anesthetic agent that exerts an antiarrhythmic effect similar to procainamide. It suppresses ventricular dysrhythmias by decreasing automaticity and excitability via attenuation of phase IV diastolic depolarization. It decreases cell membrane permeability and prevents loss of sodium and potassium ions. Lidocaine raises the ventricular fibrillation threshold. It has been shown to cause little or no decrease in ventricular contractility, cardiac output, arterial pressure, or heart rate. Lidocaine readily crosses the placenta and blood brain barriers.
Onset:	IV = 45 to 90 seconds
Peak:	1 to 2 minutes
Duration:	10 to 20 minutes
Indications:	Treatment of ventricular arrhythmia and wide-complex paroxysmal supraventricular tachycardia.
Contraindications:	Known hypersensitivity to amide local anesthetics. Lidocaine is contraindicated in Stokes-Adams syndrome and Wolff-Parkinson-White syndrome. Severe degrees of sinoatrial, atrioventricular, or intraventricular block may occur in the absence of an artificial pacemaker.
Protein Binding:	55%
Half-Life:	1.5 to 2 hours; may be increased two to three times for patients with liver dysfunction.
Considerations:	Dosage should be reduced in children and debilitated and elderly patients. Accumulation may occur in the presence of liver or kidney disease. Caution should be exercised when utilizing lidocaine in the presence of hypovolemia, severe congestive heart failure, shock, and heart block.

In patients with sinus bradycardia or incomplete heart block, the administration of IV lidocaine for the elimination of ventricular ectopy may result in more frequent and serious ventricular arrhythmia or complete heart block. Use caution in severe liver or renal disease, hypovolemia, shock, and all forms of heart block. |
| **Drug Interactions:** | Lidocaine should be used with caution in patients with digitalis toxicity. Cross-sensitivity and/or potentiation may occur with other antiarrhythmics (procainamide or quinidine). |

Lidocaine may produce excessive cardiac depression with phenytoin (Dilantin). Clearance is reduced with concomitant use of beta blockers and cimetidine.

Respiratory Effects: Respiratory depression, arrest.

CV Effects: Hypotension, bradycardia, arrhythmias, cardiovascular collapse, and heart block.

CNS Effects: Excitatory phenomena include light headedness, nervousness, dizziness, apprehension, euphoria, confusion, drowsiness, tinnitus, blurred or double vision, vomiting, sensation of heat, cold, or numbness, twitching, tremors, convulsions, and/or unconsciousness.

Metabolism: Lidocaine is rapidly metabolized by the liver.

Excretion: Ten percent of the administered dose is excreted unchanged in the urine.

Overdose: Generally results in CNS or cardiovascular toxic manifestations. In the presence of convulsions, respiratory depression or cardiac arrest requires intubation and cardiovascular support. Utilization of benzodiazepines or barbiturates is effective in the treatment of convulsions.

Dosage: *Refractory ventricular fibrillation or ventricular tachycardia:* 1 to 1.5 mg/kg of body weight (50 to 100 mg) as a loading dose. May repeat 0.5 to 1.5 mg/kg every 5 to 10 minutes to desired effect, up to a total of 3 mg/kg. Should not exceed 200 to 300 mg/hr. American Heart Association recommends repeat doses of 0.5 to 0.75 mg/kg.

Supplied: 10 mg/mL in 5 mL vial/ampule; 10 mg/mL in 10 mL vial/ampule; 20 mg/mL in 5 mL ampule

LEARNER SELF-ASSESSMENT

In order to achieve maximal educational benefit from this chapter, please complete the Learner Self-Assessment below. This self-assessment tool provides the ability to identify areas requiring additional review. Reference material for each question is provided in Appendix F.

1. Healthcare practitioner considerations associated with **JCAHO Standards** related to sedation/analgesic medication administration include:

2. **Practice Guidelines for Sedation and Analgesia by Non-Anesthesiologists** promulgated by the ASA Task Force on Sedation **related to sedation/analgesic medication administration** include:

3. The **pharmacokinetic profile** associated with sedative, analgesic, and hypnotic medications utilized in the sedation setting include:

4. The **pharmacodynamic profile** associated with sedative, analgesic, and hypnotic medications utilized in the sedation setting include:

5. **Indications, side effects, contraindications, and clinical pharmacology** associated with sedative, hypnotic, and analgesic medications include:

6. **Cardiovascular, respiratory, and central nervous system effects** associated with sedative, hypnotic, and analgesic medications include:

Please note: If you are applying for CE credit, you must contact Specialty Health Education, Inc. @ 800-694-8041 for a CE Application Packet.

1. Which benzodiazepine has a half-life of 30 to 50 hours? _____
   A. Diazepam
   B. Midazolam
   C. Ativan
   D. Bromazepam

2. Which of the following benzodiazepines has no active metabolites? _____
   A. Diazepam
   B. Midazolam
   C. Ativan
   D. Bromazepam

3. Which of the following benzodiazepines has an active metabolite "desmethyldiazepam"? _____
   A. Diazepam
   B. Midazolam
   C. Ativan
   D. Bromazepam

4. The opioid analgesic that is 75 to 125 times more potent than morphine sulfate and has a rapid onset and short duration of action is _____?
   A. Morphine
   B. Ketorolac
   C. Hydromorphone
   D. Fentanyl

5. Which pharmacologic antagonist "reverses" the clinical effects associated with benzodiazepine overdose? _____
   A. Ropivacaine
   B. Bromazepam
   C. Naloxone
   D. Flumazenil

6. Which opioid agonist possesses therapeutic actions with less spasm of smooth muscle, constipation, and suppression of the cough reflex than morphine? _____
   A. Hydromorphone
   B. Sufentanil
   C. Meperidine
   D. Naloxone

7. Which opioid agonist produces a significant amount of histamine release? _____
   A. Hydromorphone
   B. Meperidine
   C. Morphine
   D. Fentanyl

8. Which sedative/hypnotic agent produces augmentation of sedation and rapid hypnosis and possesses intrinsic antiemetic effects? _____
   A. Thiopental
   B. Brevital
   C. Ketamine
   D. Propofol

9. Which sedative/hypnotic agent should only be utilized by healthcare providers skilled in advanced airway management and cardiac life support secondary to its ability to produce the development of deep sedative states and general anesthesia? _____
   A. Midazolam
   B. Diazepam
   C. Meperidine
   D. Propofol

10. A specific opiate receptor antagonist that reverses the respiratory depressant effects associated with narcotic use is identified as _____?
    A. Bromazepam
    B. Naloxone
    C. Flumazenil
    D. Ropivacaine

REFERENCES

1. Biddle C, Aker J. Conscious sedation: Between Scylla and Carybdis. *Quality of Life—A Nursing Challenge* 1995;4(4):107.
2. Spitalnic S, Blazes C, Anderson A. Conscious sedation: A primer for outpatient procedures. *Hospital Physician.* 2000 (May):25.
3. Messinger J, Hoffman L, O'Donnell J, Dunworth B. Getting conscious sedation right. *Am J Nurs.* 1999;99:47.

ADDITIONAL RESOURCES

Barash P, Cullen B, Stoelting R. *Clinical Anesthesia.* 4th ed. Philadelphia: Lippincott Williams & Wilkins; 2001.

Faust R. *Anesthesiology Review.* 3rd ed. New York: Churchill-Livingstone; 2002.

Gahart B, Nazareno A. *2003 Intravenous Medications.* Philadelphia: Mosby; 2003.

Goodwin S. Pharmacologic management of patients undergoing conscious sedation. *Clin Nurs Specialist.* 2001;15:269-271.

Guyton A. *Textbook of Medical Physiology.* 11th ed. Philadelphia: WB Saunders; 2001.

Hardman J, Limbirch L, Goodman-Gilman A. *Goodman & Gilman's The Pharmacologic Basis of Therapeutics.* 10th ed. New York: McGraw-Hill; 2001.

Miller R. *Anesthesia.* 5th ed. New York: Churchill Livingstone; 2000.

Nagelhout J, Zaglaniczny K. *Nurse Anesthesia.* 2nd ed. Philadelphia: WB Saunders; 2001.

Physicians' Desk Reference. 57th ed. Montvale, NJ: Thompson PDR; 2003.

Spitalnic S, Blazes C, Anderson, A. Conscious sedation: A primer for outpatient procedures. *Hospital Physician,* Wayne, Pennsylvania: Turner White Communications, 2000:22–32.

Stoelting R, Dierdorf S. *Anesthesia and Co-existing Disease.* 4th ed. New York: Churchill Livingstone; 2002.

BIBLIOGRAPHY

Barash P. *Clinical Anesthesia.* 2nd ed. Philadelphia: Lippincott Williams & Wilkins; 1992.

Cummins R. *Textbook of Advanced Cardiac Life Support.* Dallas: American Heart Association; 1994.

Davidson J, Eckhardt W, Perese D. *Clinical Anesthesia Procedures of the Massachusetts General Hospital.* 4th ed. Boston: Little, Brown; 1993.

Duke J, Rosenberg S. *Anesthesia Secrets.* St. Louis: Mosby; 1996.

Estafanous F. *Opioids in Anesthesia.* 2nd ed. Boston: Butterworth-Heinemann; 1991.

Furniss S, Munger M. Understanding ACLS pharmacotherapy. *Anesth Today.* 1996;7:1.

Jacobs E. *Saunders Review for NCLEX-RN.* 2nd ed. Philadelphia: WB Saunders; 1994.

Kanarek B. *Glaxo Wellcome Announces New ULTIVA: Remifentanil HCl for Injection.* Research Triangle Park, NC: Glaxo Wellcome; 1996.

Katz J. *Anesthesiology: A Comprehensive Study Guide.* New York: McGraw-Hill; 1997.

Miller R. *Anesthesia.* 4th ed. New York: Churchill Livingstone; 1994.

Morgan E, Mikhail M. *Clinical Anesthesiology.* 2nd ed. Stamford, CT: Appleton & Lange; 1996.

Omoigui S. *The Anesthesia Drugs Handbook.* 2nd ed. St. Louis: Mosby; 1995.

Rice T. *The Physician's Desk Reference.* 50th ed. Montvale, NJ: Medical Economics Company; 1996.

Roizen M, Fleisher L. *The Essence of Anesthesia Practice.* Philadelphia: WB Saunders; 1997.

CHAPTER 6

Procedural Patient Monitoring

At the completion of this chapter, the learner shall:

◆ Identify JCAHO standards and intents related to physiologic monitoring requirements for patients presenting for sedation/analgesia clinical services.

◆ Identify Practice Guidelines for Sedation and Analgesia by Non-Anesthesiologists related to physiologic monitoring for the sedation patient.

◆ Identify the rationale, advantages, and disadvantages associated with the following monitoring parameters utilized during sedation procedures:

- ECG
- Blood pressure
- Pulse oximetry
- Level of consciousness
- End-tidal carbon dioxide
- Bispectral index analysis

◆ State which ECG lead positions are best utilized in the detection of dysrhythmias versus ischemia.

◆ Identify three types of dysrhythmias that may impact on the patient's physiologic status during a sedation procedure.

◆ List three factors that contribute to the development of hypotension.

◆ Outline recommended treatment protocols for hypotension/hypertension.

◆ State the advantages associated with the use of end-tidal carbon dioxide monitoring during sedation procedures.

◆ Identify components of the sedation/analgesia record.

Joint Commission on Accreditation of Healthcare Organizations Standards for Operative or Other High-Risk Procedures and/or the Administration of Moderate or Deep Sedation or Anesthesia

Standard PC.13.20
Operative or other procedures and/or the administration of moderate or deep sedation or anesthesia are planned.

Rationale for PC.13.20
Because the response to procedures is not always predictable and sedation-to-anesthesia is a continuum, it is not always possible to predict how an individual patient will respond.

Therefore, qualified individuals are trained in professional standards and techniques to manage patients in the case of a potentially harmful event.

Elements of Performance for PC.13.20

1. Sufficient numbers of qualified staff are available* to evaluate the patient, perform the procedure, monitor, and recover the patient.

2. *Individuals administering moderate or deep sedation and anesthesia are qualified† and have the appropriate credentials to manage patients at whatever level of sedation or anesthesia is achieved, either intentionally or unintentionally.*

3. *A registered nurse supervises perioperative nursing care.*

4. *Appropriate equipment to monitor the patient's physiologic status is available.*

5. *Appropriate equipment to administer intravenous fluids and drugs, including blood and blood components, is available as needed.*

6. *Resuscitation capabilities are available.*

Before operative and other procedures or the administration of moderate or deep sedation or anesthesia:

7. Patient acuity is assessed to plan for the appropriate level of postprocedure care.

8. Preprocedural education, treatments, and services are provided according to the plan for care, treatment, and services.

9. The site, procedure, and patient are accurately identified and clearly communicated, using active communication techniques, during a final verification process, such as "time out," prior to the start of any surgical or invasive procedure.

10. A presedation or preanesthesia assessment is conducted.

11. *Before sedating or anesthetizing a patient, a licensed independent practitioner with appropriate clinical privileges plans or concurs with the planned anesthesia.*

12. *The patient is reevaluated immediately before moderate or deep sedation and before anesthesia induction.*

Standard PC.13.30
Patients are monitored during the procedure and/or administration of moderate or deep sedation or anesthesia.

Elements of Performance for PC.13.30

1. *Appropriate methods are used to continuously monitor oxygenation, ventilation, and circulation during procedures that may affect the patient's physiological status.*

2. *The procedure and/or administration of moderate or deep sedation or anesthesia for each patient are documented in the medical record.*

---

*For hospitals providing obstetric or emergency operative services, this means they can provide anesthesia services as required by law and regulation.

†**Qualified** The individuals providing moderate or deep sedation and anesthesia have at a minimum had competency-based education, training, and experience in the following:

1. Evaluating patients before moderate or deep sedation and anesthesia.

2. Performing the moderate or deep sedation and anesthesia, including rescuing patients who slip into a deeper-than-desired level of sedation or analgesia. This includes the following:

 a. *Moderate* sedation – are qualified to rescue patients from deep sedation and are competent to manage a compromised airway and to provide adequate oxygenation and ventilation.

 b. *Deep* sedation – are qualified to rescue patients from general anesthesia and are competent to manage an unstable cardiovascular system as well as a compromised airway and inadequate oxygenation and ventilation.

© Joint Commission: Standards for Operative or Other High-Risk Procedures and/or the Administration of Moderate or Deep Sedation or Anesthesia, January, 2004. Reprinted with permission.

Practice Guidelines for Sedation and Analgesia by Non-Anesthesiologists
American Society of Anesthesiologists Task Force on Sedation and Analgesia by Non-Anesthesiologists

Recommendations. Monitoring of patient response to verbal commands should be routine during moderate sedation, except in patients who are unable to respond appropriately (e.g., young children, mentally impaired or uncooperative patients), or during procedures where movement could be detrimental. During deep sedation, patient responsiveness to a more profound stimulus should be sought, unless contraindicated, to ensure that the patient has not drifted into a state of general anesthesia. During procedures where a verbal response is not possible (e.g., oral surgery, upper endoscopy), the ability to give a "thumbs up" or other indication of consciousness in response to verbal or tactile (light tap) stimulation suggests that the patient will be able to control his airway and take deep breaths if necessary, corresponding to a state of moderate sedation. Note that a response limited to reflex withdrawal from a painful stimulus is not considered a purposeful response and thus represents a state of general anesthesia.

All patients undergoing sedation/analgesia should be monitored by pulse oximetry with appropriate alarms. If available, the variable pitch "beep," which gives a continuous audible indication of the oxygen saturation reading, may be helpful. In addition, ventilatory function should be continually monitored by observation or auscultation. Monitoring of exhaled carbon dioxide should be considered for all patients receiving deep sedation and for patients whose ventilation cannot be directly observed during moderate sedation. When possible, blood pressure should be determined before sedation/analgesia is initiated. Once sedation/analgesia is established, blood pressure should be measured at 5-minute intervals during the procedure, unless such monitoring interferes with the procedure (e.g., pediatric magnetic resonance imaging, where stimulation from the blood pressure cuff could arouse an appropriately sedated patient). Electrocardiographic monitoring should be used in all patients undergoing deep sedation. It should also be used during moderate sedation in patients with significant cardiovascular disease or those who are undergoing procedures where dysrhythmias are anticipated.

Recommendations. For both moderate and deep sedation, patients' level of consciousness, ventilatory and oxygenation status, and hemodynamic variables should be assessed and recorded at a frequency that depends on the type and amount of medication administered, the length of the procedure, and the general condition of the patient. At a minimum this should be: (1) before the beginning of the procedure; (2) after the administration of sedative/analgesic agents; (3) at regular intervals during the procedure; (4) during initial recovery; and (5) just before discharge. If recording is performed automatically, device alarms should be set to alert the care team to critical changes in patient status.

Recommendation. A designated individual, other than the practitioner performing the procedure, should be present to monitor the patient throughout procedures performed with sedation/analgesia. During deep sedation, this individual should have no other responsibilities. However, during moderate sedation, this individual may assist with minor, interruptible tasks once the patient's level of sedation/analgesia and vital signs have stabilized, provided that adequate monitoring for the patient's level of sedation is maintained.

Recommendations. Individuals responsible for patients receiving sedation/analgesia should understand the pharmacology of the agents that are administered as well as the role of pharmacologic antagonists for opioids and benzodiazepines. Individuals monitoring patients receiving sedation/analgesia should be able to recognize the associated complications. At least one individual capable of establishing a patent airway and positive-pressure ventilation, as well as a means for summoning additional assistance, should be present whenever sedation/analgesia is administered. It is recommended that an individual with advanced life support skills be immediately available (within 5 minutes) for moderate sedation and within the procedure room for deep sedation.

Recommendations. Pharmacologic antagonists as well as appropriately sized equipment for establishing a patent airway and providing positive-pressure ventilation with supplemental oxygenation should be present whenever sedation/analgesia is administered. Suction, advanced airway equipment, and resuscitation medications should be immediately available and in good working order. A functional defibrillator should be immediately available whenever deep sedation is administered and when moderate sedation is administered to patients with mild or severe cardiovascular disease.

Recommendations. Equipment to administer supplemental oxygen should be present when sedation/analgesia is administered. Supplemental oxygen should be considered for moderate sedation and should be administered during deep sedation unless specifically contraindicated for a particular patient or procedure. If hypoxemia is anticipated or develops during sedation/analgesia, supplemental oxygen should be administered.

Recommendations. Specific antagonists should be available whenever opioid analgesics or benzodiazepines are administered for sedation/analgesia. Naloxone or flumazenil may be administered to improve spontaneous ventilatory efforts in patients who have received opioids or benzodiazepines, respectively. This may be especially helpful in cases where airway control and positive-pressure ventilation are difficult. Before or concomitantly with pharmacologic reversal, patients who become hypoxemic or apneic during sedation/analgesia should: (1) be encouraged or stimulated to breathe deeply; (2) receive supplemental oxygen; and (3) receive positive-pressure ventilation if spontaneous ventilation is inadequate. After pharmacologic reversal, patients should be observed long enough to ensure that sedation and cardiorespiratory depression does not recur once the effect of the antagonist dissipates. The use of sedation regimens that include routine reversal of sedative or analgesic agents is discouraged.

From American Society of Anesthesiologists Task Force on Sedation and Analgesia by Non-Anesthesiologists. Practice guidelines for sedation and analgesia by non-anesthesiologists. *Anesthesiology.* 2002;96(4):1008-1012. Reprinted with permission.

Once the presedation assessment is completed, the patient is readied for the procedure. To avoid catastrophic mishaps and to comply with promulgated practice standards, practice guidelines, position statements, and specific state statutes, familiarity with monitoring equipment and interpretation of data is required. The monitoring process involves the following:

◆ Observation and vigilance
◆ Interpretation of data
◆ Initiation of corrective action when required

Therefore, it is important that the practitioner administering sedation/analgesia is educated and competent in the use of monitoring devices while incorporating his or her objective and subjective clinical assessment skills.

ELECTROCARDIOGRAM

The ECG is used during sedation/analgesia procedures to assist in the detection of the following conditions:

◆ Dysrhythmias
◆ Myocardial ischemia
◆ Electrolyte disturbance
◆ Pacemaker function

ECG Leads

The ECG reflects the electrical activity of the heart in graphic form. Electrodes pick up electrical signals generated by the heart's conduction system. Electrodes may be placed on the four limbs and six areas on the chest. ECG monitoring is useful in the evaluation of the pathophysiologic condition of the entire heart, with detection of cardiac rhythm disturbances and conduction disorders. The majority of ECG monitors depict cardiac electrical activity through a single lead. Lead position is determined by placement of positive and negative electrodes secured to the patient. The standard leads view the frontal plane of the heart with differences in electrical potential recorded in the left arm, the right arm, and the left leg.[1] Standard bipolar limb leads include the following:

◆ Lead I: Difference in electrical potential between the left arm and the right arm.
◆ Lead II: Difference in electrical potential between the left leg and the right arm.
◆ Lead III: Difference in electrical potential between the left leg and the left arm.

Figure 6-1 depicts the electrical potential for each bipolar limb lead.

Unipolar leads (Fig. 6-2) reflect the electrical potential between the designated extremity lead and a neutral electrical point at the center of the heart.[1] The three augmented leads view the heart in the frontal plane by means of the same three limbs in different combinations. The augmented or unipolar limb leads include the following:

◆ aVR: Augmented voltage of the right arm. The right arm is positive compared with the left arm and the left leg.
◆ aVL: Augmented voltage of the left arm. The left arm is positive compared with the right arm and the left leg.

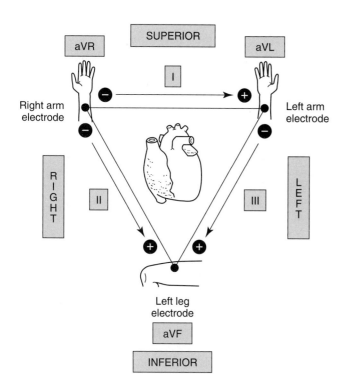

FIGURE 6-1 Electrical potential for bipolar limb leads.

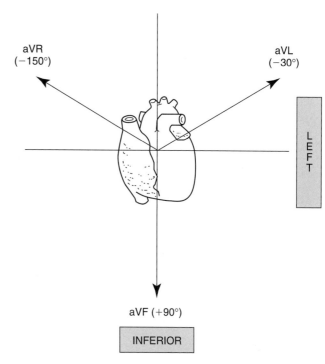

FIGURE 6-2 Electrical activity of unipolar limb leads.

◆ aVF: Augmented voltage of the left foot. The left foot is positive compared with the right arm and the left arm.

The unipolar precordial leads measure the heart's electrical activity in the horizontal planes.

◆ Leads V_1 and V_2 are placed over the right ventricle.
◆ V_3 and V_4 are placed over the interventricular septum.
◆ V_5 and V_6 are placed over the left ventricle.

Positioning of the precordial leads is depicted in Figure 6-3.

One lead (lead I, II, or III) of the standard bipolar limb leads is generally selected for procedural monitoring and recovery. Optimal ECG tracings depend on proper placement of two sensory electrodes and a ground or reference electrode. To obtain an accurate recording, gelled electrodes must be applied to clean, dry skin. **For sedation procedures, lead II is beneficial to detect the presence of dysrhythmias, primarily because of the increased visibility of the P wave in this lead.** An important rationale for use of the ECG is to assess for the presence of myocardial ischemia. Indicators for myocardial ischemia are depicted in Box 6-1. In situations that afford only three lead monitoring systems, a modified chest lead (MCL) may be used to monitor for the presence of myocardial ischemia. MCL electrode placement is depicted in Figure 6-4.

When indicated (coronary artery disease, angina, left ventricular dysfunction), lead V_5 is used to detect ischemia. Because a large portion of the left ventricle is located beneath the V_5 position, it is a useful lead for detection of myocardial ischemia.

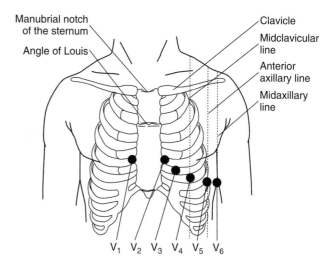

FIGURE 6-3 Placement of precordial leads.

BOX 6-1

Indicators of Myocardial Ischemia

Another important rationale for utilization of the ECG is to assess for the presence of myocardial ischemia. Myocardial ischemic indicators include:

ST-Segment Elevation
Acute myocardial infarction may be associated with ST-segment elevation. ST-segment changes may range from minor peaking or widening of the T wave to pronounced ST-segment elevation. ST-segment elevation is associated with acute ischemic injury.

ST-Segment Depression
Ischemia of the subendocardial layer of the myocardium results in ST-segment depression. Ischemia is reflected as depression of the ST-segment because the chest electrodes do not face the subendocardial layers of the heart.

T-Wave Inversion
T-wave inversion generally follows ST-segment elevation and is associated with continued myocardial ischemia.

Cardiac Rhythm and Dysrhythmias

The cardiac cycle is associated with five distinct waves or deflections as defined in Box 6-2 and depicted in Figure 6-5. Figure 6-6 compares the cardiac cycle and ECG time measurements. Alterations or variations of this cardiac cycle may represent dysrhythmias and lead to the associated symptoms presented in this chapter. The presentation of cardiac rhythms on pages 137 to 146 is intended to serve as a review of common and life-threatening dysrhythmias. A summary of these rhythm disturbances and their treatment protocol is provided in Table 6-1. It is strongly recommended that these materials be used as a reference tool and as a supplement to Advanced Cardiac Life Support (ACLS) training and treatment protocols. Although many state statutes require ACLS course completion and many specialty organizations recommend ACLS training, it is not a uniform requirement in all facilities. As Dr. Richard Cummins, chairman of the Subcommittee on Advanced Cardiac Life Support, stated: *"ACLS is about preparing yourself to provide the best possible care for the most dramatic and emotional moment of a person's life."*[2]

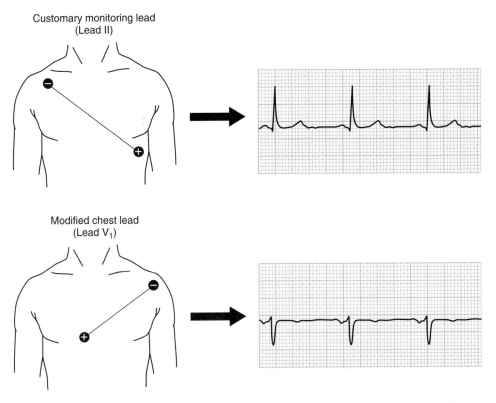

Customary monitoring lead
(Lead II)

Modified chest lead
(Lead V₁)

FIGURE 6-4 MCL electrode positioning places the right arm lead under the left clavicle and the left arm in the V₅ position. The left leg lead is placed in the standard V₁ position. (From Meltzer L. *Intensive Coronary Care: A Manual for Nurses.* 4th ed. East Norwalk, CT: Appleton & Lange; 1983:121.)

BOX 6-2

Cardiac Cycle

- **P wave:** Represents atrial depolarization and impulse generation from the sinoatrial node through the atrioventricular node.
- **PR interval:** Represents the length of time required for the atria to depolarize and delay of the impulse through the atrioventricular junction. Normally measures 0.12 to 0.20 second.
- **QRS complex:** Represents ventricular depolarization (phase 0 of the action potential).
    - Q wave = first negative deflection after P wave.
    - R wave = first positive deflection after P wave.
    - The QRS normally measures 0.04 to 1 second.
    - S wave = the negative deflection following the R wave.
- **ST-segment:** Represents early repolarization of the right and left ventricles. Begins at the end of the QRS complex and ends with onset of the T wave.
- **T wave:** Represents ventricular repolarization. Peaked T waves are seen in patients with hyperkalemia.
- **QT interval:** Represents total ventricular activity (depolarization and repolarization). Measured from the beginning of the QRS complex to the end of the T wave. Normally measures 0.36 to 0.44 second (varies with heart rate, age, and sex).

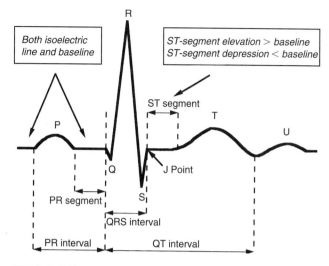

FIGURE 6-5 Waveforms of the cardiac cycle. The small boxes represent 0.04 second. Each large box is made of five small boxes and represents 0.20 second. An event that takes 0.08 second would create a line two small boxes long. (From Atlee J. *Arrhythmias and Pacemakers.* Philadelphia: WB Saunders; 1996:108.)

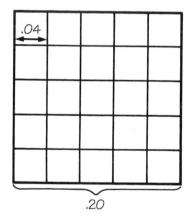

The small boxes represent 0.04 second. Each large box is made of five small boxes and represents 0.20 second.

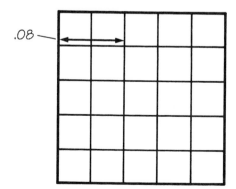

An event that takes 0.08 second would create a line two small boxes long.

FIGURE 6-6 The cardiac cycle and electrocardiograph time measurements. (From Cohn E, Gilroy-Doohan M. *Flip and See ECG.* Philadelphia: WB Saunders; 1996:44.)

TABLE 6-1

Causes and Treatments of Cardiac Dysrhythmias

RHYTHM AND CHARACTERISTICS	CONTRIBUTING/PREDISPOSING FACTORS	CLINICAL SYMPTOMS AND SIGNS	TREATMENTS/NOTES
Sinus Tachycardia (ST) Normal complex sinus rate of 100-150 bpm. Usually secondary to factors outside the heart.	Exercise, fever, anxiety, hypovolemia	Palpitations, hypotension, signs and symptoms of congestive heart failure, decreased level of consciousness, persistent chest pain	Never treat tachycardia, treat the cause of it. Fluid/electrolyte replacement, analgesics, sedation, emotional support Dangerous to give drug therapy without determining cause because severe hypotension may occur. Propranolol if cardiac ischemia. Do NOT give digitalis unless cause is CHF.
Premature Atrial Contractions (PACs) Beat initiated by an ectopic atrial focus and appears early in the cycle (before the next sinus beat is expected). P waves differ in shape because the impulse is from a site other than the sinus node and the PR interval may vary.	May be indicative of atrial irritability from distention, stress, or heart disease. May initiate atrial tachydysrhythmias. Electrolyte imbalance, COPD, nicotine, anxiety, caffeine, drug toxicity.	Usually asymptomatic	Asymptomatic patients need no treatment. Occasionally procainamide, quinidine, propranolol, and digitalis are used.
Paroxysmal Supraventricular Tachycardia (PSVT)/Paroxysmal Atrial Tachycardia (PAT) A re-entry phenomenon with abrupt episodes of tachycardia, usually between 150-250 bpm, averaging around 180 bpm. P waves may be abnormally shaped because of ectopic atrial site or may be buried in preceding T wave. May appear as VT if bundle branch block is present.	Wolff-Parkinson-White syndrome, chronic lung disease, digitalis toxicity, thyrotoxicosis. Anxiety, stress, caffeine, nicotine	Reduction in cardiac output, palpitations, dyspnea, faintness, CHF, hypotension	Vagal stimulation from a cough, Valsalva maneuver, or carotid message may terminate this. Adenosine, 6 mg IVP over 1-3 sec, should be initiated if above measures are not effective; a second or third dose of 12 mg may be tried after 1-2 min. Verapamil, 2.5-10 mg IVP (up to 10 mg). Digitalis, procainamide, and beta blockers may be used. If not effective and symptoms of myocardial ischemia, CHF, hypotension, pulmonary edema are evident, consider cardioversion. Amiodarone, 150 mg/50 mL.
Atrial Fibrillation Very fast atrial rate arising from many ectopic foci. P waves are irregularly shaped, and ventricular response is irregular. Pulse rate is rapid	Sick sinus syndrome, hypoxia, increased atrial pressure, pericarditis, COPD, atheroslerotic heart disease, pulmonary embolism, hyperthyroidism, CHF	CHF, hypotension, angina	Rate control is initial treatment: diltiazem, verapamil, beta blockers, or digoxin. Chemical cardioversion after anticoagulation can be achieved with procainamide or quinidine.

TABLE 6-1

Causes and Treatments of Cardiac Dysrhythmias—cont'd

RHYTHM AND CHARACTERISTICS	CONTRIBUTING/PREDISPOSING FACTORS	CLINICAL SYMPTOMS AND SIGNS	TREATMENTS/NOTES
Atrial Fibrillation—cont'd (160-220 bpm) or slow, depending on ventricular response.			Electrical cardioversion is the third alternative; however, in symptomatic patients with new onset of short duration (1-3 days), this is treatment of choice. Amiodarone, 150 mg/50 mL over 10-30 min.
Atrial Flutter P waves have characteristic "sawtooth" appearance. A result of re-entry circuit within atria. QRS usually regular with an AV block at 2:1, 3:1, 4:1 ratio.	Less common than atrial fibrillation. Anxiety, movement, and excitement can trigger this.	Hypotension, CHF, decreased cardiac output, dizziness, faintness	Digitalis often used to decrease ventricular rate by blocking AV node. Synchronized cardioversion is treatment of choice in unstable patients.
1st Degree AV Block A delay in passage of impulse from atria to ventricles. PR interval is >0.21 sec.		Usually asymptomatic	No treatment except observation.
Mobitz Type I Second-Degree AV Block (Wenckebach's Block) PR intervals become progressively longer until a ventricular beat is missed, in a consistent pattern. PR interval is irregular and there are more P waves than QRS complexes.	Increased parasympathetic tone or drug effect (digitalis, propranolol, or verapamil). May be caused by inferior wall MI causing AV node ischemia	Usually asymptomatic	Treatment rarely needed unless symptoms are present.
Mobitz Type II Second-Degree AV Block Occurs below the AV node at either the Bundle of His (uncommon) or the bundle branches (common). Some beats are conducted while others are not, often in a ratio of atrial to ventricular beats of 2:1 or 3:1. Conducted beats have consistent PR interval; in blocked beats, there is a P wave not followed by a QRS complex.	Organic lesion in the conduction system; rarely the result of increased parasympathetic tone or drug effect	May be faint, weak, tired	Atropine is often ineffective. Artificial pacemaker is first line of therapy.

TABLE 6-1

Causes and Treatments of Cardiac Dysrhythmias—cont'd

RHYTHM AND CHARACTERISTICS	CONTRIBUTING/PREDISPOSING FACTORS	CLINICAL SYMPTOMS AND SIGNS	TREATMENTS/NOTES
Third-Degree AV Block/Complete Heart Block			
No connection between atria and ventricles. Atrial rate is always equal or faster than ventricular rate. Rate depends on whether the heart is being driven by nodal (40-50 bpm) or ventricular (30-40 bpm) area.	Infranodal conduction system disease, atherosclerosis, extensive anterior wall MI	Hypotension, decreased cardiac output, weakness	Atropine, transcutaneous pacemaker, catecholamine infusions (dopamine or epinephrine). Isoproterenol is rarely indicated.
Premature Ventricular Contractions (PVCs)			
Sign of irritability in the ventricles. Appear as wide, bizarre QRS complexes, occurring early in the cycle and not preceded by a P wave. T wave is usually in opposite direction and followed by full compensatory pause (the duration of two cycles, including the PVC, is the same as the duration of two normal cycles). Unifocal PVCs originate from same site and have same configuration; multifocal PVCs arise from different sites and have different appearance from each other.	Hypoxia, cardiac disease, anxiety, pain, hypercarbia, mitral valve prolapse, nicotine, hypokalemia, halothane, succinylcholine, digitalis toxicity, irritation from endotracheal tube		Lidocaine is drug of choice. Procainamide may be used. Acute onset should be monitored for underlying cause. Chronic PVCs, usually related to underlying heart disease and producing no symptoms, do not require treatment
Ventricular Tachycardia (VT)			
Series of three or more consecutive PVCs occurring at a rate of 150-200 bpm	Myocardial irritability	Decreases cardiac output, may lead to ventricular fibrillation, especially if PVC falls on the T wave	In hemodynamically stable patient, treat with lidocaine bolus of 1-1.5 mg/kg. A second bolus may be given after 5 min for total of 3 mg/kg. Procainamide, 20 mg/min up to 17 mg/kg, or amiodarone, 150 mg/50 mL over 10 to 30 minutes. In unstable patient with a pulse, synchronized cardioversion often suppresses VT. In pulseless VT, follow the V-fib algorithm.

TABLE 6-1

Causes and Treatments of Cardiac Dysrhythmias—cont'd

RHYTHM AND CHARACTERISTICS	CONTRIBUTING/PREDISPOSING FACTORS	CLINICAL SYMPTOMS AND SIGNS	TREATMENTS/NOTES
Ventricular Fibrillation (V-fib)			
Most common dysrhythmia in adult cardiac arrest. Uncoordinated, irregular, chaotic rhythm; no P wave, and QRS complexes are bizarre waves with no relationship to each other	Myocardial irritability R on T phenomenon	Pulseless state No cardiac output	Defibrillate with 200 J (watt-sec) to start, increase to 300 and 360 J. Alternate defibrillation with drug therapy; epinephrine or vasopressin followed by amiodarone, lidocaine, magnesium, or procainamide. Calcium and magnesium are given when a deficiency is suspected.
Asystole			
No electrical activity noted on ECG; may be slightly wavy line	Alfentanil toxicity may be transient with second dose of succinylcholine	Pulseless state Must be verified in two ECG leads	Initiate CPR. Apply pacemaker as soon as possible. Atropine and epinephrine are drugs of choice. Look for possible causes.
Pulseless Electrical Activity (PEA)			
Electrical conduction present but no mechanical action of the heart is detectable	Massive MI, drug overdose, pulmonary embolus, acidosis, tension pneumothorax, cardiac tamponade, hypothermia, hypoxemia, hyperkalemia, hypovolemia	No palpable pulse	Identify and treat initial cause. Initiate CPR. Epinephrine and atropine are first-line drugs.

bpm, beats per minute; *CHF,* congestive heart failure; *VT,* ventricular tachycardia; *COPD,* chronic obstructive pulmonary disease; *AV,* atrioventricular; *MI,* myocardial infarction; *CPR,* cardiopulmonary resuscitation.
From Burden N: *Ambulatory Surgical Nursing,* ed 2. Data from *Cummins* R (ed). *Advanced Cardiac Life Support.* Dallas: American Heart Association; 2000.

RHYTHMS
Normal Sinus Rhythm (NSR)

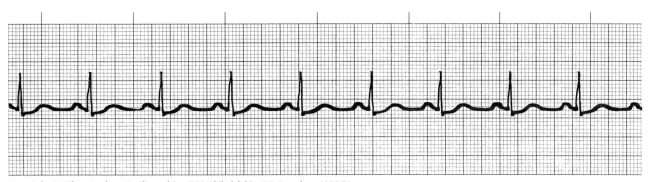

From Cohn E, Gilroy-Doohan M. *Flip and See ECG.* Philadelphia: WB Saunders; 1996:71.

Etiology: Each complex is complete and consists of one P wave, QRS complex, and T wave. There are no wide, bizarre, ectopic, late, or premature complexes.

Rate: 60 to 100 beats per minute

Rhythm: Regular

P waves: Uniform and upright in appearance. One P wave precedes each QRS complex, and the interval between P waves is constant.

PR interval: 0.12 to 0.20 second

QRS: 0.04 to 0.10 second

Treatment: None required

Sinus Tachycardia (ST)

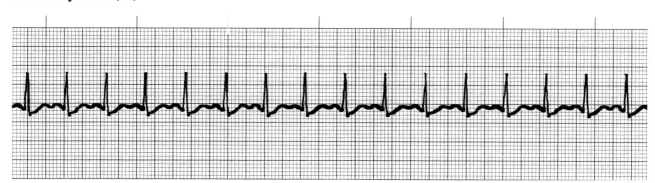

From Cohn E, Gilroy-Doohan M. *Flip and See ECG.* Philadelphia: WB Saunders; 1996:77.

Etiology: The sinoatrial (SA) node in the atria discharges at a rate greater than 100 beats per minute. Very rapid rates decrease cardiac output secondary to reduced cardiac filling. Factors that increase heart rate include fever, pain, hypoxia, sepsis, anxiety, myocardial ischemia, exercise, or increased sympathetic nervous system activity. Each complex is complete, consisting of a P wave, a QRS complex, and a T wave. The P wave may be buried in the previous T wave. There are no bizarre, wide, ectopic, early, or late complexes.

Rate: 100 to 160 beats per minute

Rhythm: Regular

P waves: Uniform and upright in appearance. One P wave precedes each QRS complex. 1:1 with QRS complex. The interval between P waves is constant.

PR interval: 0.12 to 0.20 second

QRS: 0.04 to 0.10 second

Comments: Normal response to increased demand for O_2 due to fever, pain, anxiety, hypoxia, congestive heart failure (CHF), fright, stress, and so on.

Signs/Symptoms: In most cases, sinus tachycardia is asymptomatic. An attempt must be made to ascertain the underlying cause. Once recognized, treatment is directed at the causative factor (e.g., fever, anxiety, hypovolemia).

Treatment: Directed at correcting the underlying cause. *Fever:* acetylsalicylic acid (ASA), acetaminophen, cooling. *Pain:* opioids, nonsteroidal anti-inflammatory drugs (NSAIDs). *Hypovolemia:* volume infusion. *Medications:* reversal or washout.

Sinus Bradycardia (SB)

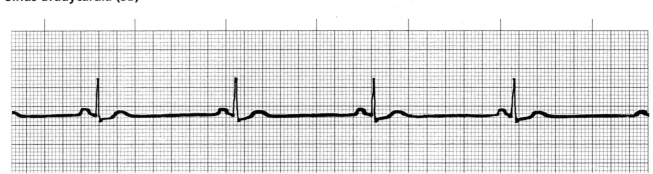

From Cohn E, Gilroy-Doohan M. *Flip and See ECG.* Philadelphia: WB Saunders; 1996:75.

Etiology: The SA node emits impulses at a rate less than 60 beats per minute. Each complex is complete, consisting of a P wave, a QRS complex, and a T wave. All intervals are within normal limits except heart rate. Parasympathetic dominance of the autonomic nervous system occurs. Sinus bradycardia is associated with pain, beta blockade, vagal stimulation, and myocardial infarction.

Rate: Less than 60 beats per minute

Rhythm: Regular

P waves: Uniform and upright in appearance. One P wave precedes each QRS complex. 1:1 with each QRS complex. The interval between the P waves is constant.

PR interval: 0.12 to 0.20 second

QRS: 0.04 to 0.10 second

Comments: Normal in conditioned athletes. May be due to a variety of factors, which include enhanced vagal tone, parasympathetic dominance of the autonomic nervous system, vomiting, straining, sinoatrial nodal disease, increased intraocular pressure, or increased intracranial pressure. Often seen after acute inferior myocardial infarction or in patients taking beta blockers, quinidine, or verapamil and some calcium channel blockers.

Signs/Symptoms: May be asymptomatic. Fatigue, hypotension, and syncope are associated with decreased cardiac output.

Treatment: Sinus bradycardia should be treated when signs and symptoms of decreased cardiac output occur (syncope, unconsciousness) or ventricular ectopy develops. If symptomatic:

◆ Assess airway
◆ Discontinue procedural or diagnostic stimulation (e.g., colonoscopy, endoscopy, hypoxia), which may correlate with the onset of bradycardia.
◆ The presence of severe pain may also enhance vagal tone. Stimulation may need to be decreased or discontinued, or additional analgesia may have to be administered. For additional treatment modalities, see Table 6-1.

Sinus Arrhythmia (SA)

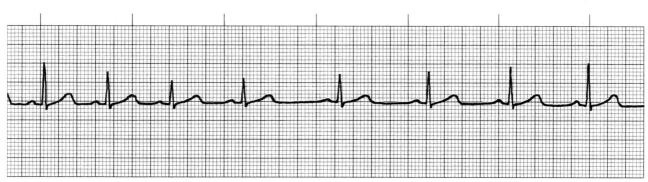

From Cohn E, Gilroy-Doohan M. *Flip and See ECG.* Philadelphia: WB Saunders; 1996:73.

Etiology: The sinoatrial node discharges at an irregular rate. The rate of discharge is influenced by the respiratory pattern and the degree of parasympathetic nervous system (vagal) control over the SA node. Each complex is complete, consisting of a P wave, a QRS complex, and a T wave. All intervals are within normal limits except the RR interval.

Rate: Usually 60 to 100 beats per minute; however, the rate may be faster or slower. During inspiration the heart rate increases, whereas expiration produces a decrease in heart rate.

Rhythm: Irregular

P waves: Uniform and upright in appearance. One P wave precedes each QRS complex. The interval between P waves is not constant.

PR interval: 0.12 to 0.20 second

QRS: Less than 0.10 second

Comments: Common in children and physically fit adults. Reflex vagal stimulation is related to the normal respiratory cycle. Sinus arrhythmia is a natural variation caused by normal breathing.

Signs/Symptoms: The patient is generally unaware of the underlying rhythm. Although characterized by its irregularity, the rhythm possesses essentially normal waveform morphology.

Treatment: Generally, no treatment is required. Continued procedural and postsedation monitoring is warranted by patient condition.

Premature Atrial Complexes/Contractions (PACs)

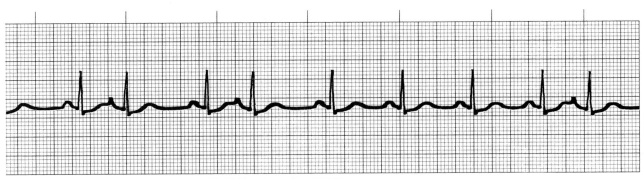

From Cohn E, Gilroy-Doohan M. *Flip and See ECG*. Philadelphia: WB Saunders; 1996:79.

Etiology:	PACs occur secondary to irritable ectopic foci in the atrium discharging prior to the SA node. Isolated PACs are frequently inconsequential. An increase in the rate of PACs may signify impending atrial fibrillation or flutter secondary to irritability of the atrial musculature.
Rate:	Usually normal, but varies depending on the number of extra atrial beats that are created and the rate of the underlying rhythm.
Rhythm:	Irregular because of the PAC.
P wave:	P wave of the early beat differs from the sinus P waves. The wave is premature and may be lost in the preceding T wave. 1:1 with the QRS complex.
PR interval:	Varies from 0.12 to 0.20 second when the pacemaker site is near the SA node to 0.23 second when the pacemaker site is closer to the atrioventricular (AV) node.
QRS:	Usually less than 0.12 second but may be prolonged if underlying bundle branch block or aberrant conduction.
Comments:	The most distinguishing feature of an ectopic beat arising in the atria (PAC) is that the configuration of

the premature P wave differs from the other P waves. The P wave may also be obscured by the preceding T waves, particularly if the PAC occurs soon after the previous beat.

Signs/Symptoms:	The patient may be unaware of the underlying rhythm. Premature atrial complexes are frequently diagnosed when ECG monitoring commences immediately before the procedure. PACs may be elicited by ingestion of caffeine, tobacco, or alcohol; hypoxia; anxiety; or atrial enlargement.
Treatment:	Identification of underlying cause. Rare PACs require no treatment. If PACs are increasing in frequency (>6 per minute), it may be beneficial to complete the procedure as soon as feasible. Medical consultation may be indicated to prevent the development of atrial tachycardia or atrial fibrillation/flutter and to ascertain the cause of the atrial irritability. For additional treatment modalities, see Table 6-1.

Supraventricular Tachycardia (SVT)

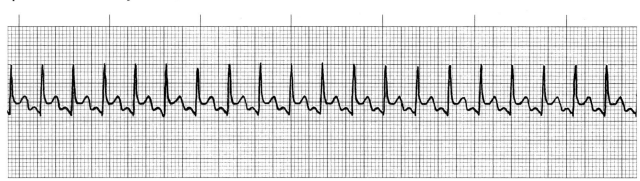

From Cohn E, Gilroy-Doohan M. *Flip and See ECG*. Philadelphia: WB Saunders; 1996:87.

Etiology: Like PACs, SVT occurs secondary to atrial irritability. SVT occurs at an atrial discharge rate between 150 and 250 beats per minute. Ectopic foci override the sinoatrial node with a corresponding ventricular response for each atrial impulse conducted.

Rate: 150 to 250 beats per minute

Rhythm: Regular

P waves: Atrial P waves differ from sinus P waves. P waves are generally identified at the lower end of the rate range but seldom are identified at rates greater than 200 beats per minute.

PR interval: Usually not measurable because the P wave is difficult to distinguish from the preceding T wave. If measurable, the PR interval is 0.12 to 0.20 second.

QRS: Less than 0.12 second but may be prolonged if bundle branch block or aberrant conduction.

Comments: Common causes are physical or psychologic stress, hypoxia, epinephrine in the local anesthetic solution, and excessive caffeine intake. Also may occur in patients with rheumatic heart disease, coronary artery disease, digitalis toxicity, and respiratory failure.

Signs/Symptoms: Because of decreased ventricular filling time, signs and symptoms of decreased cardiac output (hypotension, syncope) may occur. Sudden feelings of palpitations, lightheadedness, and severe anxiety are common. In patients with underlying heart disease, congestive heart failure, angina, or shock may occur as a result of decreased cardiac output. Myocardial oxygen consumption increases in response to the tachycardic state.

Treatment: Monitor patient for signs and symptoms of congestive heart failure or shock. *Stable:* Administer oxygen, establish intravenous line, vagal maneuvers, pharmacologic intervention. *Unstable:* Administer oxygen, intravenous medications. Additional treatment modalities are identified in Table 6-1.

Atrial Flutter (A-Flutter)

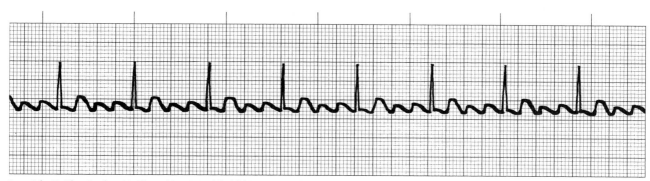

From Cohn E, Gilroy-Doohan M. *Flip and See ECG.* Philadelphia: WB Saunders; 1996:83.

Etiology: Atrial flutter occurs secondary to rapid ectopic atrial discharge at a rate of 250 to 350 beats per minute. Because of this rapid ectopic rate, the ventricle cannot respond to each impulse. However, the ventricle will selectively respond to impulses and contract. According to the number of atrial impulses discharged before ventricular contraction, atrial flutter is referred to as 2:1, 3:1, or 4:1 flutter.

Rate: Atrial rate is 250 to 350 beats per minute. Ventricular rate is variable, depending on conduction through to the ventricle.

Rhythm: Atrial rhythm is regular. Ventricular rhythm is usually regular with constant conduction ratio but may be irregular.

P waves: Saw-toothed *"F"* or *"flutter waves."*

PR interval: None, not measurable.

QRS: Usually 0.04 to 0.12 second but may be widened. Flutter waves are buried in the QRS complex.

Comments: Clinical significance of this rhythm depends on the ventricular response rate. The more rapid the rate, the more serious the dysrhythmia. Seldom occurs in the absence of organic heart disease. Seen in association with mitral or tricuspid valve disorders, digitalis toxicity, pericarditis, and inferior wall myocardial infarction.

Signs/Symptoms: The patient may report a sense of palpitations. If ventricular filling and coronary artery blood flow are compromised, symptoms of decreased cardiac output may become clinically evident.

Treatment: Hemodynamically stable patients generally require no initial treatment. Ventricular rates that are rapid may be terminated with cardioversion (50 watt sec), digitalis, or beta blockade. For additional treatment modalities, see Table 6-1.

Atrial Fibrillation (A-Fib)

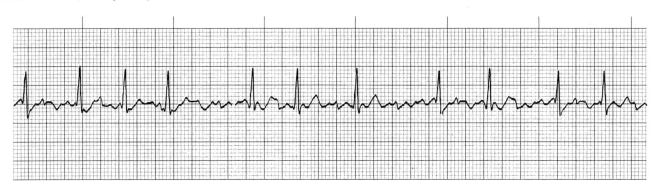

From Cohn E, Gilroy-Doohan M. *Flip and See ECG.* Philadelphia: WB Saunders; 1996:85.

Etiology: Rapid atrial ectopic foci discharge at a rate of 350 to 600 bpm. The atria fibrillate in an unsynchronized fashion. This fibrillation can result in a 20% to 30% reduction in cardiac output secondary to decreased diastolic filling time and loss of atrial contribution.

Rate: Atrial rate usually greater than 400. Ventricular rate variable: less than 100 = controlled, greater than 100 = uncontrolled.

Rhythm: Atrial and ventricular rhythm is very irregular (regular, bradycardic ventricular rhythm may occur as a result of digitalis toxicity).

P waves: No identifiable P waves; erratic, wavy baseline

PR interval: None

QRS: Usually 0.04 to 0.12 second

Comments: Erratic, wavy, chaotic baseline. Inefficient movement of blood in the atria predisposes the patient to stroke secondary to cardioemboli. It may occur intermittently or as a chronic rhythm. Additional predisposing factors include myocardial infarction, chronic obstructive pulmonary disease, coronary artery disease, congestive heart failure, cardiac valve disorders, rheumatic heart disease.

Signs/Symptoms: Asymptomatic, or the patient may sense palpitations. If underlying heart disease exists, then signs of decreased cardiac output may be present. In patients with a history of coronary artery disease, angina may manifest as the primary patient complaint.

Treatment: Treatment is dependent on clinical presentation and ventricular rate. The goal of therapy is to convert to normal sinus rhythm, reduction of the ventricular rate to less than 100, and restoration of atrial kick. Additional treatment modalities are identified in Table 6-1.

Junctional Rhythm

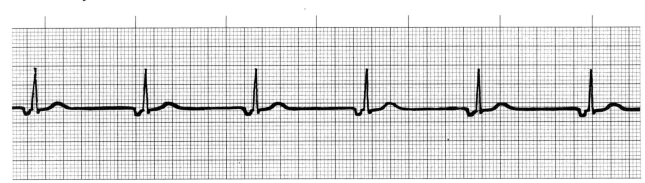

From Cohn E, Gilroy-Doohan M. *Flip and See ECG.* Philadelphia: WB Saunders; 1996:93.

Etiology: Junctional tissue surrounding the AV node will discharge when the intrinsic rate of the SA node or atria is less than 40 to 60 beats per minute.

Rate: 40 to 60 beats per minute.

Rhythm: *Atrial:* regular when present. *Ventricular:* regular.

P waves: May occur before, during, or after the QRS complex. If P waves are present, they are often inverted (retrograde) in lead II.

PR interval: Not measurable unless P wave precedes the QRS complex. When present, generally measures 0.12 second or less.

QRS: Less than 0.12 second

Comments: The presence of a junctional rhythm (at a rate of approximately 40 beats per minute) indicates that the SA node is no longer discharging or is firing at a rate of less than 40 beats per minute. A junctional rhythm is a safety mechanism that preserves the heart rate if higher pacemaker sites fail. The suppression of SA nodal discharge activity may permit lower pacemaker sites to develop. Junctional rhythm often results in response to excessive vagal activity. Additional factors include ischemic damage to the SA node and digitalis or quinidine toxicity.

Signs/Symptoms: A junctional rhythm seldom produces symptoms unless the rate is very slow (<40 beats per minute).

Treatment: Generally, no special drug therapy is indicated. Atropine may be successful in increasing the discharge rate of the sinoatrial node. If the slow heart rate compromises circulation, a transvenous pacemaker may be required to increase the ventricular rate and cardiac output. If ventricular ectopy develops with a junctional rhythm, rate control (atropine, cardiac pacing) can be efficacious.

Premature Ventricular Contractions (PVCs)

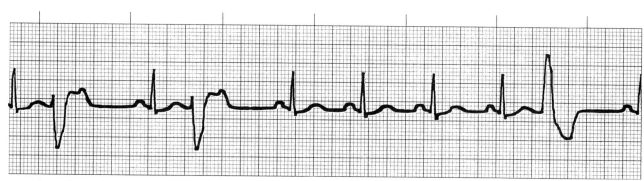

From Cohn E, Gilroy-Doohan M. *Flip and See ECG.* Philadelphia: WB Saunders; 1996:81.

Etiology: Discharge from an irritable ventricular focus before discharge of the next impulse from the SA node. The resultant wide, distorted, and bizarre ventricular complex is a result of ventricular contraction outside the normal conduction pathway.

Rate: Atrial and ventricular rate is dependent on underlying rhythm.

Rhythm: Irregular because of the premature ventricular complex.

P waves: There are no P waves associated with the PVC.

PR interval: None because the ectopic beat originates in the ventricle.

QRS: Less than 0.12 second. Wide and bizarre configuration is frequently in the opposite direction of the QRS complex.

Comments: PVCs are among the most common of all arrhythmias associated with acute myocardial infarction. PVCs signify ventricular irritability. PVCs are associated with hypoxia, electrolyte imbalance (hypokalemia), myocardial infarction, stress, chronic heart disease, and medication overdosage. It is important to treat the underlying cause, not merely the symptom (PVC). Complications associated with PVCs rest in their ability to initiate ventricular tachycardia or fibrillation.

Signs/Symptoms: Many patients are aware of PVCs and describe the sensation as "palpitations" or "skipping of the heart." When one is auscultating the heart or taking the pulse, a relatively long pause is noted immediately after the premature beat. This delay (complete compensatory pause) is characteristic and is particularly diagnostic of the arrhythmia.

Treatment: Treatment of PVCs should be considered if (1) they occur at a rate of more than six per minute; (2) they are multifocal in appearance; (3) there are two or more in a row; or (4) an R on T phenomenon occurs (PVC falls on the T wave of the preceding beat).

Continued

Supportive care is aimed at the cause of the PVCs. Treatment protocol during sedation procedures requires airway assessment, procedural correlation, frequency of PVCs, and evaluation of the patient's pain threshold. For frequent PVCs (>six per minute), common causative factors must be ruled out. The administration of lidocaine, 1 to 1.5 mg/kg (at a rate of 50 mg/min) may decrease the incidence of PVCs for a brief period of time until additional studies may ensue. For additional treatment see Table 6-1.

Ventricular Tachycardia (V-Tach, Monomorphic VT)

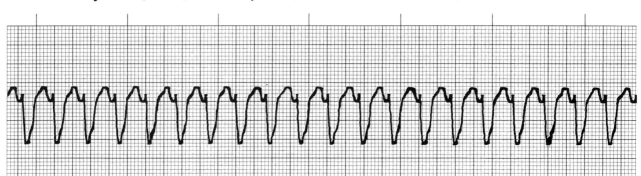

From Cohn E, Gilroy-Doohan M. *Flip and See ECG.* Philadelphia: WB Saunders; 1996:89.

Etiology:	Ventricular tachycardia occurs when three or more PVCs occur at a rate greater than 100 beats per minute. These consecutive beats signify pronounced ventricular irritability. Persistent ventricular tachycardia leads to ventricular failure, cardiogenic shock, and decreased cardiac output and cerebral blood flow with resultant cerebral ischemia.
Rate:	Atrial not discernible; ventricular 100 to 250 beats per minute.
Rhythm:	Atrial not discernible, ventricular rhythm is essentially regular.
P waves:	May be present or absent. If present, there is no set relationship to the QRS complexes. AV dissociation may be present during the ventricular tachycardia.
PR interval:	None
QRS:	Greater than 0.12 second with a bizarre configuration. Often difficult to differentiate between the QRS complex and the T wave. Three or more PVCs

occurring sequentially are referred to as a "run" of ventricular tachycardia.

Comments: May result in decreased cardiac output with potential deterioration to ventricular fibrillation. Often precipitated by R on T phenomenon, PVC, myocardial irritability due to acute myocardial infarction, coronary artery disease, congestive heart failure, or electrolyte imbalance. Development of ventricular tachycardia is also associated with toxicity from digitalis, quinidine, or procainamide.

Signs/Symptoms: If conscious, the patient may complain of palpitations, chest pain, or shortness of breath. If ventricular tachycardia is prolonged or sustained, signs and symptoms of decreased cardiac output generally occur.

Treatment: Lidocaine, 1 to 1.5 mg/kg. For additional treatment modalities, see Table 6-1.

Ventricular Fibrillation (V-Fib)

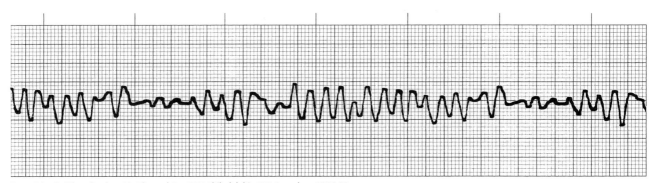

From Cohn E, Gilroy-Doohan M. *Flip and See ECG.* Philadelphia: WB Saunders; 1996:91.

Etiology: Ventricular muscle fibers, which normally contract as a single unit, lose this inherent ability. Individual ventricular muscle fibers are stimulated so rapidly that there is no recovery phase between ventricular contractions. Fibrillation is ineffective in moving blood out of the ventricles, and circulation stops. If not corrected immediately, death ensues within minutes.

Rate: Cannot be determined because there are no discernible waveforms or complexes to measure.

Rhythm: Rapid and chaotic, with no pattern or regularity.

P waves: Not discernible.

PR interval: Not discernible.

QRS: Not discernible.

Comments: Life-threatening arrhythmia. If not converted, causes death within minutes.

Signs/Symptoms: Unconsciousness, absence of pulse.

Treatment: Check vital signs; if none present, defibrillate immediately, begin cardiopulmonary resuscitation, establish intravenous line, and institute ACLS protocol. For additional treatment modalities, see Table 6-1.

Asystole ("Flat Line")

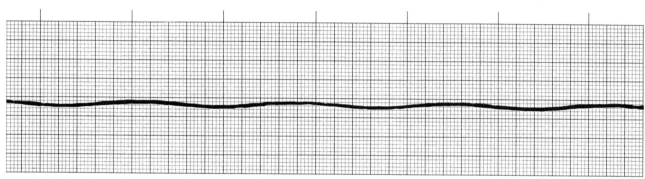

From Cohn E, Gilroy-Doohan M. *Flip and See ECG.* Philadelphia: WB Saunders; 1996:95.

Etiology: The absence of electrical impulse activity within the myocardium signifies massive myocardial ischemia. Development of asystole may be attributed to acute respiratory failure, myocardial rupture, or extensive ischemic damage.

Rate: None

Rhythm: None

P wave: None

QRS: None

PR interval: None

Comments: Always check "absence" of a rhythm in two leads and verification of lead placement.

Signs/Symptoms: Absence of pulse (check for carotid pulse), apnea, "no signs of life."

Treatment: Cardiopulmonary resuscitation; again verify rhythm in two leads; consider other causes, pacing, and pharmacologic therapy. For additional treatment modalities, see Table 6-1.

Pacemaker with Capture

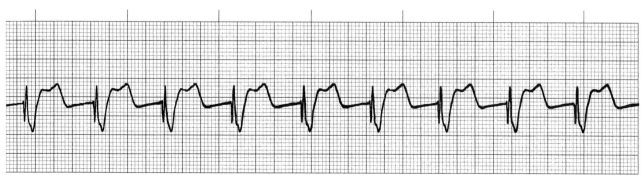

From Cohn E, Gilroy-Doohan M. *Flip and See ECG.* Philadelphia: WB Saunders; 1996:105.

Etiology: Cardiac pacemakers deliver an electrical stimulus to the heart with resultant electronic depolarization and cardiac contraction.

Rate: Overdrive pacing is used occasionally for severe tachycardia. Demand pacing is activated if the heart drops below a preset rate.

Rhythm: A variety of rhythms may occur in patients with pacemakers.

P waves: May be present or absent. P waves may or may not be associated with the QRS complex. Functional pacemakers produce spikes followed by a wide QRS complex and T wave.

Comments: A variety of pacemakers for use:
- Transcutaneous: through the skin
- Transvenous: tip of venous catheter in the right ventricle, right atrium, or both
- Transthoracic: through the anterior chest wall into the heart
- Epicardial: on the surface of the heart
- Permanent: surgically implanted inside the heart

Signs/Symptoms: Patients presenting for pacemaker insertion may have a compromised hemodynamic profile.

Treatment: Indications for pacemaker insertion include complete heart block, sick sinus syndrome, and symptomatic bradycardia.

It is strongly recommended that all team members participating in the administration of sedation and analgesia have ACLS course completion and a working knowledge of treatment algorithms.

BLOOD PRESSURE MONITORING (NONINVASIVE)

The manual blood pressure cuff applied externally provides an estimation of systolic and diastolic blood pressure. Systolic blood pressure is ascertained once the first Korotkoff sound is detected. Korotkoff sounds are a result of turbulent blood flow detected during deflation of the blood pressure cuff. Diastolic blood pressure is ascertained when the Korotkoff sounds change or disappear. Oscillotonometers are small microprocessor units that measure systolic (SBP), diastolic (DBP), and mean arterial pressure (MAP).[3]

$$MAP = (SBP + [2 \times DBP]) \div 3$$

Cuff oscillations are obtained through the sensing unit at approximately 3-mm Hg increments. The sensory unit directly measures mean blood pressure by maximal changes in cuff pressure during the deflation phase of the cycle. It is important to select the correct size cuff for the monitoring of patients receiving sedation/analgesia. The effect of blood pressure cuff width on accuracy is represented in Figure 6-7. Additional healthcare implications related to automated blood pressure cuffs are listed in Box 6-3.

Hypotension

Significant hypotension is defined as a decrease in systemic arterial blood pressure of 20% to 30%.[4] Hypotension may be caused by a variety of factors, which include:
- Hypovolemia
- Myocardial ischemia
- Myocardial depressant effects of pharmacologic agents
- Acidosis
- Parasympathetic stimulation (pain, vagal response)

Definitive treatment for hypotension includes the following:
- Administration of oxygen
- Administration of fluid challenge (300 to 500 mL of crystalloid)
- Correction of acidosis or hypoxemia
- Relief of myocardial ischemia

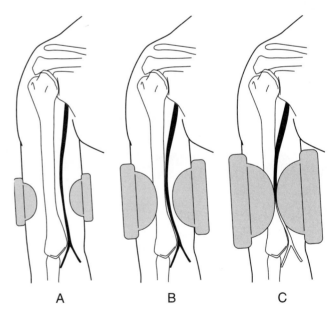

A   B   C

FIGURE 6-7 Effects of blood pressure cuff size. Blood pressure cuff width influences the pressure readings. Three cuffs, all inflated to the same pressure, are shown. The narrowest cuff (**A**) will require more pressure and the widest cuff (**C**) less pressure to occlude the brachial artery for determination of systolic pressure. Too narrow a cuff may produce a large overestimation of systolic pressure. Whereas the wider cuff may underestimate the systolic pressure, the error with a cuff 20% too wide is not as significant as that with a cuff 20% too narrow. (Reproduced with permission from Gravenstein JS, Paulus DA. *Monitoring Practice in Clinical Anesthesia,* 2nd ed. Philadelphia: JB Lippincott; 1987:58.)

BOX 6-3

Healthcare Provider Considerations: Automated Blood Pressure Cuffs

- Requires several cardiac cycles to adapt to respiratory patterns and motion artifact.
- Erratic cuff movement alters the accuracy of pressure output.
- Inappropriate cuff size = erroneous readings:
  - Narrow cuffs = elevated readings
  - Wide cuffs = decreased readings
- Appropriately sized blood pressure cuffs should fit approximately two thirds of the extremity or offer a width that is 20% greater than the diameter of the limb.
- Vascular congestion may occur when frequent blood pressures are cycled.
- To avoid low readings for manual cuffs, recommended inflation rate is 3 to 5 mm Hg per second.
- One layer of Webril may be used to protect friable skin (geriatric patients) against abrasion and bruising without greatly influencing the accuracy of cuff pressure.

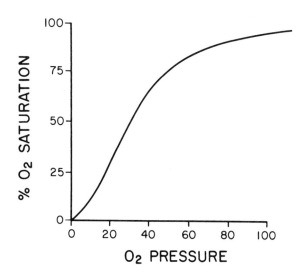

FIGURE 6-8 Oxyhemoglobin dissociation curve. The relationship between oxygen saturation and P_{O_2} is important in clinical practice. A general rule of thumb equates:

| P_{O_2} (mm Hg): | 40 | 50 | 60 |
| Saturation (%): | 70 | 80 | 90 |

(From Lake C. *Clinical Monitoring.* Philadelphia: WB Saunders; 1991:587.)

- Titration of sympathomimetic medications:
  - Beta agonists (ephedrine)
  - Alpha agonists (phenylephrine)
  - Alpha and beta agonists (epinephrine, dopamine)
- Titration of inotropic agents:
  - Calcium chloride

In the presence of hypotension, it is important for the healthcare provider monitoring the patient and the licensed independent practitioner to arrive at a timely diagnosis. Close communication is required of all team members to identify and treat the underlying causative factor.

Hypertension

Hypertension is defined as a systolic blood pressure greater than 140 mm Hg or a diastolic blood pressure greater than 90 mm Hg.[5] To prevent complications, hypertension must be treated in a timely fashion. Hypertension increases bleeding, predisposes the patient to hemorrhage, may lead to cardiac dysrhythmias, and increases myocardial oxygen consumption. Activation of the sympathetic nervous system (alpha- and beta-agonist stimulation) results in increased systemic vascular resistance and heart rate. Identification of the cause of hypertension is required to effectively return the blood pressure to baseline or normal values:

- Fluid overload requires diuresis
- Noxious stimuli require analgesia or discontinuation of stimulation
- Sympathetic nervous stimulation activation may require alpha and/or beta blockade
- Myocardial ischemia may require nitrates and analgesia

PULSE OXIMETRY

The advent of pulse oximetry in the 1980s has provided the clinician with a simple, safe, and inexpensive method to assess patient oxygenation. Pulse oximetry is a standard clinical assessment tool utilized to decrease the incidence of unrecognized hypoxic events. Oxygen saturation is recorded as an SpO_2 parameter. Ninety-eight percent of oxygen is transported throughout the body in combination with hemoglobin, whereas 2% is dissolved in plasma. The oxyhemoglobin dissociation curve depicted in Figure 6-8 assists the clinician in determining the correlation between oxygen saturation and P_{O_2}. Hemoglobin saturation is determined by a light-absorbance technique across a pulsating vascular bed. Examination of the oxyhemoglobin-dissociation curve reveals the development of hypoxemia at an SaO_2 of 90%, which equals a P_{O_2} of 60 mm Hg. Severe hypoxemia develops when SaO_2 decreases to 75% with a resultant P_{O_2} of 40 mm Hg. The height and slope of the curve depend on a variety of factors (Box 6-4). Factors that shift the curve to the left result in a decreased release of oxygen at the tissue level. Factors that shift the curve to the right result in an increase in the amount of oxygen released at the tissue level. During sedation procedures it is important to understand the principles of pulse oximetry to recognize the development of hypoxic episodes and to take corrective action when required.

> Pulse oximetry provides a noninvasive, continuous monitoring parameter to assess the percent of oxygen combined with hemoglobin.

BOX 6-4

Factors Affecting Hemoglobin-Oxygen Affinity

Causes of Increased Oxygen Affinity
- Hypothermia
- Respiratory alkalosis
- Metabolic alkalosis
- Decreased 2,3-diphosphoglycerate
- Decreased serum phosphate
- Anemia
- Hypothyroidism

Factors that Decrease Oxygen Affinity
- Fever
- Respiratory acidosis
- Metabolic acidosis
- Increased 2,3-diphosphoglycerate
- Corticosteroid administration
- Hyperaldosteronism
- Hyperthyroidism
- Polycythemia

From Lake C. *Clinical Monitoring*. Philadelphia: WB Saunders; 1991:589.

BOX 6-5

Optical Plethysmography and Spectrophotometry Techniques

Optical plethysmography uses light absorption to reproduce waveforms produced by pulsatile blood flow. Changes that occur in the absorption of light due to vascular bed changes are reproduced by the pulse oximeter as plethysmographic waveforms. Spectrophotometry is the scientific technology that uses various wavelengths of light to perform quantitative measurements of light absorption through given substances.

Oxygen Transport

The arterial system carries oxygen to the tissue and is dependent on a balance between oxygen supply and tissue oxygen demand. Hypoxemia occurs when oxygen demand exceeds oxygen supply. An adequate balance is provided by maintenance of the following:

- Adequate blood oxygen
- Adequate hemoglobin content to carry oxygen
- Adequate cardiac output to transport oxygenated blood
- Appropriate tissue utilization of oxygen

Pulse Oximetry Technology

Pulse oximetry combines the principles of optical plethysmography and spectrophotometry to ascertain hemoglobin oxygen saturation. The technology of optical plethysmography and spectrophotometry is outlined in Box 6-5. As depicted in Figure 6-9, pulse oximeters use two light-emitting diodes (LEDs), which are placed opposite each other across an arterial vascular bed. These LEDs measure the intensity of transmitted light across the vascular bed. The critical feature of pulse oximetry is that it measures the difference in the intensity of light absorption at each wavelength caused by oxygenated and deoxygenated hemoglobin. The signal is then transmitted to the pulse oximetry unit for determination of arterial hemoglobin oxygen saturation. Pulse oximeter sensors come in a variety of types and include adhesive sensors (adult, neonatal, infant, pediatric, and adult nasal) and reusable sensors (adult, adult/neonatal, pediatric/infant, reflectance, multisite, and ear clip) (Fig. 6-10). Sensors are chosen according to the patient's body weight, exposed site of application, patient activity level, and expected duration of patient monitoring. Factors that contribute to pulse oximetry interference are shown in Figure 6-11.

END-TIDAL CARBON DIOXIDE MONITORING

Monitoring of CO_2 provides a useful objective clinical assessment parameter. Although it is not yet considered standard of care monitoring, it is a useful physiologic indicator that demonstrates:

- Ventilation is sufficient to carry oxygen into the lungs
- Oxygen is being transported to the mitochondria (cardiovascular function)

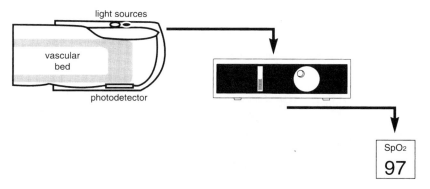

FIGURE 6-9 Pulse oximeter technology. Two light-emitting diodes measure the intensity of transmitted light across the vascular bed. (Courtesy of Nellcor, Inc., Pleasanton, CA.)

NELLCOR SENSOR SELECTION GUIDE

Adhesive Sensors

Check site at least every 8 hours as directed.

Sterile in unopened, undamaged package.

Patient Size	D-25*/D-25L* Oxisensor® II Adult	N-25* Oxisensor II Neonatal/Adult	I-20* Oxisensor II Infant	D-20* Oxisensor II Pediatric	R-15* Oxisensor II Adult Nasal
	>30 kg	<3 kg or >40 kg	3–20 kg	10–50 kg	>50 kg

Check site at least every 8 hours as directed.

Sterile in unopened, undamaged package.

Patient Size	A* OxiCliq® Adult	N OxiCliq Neonatal/Adult	I OxiCliq Infant	P* OxiCliq Pediatric
	>30 kg	<3 kg or >40 kg	3–20 kg	10–50 kg

* Latex free.

⊛ These sensors are eligible for the Sensor Recycling Program. For more information on enrolling in the program, contact your local Nellcor representative. Currently available in the U.S. only.

Reusable Sensors

Warning: Carefully read the directions for use provided with Nellcor® sensors for complete description, instructions, warnings, cautions and specifications.

Change site at least every 4 hours as directed.

Patient Size	DS-100A* Durasensor® Adult	OXI-A/N* Oxiband® Adult/Neonatal	OXI-P/I* Oxiband Pediatric/Infant	RS-10 RS-10 Adult Reflectance
	>40 kg	<3 kg or >40 kg	3–40 kg	>40 kg

Change site at least every 4 hours as directed.

PediCheck for attended spot check only (not to exceed 20 minutes).

Patient Size	D-YS* Dura-Y® Multisite	D-YSE* D-YSE Ear Clip *Use with Dura-Y sensor*	D-YSPD* PediCheck™ Pediatric Spot-Check *Use with Dura-Y sensor*
	>1 kg	>30 kg	3–40 kg

◆ NELLCOR

FIGURE 6-10 Nellcor sensor selection guide. (Courtesy of Nellcor, Inc., Pleasanton, CA.)

◆ Aerobic metabolism is consuming oxygen and producing CO_2

◆ CO_2 is being transported to the lungs (cardiovascular function)

◆ CO_2 in the expired air gives an indication of adequate ventilation

Capnography measures CO_2 in expiratory gases. The majority of capnographs utilize infrared absorption techniques.[6] Infrared absorption analysis provides quantitative respiratory monitoring data in the sedation setting.

> It is important for the sedation clinician to remember that oximeters measure the oxygen saturation of hemoglobin in peripheral blood, whereas capnography continuously, and nearly instantaneously, measures pulmonary ventilation and is able to rapidly detect small changes in cardiorespiratory function before oximeter readings change.

NELLCOR SENSORS

Basic Principles

The following considerations should be evaluated when choosing a Nellcor sensor for your patient:

- Patient's body weight

- Duration of use
  (long-term, short-term, spot-check)

- Patient activity

- Infection control concerns

Adhesive and reusable sensors are available.

Tips for Use

- Ensure that the optical components of the sensor are properly aligned as outlined in the directions for use.

- Adhesive sensor sites must be checked at least every 8 hours and moved to a new site if necessary. Reusable sensors must be moved to a new site at least every 4 hours.*

- Adhesive digit sensors may be reused on the same patient, if the adhesive portion attaches without slipping. Replace the sensor whenever the adhesive quality is depleted.

- Reusable sensors should be cleaned between patients. Refer to directions for use.

- When selecting a sensor site, priority should be given to an extremity free of an arterial catheter, blood pressure cuff, or intravascular infusion line.

  * *PediCheck* for attended spot-check only (not to exceed 20 minutes).

PULSE OXIMETRY: CLINICAL CONSIDERATIONS AND RECOMMENDATIONS

Certain conditions may result in pulse oximetry readings that are unreliable, incorrect, or less informative. These considerations and associated recommendations are listed below:

CONSIDERATION	RECOMMENDATION
Motion	Move sensor to a less active site or replace adhesive. Place reflectance sensor on the forehead if the patient is not on a ventilator or not placed in a Trendelenburg or supine position. Adjust averaging time on pulse oximeter if possible. For optimal performance in high-motion environments, use *Oxismart®* technology (N-3000, NBP-290 and NBP-295) or *C-Lock®* ECG synchronization.
Poor Perfusion	Use an adhesive digit sensor or apply an R-15 nasal sensor if the patient is immobile. Protect sensor site from heat loss or rewarm sensor site as permitted by hospital policy.
Venous Pulsation	Position digit sensor at heart level. Avoid restrictive taping. Use care when interpreting SpO_2 values in patients with elevated venous pressure.
Edema	Position the sensor on nonedematous application sites. Otherwise, the fluid in the edematous tissue may cause the light from the LEDs to scatter and affect the SpO_2 readings.
Light Interference	Cover the sensor with an opaque material in the presence of bright light sources, including direct sunlight, surgical lamps, infrared warming lamps, and phototherapy lights.
Nail Polish	Remove nail polish (especially brown, blue, green) or apply sensor to unpolished site.
Intravascular Dyes	Use care when interpreting SpO_2 values after injection of intravascular dyes, which may affect the reading.
Dyshemoglobins	Dysfunctional hemoglobins such as carboxyhemoglobin, methemoglobin or sulphhemoglobin are unable to carry oxygen. However, SpO_2 values only report functional saturation—oxygenated hemoglobin as a percentage of *functional* hemoglobin. Therefore, although the SpO_2 values reported by a pulse oximeter may appear normal when dysfunctional hemoglobins are elevated, oxygenation may be compromised due to decreased arterial oxygen content. A more complete assessment of oxygenation beyond pulse oximetry is recommended whenever dysfunctional hemoglobins are suspected.
Anemia	Anemia causes decreased arterial oxygen content by reducing the number of hemoglobins that are available to carry oxygen. Although SpO_2 percentages may be in the "normal" range, an anemic patient may be hypoxic due to reduced hemoglobin levels. The pulse oximeter may fail to provide an SpO_2 reading if hemoglobin levels fall below 5 gm/dl. Correcting anemia can improve arterial oxygen content.

U.S. Patents 4,621,643; 4,685,464; 4,700,708; 4,830,014; and 5,246,003.
© 2001 Nellcor Puritan Bennett Inc. All rights reserved. l.b.00130v1-0401

tyco

Healthcare

Nellcor

4280 Hacienda Drive
Pleasanton, CA 94588
Tel 925.463.4000
Toll Free 1.800.635.5267

Mallinckrodt
Europe BV
Hambakenwetering 1
5231 DD's-Hertogenbosch
The Netherlands
Tel +31.73.6485200

FIGURE 6-11 Pulse oximetry: clinical considerations and recommendations. (Courtesy of Nellcor, Inc., Pleasanton, CA.)

$ETCO_2$ is the partial pressure or maximal concentration of carbon dioxide (CO_2) at the end of an exhaled breath, which is expressed as a percentage of CO_2 or mm Hg.[7] The normal values are 5% to 6% CO_2, which is equivalent to 35 to 45 mm Hg.[8] CO_2 reflects cardiac output (CO) and pulmonary blood flow as the gas is transported by the venous system to the right side of the heart and then pumped to the lungs by the right ventricles.[9] When CO_2 diffuses out of the lungs into the exhaled air, a device called a capnometer measures the partial pressure or maximal concentration of CO_2 at the end of exhalation.

Sidestream Capnographs

First-generation sidestream capnographs sample a fixed amount of gas from the "side" of the main respiratory gas flow. The rate of gas sampling is generally between 50 to 500 mL (typical amounts = 150 mL, which precludes their use in neonatology and pediatrics). The gas sample is processed through sample tubes and adapters to an infrared light source and detector. Complications associated with sidestream capnographs include contamination and clogging by respiratory secretions unless sample tubes are frequently replaced.

Mainstream Capnographs

Second-generation capnographs mount the infrared head in close proximity to the endotracheal tube. Although the mainstream capnograph has resolved some of the technical problems associated with capnography use, its major limiting factor is that it can only be used on intubated patients. Additional limiting technical factors associated with mainstream capnography include optical pathway clouding and disruption by moisture and respiratory tract secretions, costly damage secondary to optical sensor mounting, and bulkiness associated with sensor assemblies, which predispose to kinking of ventilator lines. Therefore, the mainstream capnograph has no clinical use in the nonintubated sedation patient.

Microstream Capnography Technology

Microstream capnograph technology is based on molecular correlation spectroscopy (MCS) developed by Oridion (Danville, CA). Microstream technology employs a unique, laser-based technology called molecular correlation spectroscopy as the infrared emission source. Operating at room temperature, the Microstream emitter is electronically activated and self-modulating, which eliminates the need for moving parts. This new generation respiratory monitoring system is suitable for all patients including neonates and pediatric and adult patients. The comparative versatility associated with sidestream, mainstream, and Microstream capnographs is featured in Table 6-2. An advantage of Microstream capnography to the sedation clinician includes its use in nonintubated patients. It may also be utilized in a variety of clinical environments, including procedural sedation units, operating rooms, intensive care units, emergency departments, and home care. Oridion utilizes a patented Smart CapnoLine carbon dioxide circuit, which is ideal for nonintubated patients, including procedural sedation where oral ventilation can occur and cause inaccurate readings and waveforms if the patient alternates oral and nasal breathing. The Smart CapnoLine uses a unique uni-junction (Fig. 6-12), which enables a crisp continuous waveform and accurate data, regardless if the patient is a mouth or nose breather or alternates between the two modes. This "smart" design enables the cannula to collect the $ETCO_2$ from either the mouth or the nose.[10]

Capnography Waveforms

A capnogram is the graphical waveform depicting CO_2 concentration throughout respiration. $ETCO_2$ refers to the measurement of CO_2 concentration at the end of exhalation. A normal range for $ETCO_2$ is 35 to 45 mm Hg (4.5% to 6%).[11] Capnogram waveforms are featured in Figure 6-13. During each breath, the alveoli exchange carbon dioxide and oxygen. At the inhalation the alveoli receive oxygen, which diffuses into the pulmonary capillaries. Then, at exhalation, CO_2 diffuses into the alveoli and is eliminated by ventilation.

> Monitoring of the CO_2 waveform allows the sedation clinician an additional physiologic parameter coupled with an $ETCO_2$ measurement (normal 35 to 45 mm Hg) to assess for hypoventilation.[12]

Bispectral Index Analysis (BIS Monitoring)

Bispectral Index technology, introduced to the anesthesia community in 1996, became the first clinically proven and commercially available direct measure of the effects of anesthetics and sedatives on the brain. Recent clinical studies show that BIS monitoring may be an effective tool to assist in managing the sedation needs of such patients.[13,14] Although BIS monitoring is not a standard of care monitoring protocol, advantages associated with its clinical efficacy may lead to more pronounced use in the future. **Clinical advantages associated with BIS monitoring include decreased total medication dose, accurate level of consciousness (LOC) scoring (in conjunction with subjective and objective clinical parameters), and faster more predictable patient assessment.** There may prove to be additional benefits in monitoring situations where precise titration of medications is required (pediatric and geriatric patient populations). Monitoring with BIS offers the clinician the ability to utilize a monitor that will directly measure the effects of anesthetics and sedatives on the brain. This provides clinicians with the ability to customize the type and amount of medication they administer to a patient's individual needs. BIS technology is supported by more than 1000 published studies undertaken to assess its efficacy and utility. It has been used to assess more than 5.5 million patients and is utilized in operating rooms, intensive care units, and a range of sedation settings.[15]

TABLE 6-2

Comparative Versatility of Capnographs

SIDESTREAM	MAINSTREAM	MICROSTREAM
Liquid and Secretion Handling Contaminated liquids and secretions drawn into sample line require frequent sample line replacement, water trap emptying, and instrument decontamination.	Position-sensitive adapters must be routinely cleared to prevent optical path shadowing. Adapters must be sterilized between uses.	Position-independent adapters, vapor-permeable tubing, and sub-micron, multisurface filters minimize the frequency of filter line replacement and instrument contamination. There are no water traps to service.
Transportability and Ruggedness Usable with intubated or nonintubated patients. Monitors with water traps cannot be tilted. Those without traps require bulky filters. Black-body IR source and larger air pump require more power.	Not practical for use with nonintubated patients, especially children. Airway-mounted, position-dependent CO_2 sensors are frequently damaged. Black-body IR source and window heating require more power.	Usable with intubated or nonintubated patients. Rugged, compact units are highly mobile and are not position-dependent. Low-power $ETCO_2$ sensor is protected within the instrument and requires a small battery with up to 6 hours of battery life. No bulky water traps or filters.
Cross Sensitivity to Non-CO_2 Gases Narrow-band IR filters are not CO_2-specific. Compensation for non-CO_2 gases requires either user intervention or N_2O calibration and is only approximate.	Narrow-band IR filters are not CO_2-specific. User corrections for non-CO_2 gases are only approximate.	Microbeam IR sensor is inherently specific for CO_2 and does not require user corrections, recalibration, or software compensation for N_2O, O_2, or other common anesthetic gases.
Support for Neonatal Applications Large measuring cell volume requires sample flow rates as high as 300 mL/min. Not (generally) suitable for neonates.	Sensors are heavy, bulky, and difficult to use for neonates. Heated sensors are uncomfortable and may be risky.	Measuring cell volume is that of other technologies, making Microstream capnographs inherently suitable for low flow, for many neonatal applications as well as adult use.
Sample Line Compatibility Sample lines are compatible with units from only one manufacturer.	Adapters/sensors are incompatible with units from other manufacturers.	Microstream adapters and filter lines can be used with inpatients and outpatients whether intubated or not, and thus allow for standardization of patient connections.

BIS Technology

The Bispectral Index (BIS) is a processed EEG parameter that measures the hypnotic effects of anesthetic and sedative agents on the brain. Its measurements are derived from the frequency, amplitude, and coherence of the EEG, which have been shown statistically to relate to consciousness and unconsciousness. BIS values are represented as single numbers, which range from 100 for patients who are wide awake to 0 in the absence of brain activity. As demonstrated in Figure 6-14, the BIS Range Guidelines are based on results from a multicenter study of the BIS involving the administration of four commonly used anesthetics: propofol, midazolam, alfentanil, and isoflurane.[16] Clinical judgment is utilized when interpreting the BIS in conjunction with other available objective and subjective clinical monitoring parameters. **BIS measures the hypnotic component of anesthesia, with hypnosis defined as the state of consciousness, level of awareness, and memory.**

BIS monitoring may be an effective titration guide for dosing without increasing the risk of awareness and can allow a better balance of hypnotic and analgesic medications.

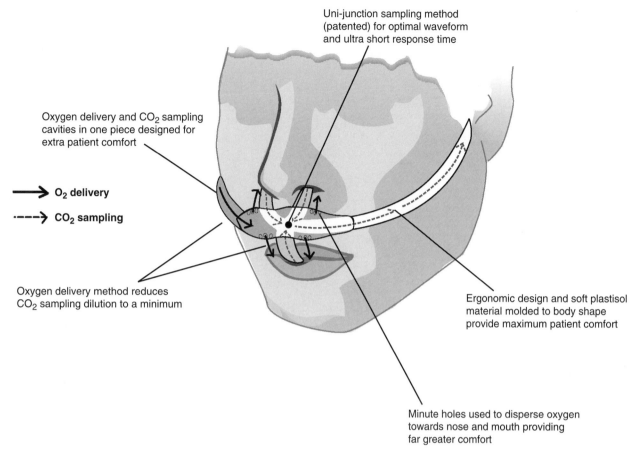

Uni-junction sampling method
(patented) for optimal waveform
and ultra short response time

Oxygen delivery and CO_2 sampling
cavities in one piece designed for
extra patient comfort

→ O_2 delivery

- - → CO_2 sampling

Oxygen delivery method reduces
CO_2 sampling dilution to a minimum

Ergonomic design and soft plastisol
material molded to body shape
provide maximum patient comfort

Minute holes used to disperse oxygen
towards nose and mouth providing
far greater comfort

FIGURE 6-12 O_2/CO_2 Nasal FilterLine by Oridion. The end-tidal CO_2 sampling cannula by Oridion minimizes dilution of sample from O_2 flow, removes dead space to improve waveform integrity, samples both nares, and meets at a single junction simultaneously to provide O_2 delivery to mouth and nose for maximum versatility and comfort. (Courtesy of Oridion, Danville, CA.)

The conventional processed electroencephalographic (EEG) parameters, such as Spectral Edge Frequency (SEF), are based solely on power spectral analysis. SEF quantifies the gross EEG shift to lower frequencies, which occurs as anesthesia deepens, but it does not correlate well with the level of sedation.[17] The BIS value is mathematically derived utilizing several complementary signal processing techniques including bispectral analysis, an advanced processing technology that incorporates EEG data inaccessible to conventional power spectral analysis. The BIS has undergone more clinical validation than any other EEG parameter and is strongly correlated with clinical measurements of sedation and hypnosis. It is currently the only measure of anesthetic effect that has received clearance by the U.S. Food and Drug Administration for its demonstrated clinical utility in the management of anesthesia. BIS monitor screen regions are featured in Figure 6-15, and a BIS sensor is identified in Figure 6-16.

> The BIS is the only monitoring parameter specifically created to describe changes in the EEG that relate to levels of sedation and consciousness.

DOCUMENTATION AND RECORD KEEPING

The purpose of the medical record (see Procedural Record for Sedation/Analgesia Figure 6-17 on p. 157) is to provide a legible, complete record of patient care during the administration of sedation. The record should be:

◆ Neat
◆ Accurate
◆ Clear
◆ Concise

The sedation/analgesia flowsheet should provide proof of continuous care reflective of medical and nursing standards

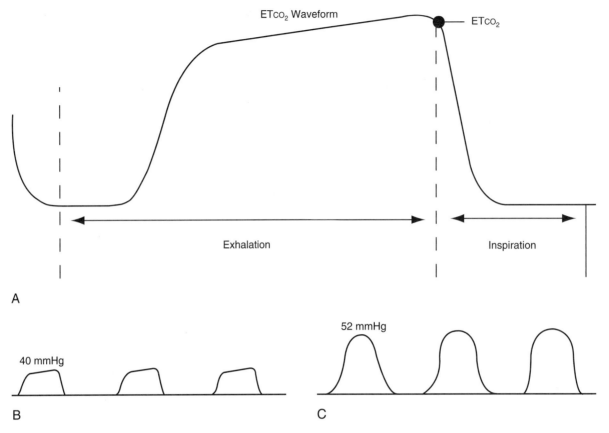

FIGURE 6-13 End-tidal carbon dioxide waveforms. **A,** End-tidal CO_2 waveform. **B,** End-tidal carbon dioxide waveform and value are normal, indicating adequate ventilation. **C,** End-tidal carbon dioxide waveform is rounded and value is elevated, which indicates hypoventilation. Left untreated, impending respiratory insufficiency will ensue.

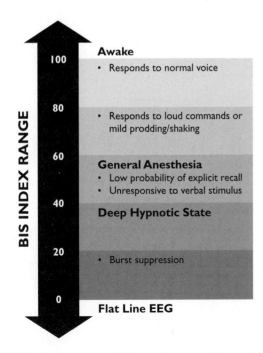

FIGURE 6-14 BIS range guidelines. (Courtesy of Aspect Medical Systems, Inc., Newton, MA.)

of care. The components of any sedation flowsheet include the following:

◆ Date
◆ Patient name
◆ Physical characteristics (age, height, weight)
◆ Premedication
◆ Medications
◆ Allergies
◆ Presedation vital signs
◆ Physiologic monitors used
◆ Airway management
◆ Medications administered
◆ Administration of reversal agents
◆ Vital sign graphic flowchart
◆ Intravenous solutions administered
◆ Estimated blood loss (if applicable)
◆ Attending physician
◆ Nurse/healthcare provider signature
◆ Procedure start and stop time

Incorrect notations may be changed in the medical record as follows:

◆ Lining out the original notation
◆ Insertion of the correct data

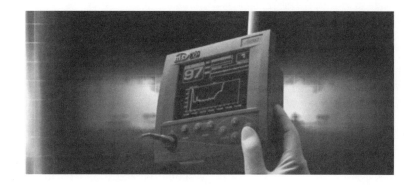

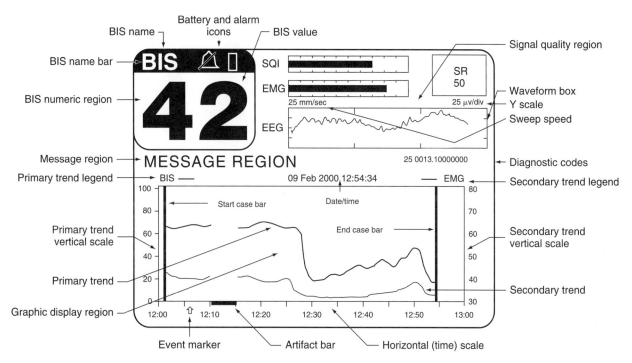

FIGURE 6-15 BIS screen region features. (Courtesy of Aspect Medical Systems, Inc., Newton, MA.)

- Initialing the change
- The original entry must remain legible.

The medical record is considered a legal document and should not be altered in any manner other than listed above.

> Spoilation of medical records refers to the illegal alteration, destruction, or removal of the medical record. Any attempt to tamper with or alter the patient's medical record may be viewed as evidence that supports a plaintiff's cause.

SEDATION FLOWSHEET
Name, Date, Physical Characteristics

Basic patient identification information is initially recorded on the sedation flowsheet and includes the patient's name, address, hospital administrative identification number, and so on. Physical characteristics (height, weight) may be recorded on the flowsheet or placed in the presedation patient assessment form.

Premedication, Medications, Allergy Status

Any premedication that has been administered should be documented on the procedural sedation record prior to the start of the procedure. The effect of the sedative should be noted and is characteristically recorded as cooperative, calm, sleeping, and so on. The time of administration of the premedication should also be noted. Patient medications are recorded on the sedation record with last dose administered noted before the procedure. Allergy status should also be recorded on the flowsheet. The patient's allergies should be and the size of the catheter should be recorded. Type and amount of intravenous solution administered must be recorded and should be totaled at the conclusion of the procedure. A column for blood loss (if applicable) allows an accurate mechanism for postsedation correlation and assessment.

Medications used during the procedure are recorded on the graphic flowsheet. Depending on the pharmacologic technique used, medications are recorded in incremental doses or as a continuous infusion. Total dose administered should be added and recorded in a total dose column. If reversal agents are required to counteract the pharmacologic effects of sedative medications, dosage and time of administration must be recorded. Information on time of administration and total dose of reversal agent used assists the clinician with postprocedure monitoring and discharge planning.

Graphic Flowsheet

A graphic flowsheet for vital signs provides a quick reference and history of the patient's cardiovascular stability throughout the procedure. Vital signs should be recorded every 5 minutes and provide an accurate reflection of cardiopulmonary parameters. **In addition to the notation of cardiovascular parameters, it is important to document the patient's level of consciousness.** Objective clinical scoring systems have been developed and utilized for sedation/analgesia and monitored anesthesia care (MAC) cases.[18] Commonly utilized systems include:

Ramsay Scale

The scale was originally used to quantitate the level of drug-induced sedation and to measure patient responsiveness and drowsiness in the intensive care unit. It is however, difficult to quantify a degree of agitation and oversedation with this scale.[19] The Ramsay scale is represented in Box 6-6.

Observer's Assessment of Alertness/Sedation (OAA/S)

The OAA/S was developed to quantify the CNS effects of benzodiazepines.[20] The OAA/S assesses patient responsiveness, speech, facial expression, and ocular appearance. **The OAA/S provides a higher level of discrimination for various levels of sedation.** However, a major disadvantage of this level of consciousness assessment technique is that the patient needs to be stimulated to perform the testing procedure. The OAA/S scale is represented in Table 6-3.

Sedation Visual Analogue Scale

The sedation visual analogue scale has been used to quantify the level of sedation during monitored anesthesia care cases.[21-23] The Sedation Visual Analogue Scale utilizes a 100-mm visual analogue scale, which is displayed at one end as "awake and alert" and at the opposite end by "asleep." **A distinct disadvantage associated with this scale is that it**

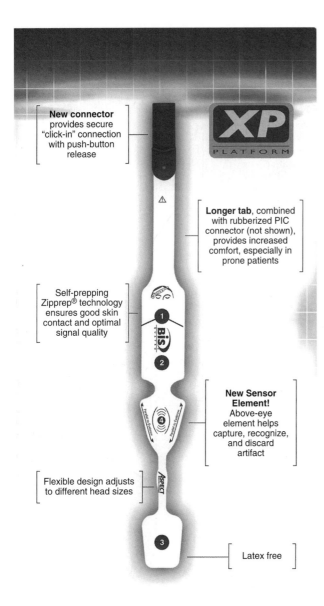

FIGURE 6-16 BIS sensor. (Courtesy of Aspect Medical Systems, Inc., Newton, MA.)

documented, and an attempt should be made to elicit the type of reaction (e.g., hives, gastrointestinal upset) with these data recorded on the flowsheet.

Presedation vital signs or the first set of vital signs obtained immediately before the procedure should be recorded on the sedation flowsheet. A presedation Aldrete score should also be recorded before commencement of the procedure. Although initial vital signs may be falsely elevated because of anxiety, they provide a baseline before the therapeutic, diagnostic, or minor surgical procedure. Monitors used and site of application are recorded before the procedure. The site of intravenous catheter insertion

SEDATIVE/ANALGESIC ADMINISTRATION FOR DIAGNOSTIC AND THERAPEUTIC PROCEDURES

Name: _____ Medical Record #: _____

Procedure/Date: _____ Physician: _____

(1) ADULT HISTORY (✔ or circle all applicable - elaborate under comments)   **NPO:** Date/Time _____

CV: ☐ MI ☐ chest pain ☐ heart failure ☐ murmurs ☐ arrhythmias ☐ hypertension ☐ heart surgery ☐ pacemaker/AICD

PULM: ☐ COPD ☐ asthma ☐ recent resp infection ☐ sleep apnea/snoring ☐ SOB ☐ home O2 ☐ smoke (____ PPD) ☐ hemoptysis

CNS: ☐ CVA/deficits ☐ TIA ☐ seizures ☐ retardation/Down's ☐ dementia ☐ head trauma ☐ psychiatric disease

GI/HEPATIC/ENDOCRINE: ☐ ETOH/abuse ☐ PUD ☐ GERD/HH ☐ hepatitis ☐ jaundice ☐ DM (glucometer _____) ☐ thyroid disease

RENAL: ☐ CRF ☐ dialysis (Hemo/PD) ☐ stones ☐ recurrent UTI's

HEM: ☐ anemia ☐ easy bleeding/bruising ☐ sickle cell disease/trait ☐ Aspirin/NSAID use ☐ heparin/coumadin

MISC: ☐ obesity ☐ dysmorphic facies ☐ previous anesthesia/sedation problems ☐ LMP _____ ☐ illicit drugs ☐ glaucoma

(2) ADDITIONAL PEDIATRIC HISTORY (✔ or circle all applicable - elaborate under comments)

☐ premature ☐ nursery problems ☐ failure to thrive ☐ developmental delay ☐ Down's ☐ congenital airway anomaly ☐ SIDS in family

☐ breath holding ☐ apnea monitor ☐ home O2 ☐ asthma ☐ recent URI ☐ CHD

(3) OTHER HISTORY/COMMENTS (Please note when above systems are normal): _____

_____

_____

(4) CURRENT MEDICATIONS: _____

_____ **(5) ALLERGIES:** _____

(6) PHYSICAL EXAMINATION (✔ or circle all applicable - elaborate under comments)

Age _____ months/years Weight _____ kg BP _____ P _____ R _____ RA SpO2 _____ %

AIRWAY: (examined upright, head neutral, maximal mouth opening, maximal tongue protrusion - circle one)

CLASS I   CLASS II   CLASS III   CLASS IV

NECK FLEXION: ☐ FROM ☐ limited

HEAD EXTENSION ON NECK: ☐ FROM ☐ limited

TEETH: ☐ normal ☐ artificial ☐ carious ☐ loose

HEART: ☐ rhythm reg/irreg ☐ extra sounds Y/N

LUNGS: ☐ normal ☐ rales ☐ rhonchi ☐ wheezing

MISC/COMMENTS/LABS: _____

I have reviewed and confirmed key pre-assessment elements using the above form or consultation/dictation. (circle) by

Dr _____ dated _____

Attending signature/Date _____   RN/PA/Resident signature/Date _____

(7) PROCEDURE MONITORING Arrival time/mode _____ Responsible adult/location _____

☐ Crash cart checked/available   Permits signed (circle) procedure sedation contrast   IV size/site _____

Sedation start ____ end _____ Procedure start ____ end _____ Pain/anxiety scale 0 1 2 3 4 5 6 7 8 9 10

                                                                                              mild   moderate   worst

	TIME ▶										
MONITORS	OXYGEN										
	O2 SAT %										
	EKG										
	PAIN/ANXIETY SCALE										
	CONSCIOUSNESS SCORE										
DRUGS											

REMARKS:

FLUIDS/TYPE/RATE

PRESEDATION VALUES:

BP _____ 220

HR _____ 200

FiO2 _____ 180

O2 SAT% _____ 160

Consciousness Score _____ 140

SYMBOLS: 120

BP ⋁ ⋀ Pulse ● 100

Arterial Cuff
          L
          R 80
          Arm
          Leg 60

Respiration

Spon. ◯ 40

Ass't. ⊘ 20

Contr. ⊗ 0

Monitor Signature/Title _____

Attending MD Signature _____

09-017600 (6/01)

WHITE - Chart   CANARY - Department   PAGE 1 OF 3

FIGURE 6-17 Sample sedation/analgesia procedural record. (Reprinted with permission from Wake Forest University Baptist Medical Center.)

Continued

Wake Forest University Baptist
M E D I C A L   C E N T E R
The North Carolina Baptist Hospitals, Inc.
Winston-Salem, North Carolina

PREASSESSMENT, MONITORING AND RECOVERY FORM
Sedative/Analgesic Administration for Diagnostic and Therapeutic Procedures

(8) RECOVERY PERIOD

Date _____ Location _____ Procedure _____

Sedative medication summary _____

☐ Crash cart checked/available

STATUS AT ADMISSION [A]			STATUS AT DISCHARGE [D]				

COLOR	PINK [A] [D]	PALE [A] [D]	JAUNDICED [A] [D]	CYANOTIC [A] [D]	OTHER [A] [D]

AIRWAY	NATURAL [A] [D]	ENDOTUBE	NASAL [A] [D] ORAL [A] [D]	AIRWAY	NASAL [A] [D] ORAL [A] [D]	TRACH [A] [D]

RESPIRATIONS	SPONT [A] [D]	REG [A] [D]	IRREG [A] [D]	DEEP [A] [D]	SHALLOW [A] [D]	NORMAL [A] [D]	RAPID [A] [D]	SLOW [A] [D]	LABORED [A] [D]	UNLABORED [A] [D]

SKIN	COLD [A] [D]	COOL [A] [D]	WARM [A] [D]	HOT [A] [D]	DRY [A] [D]	CLAMMY [A] [D]	PERSPIRING [A] [D]

HAND GRIP STRENGTH	LEFT: STRONG [A] [D] WEAK [A] [D] ABSENT [A] [D]	RIGHT: STRONG [A] [D] WEAK [A] [D] ABSENT [A] [D]

IV SITE CONDITION	ADM:	REMOVAL TIME:	WHEELS LOCKED ☐	SIDERAILS UP ☐

TIME: / ADMIT

BP ✕

Pulse ●

220 220
200 200
180 180
160 160
140 140
120 120
100 100
80   80
60   60
40   40
20   20
0   0

MONITORS: RESPS / O₂ SAT % / FiO2 / EKG

DRUGS

FLUIDS/TYPE/RATE

RECOVERY SCORE		ADM	DISCH
ACTIVITY	MOVES 4 EXTREMITIES = 2		
	MOVES 2 EXTREMITIES = 1		
	MOVES 0 EXTREMITIES = 0		
RESPIRATION	DEEP BREATHES, COUGHS, OR CRIES = 2		
	DYSPNEIC OR LIMITED BREATHING = 1		
	APNEIC = 0		
CIRCULATION	BP ± 20% OF PRE SED LEVEL = 2		
	BP ± 20-50% OF PRE SED LEVEL = 1		
	BP ± 50% OF PRE SED LEVEL = 0		
CONSCIOUS-NESS	ALERT, ORIENTED + 3 = 3		
	AWAKE TO VERBAL STIMULUS BUT SLEEPS WHEN UNDISTURBED = 2		
	RESPONSE TO PAINFUL STIMULI = 1		
	UNCONSCIOUS, UNRESPONSIVE = 0		
COLOR	PINK (SKIN, MUCOUS MEMBRANES) = 2		
	PALE, DUSKY, BLOTCHY = 1		
	CYANOTIC = 0		

SEDATION NURSE SIGNATURE	TOTAL SCORE:		

RECOVERY NURSE INITIALS	TIME ADM	TIME DISCH	TOTAL TIME

RECOVERY DISCHARGE CHECKLIST

(1) significant bleeding/drainage Y/N/NA

(2) return of preprocedure mobility Y/N/NA

(3) return of preprocedure mental status Y/N/NA

(4) minimal or no nausea or vomiting Y/N/NA

(5) easily tolerable, minimal, or no pain Y/N/NA

(6) if ambulatory, minimal or no dizziness Y/N/NA

(7) responsible adult to accompany home Y/N/NA

(8) care instructions given to responsible adult Y/N/NA

(9) patient questions have been answered Y/N/NA

(10) phone report to floor nurse Y/N/NA

RECOVERY REMARKS/TIME

_____
_____
_____
_____
_____

Signature of recovery nurse/initials _____

The patient may be discharged from the care of _____ when they satisfactorily fulfill the above recovery discharge checklist. Please notify me to reassess the patient if this does not occur within _____ hours or if any emergency arises.

Attending MD Signature _____ Beeper _____

FIGURE 6-17, cont'd For legend, see previous page.

BOX 6-6

Ramsay Sedation Scale

Level of Sedation: Sedation/Analgesia (Conscious Sedation)
- 1 = Patient is anxious and agitated or restless or both.
- 2 = Patient is cooperative, oriented, and tranquil.
- 3 = Patient responds to commands only.

Level of Sedation: Deep
- 4 = Patient exhibits brisk response to light glabellar tap or loud auditory stimulus.
- 5 = Patient exhibits a sluggish response to light glabellar tap or loud response.
- 6 = Patient exhibits no response.

Data from Ramsay MAE, Savage TM, Simpson BRJ, Goodwin R. Controlled sedation with alphaxalone-alphadolone. *BMJ.* 1974;2:656-659.

requires the patient to be alert and stimulated throughout the procedure. A sample of the Sedation Visual Analogue Scale is represented in Figure 6-18.

Utilization of a level of consciousness scoring tool or monitor (Ramsay Scale, Observer's Assessment of Alertness/Sedation, Sedation Visual Analogue Scale, BIS monitor) provides the clinician with the ability to more objectively monitor levels of central nervous system depression in an attempt to adhere to the goals and objectives of sedation/analgesia. Additional information recorded on the sedation flowsheet includes name or signature of the attending physician, healthcare provider monitoring the patient, diagnosis, procedure, and start and stop time.

SUMMARY

Patients receiving sedation are monitored on a continuous basis. Although vital sign parameters are recorded at regular intervals (every 5 minutes is most common), subjective and objective monitoring is conducted on a continuum. Differential diagnoses associated with sedation and postsedation complications are outlined in Box 6-7. Monitoring parameters outlined in this chapter are effective tools when used in conjunction with healthcare provider assessment strategies. Monitoring practices that are congruent with practice standards, recommended practice guidelines, position statements, state statute, and hospital policy and procedure promote quality patient care.

Faulty equipment requires immediate intervention. Rescheduling of procedures may be inconvenient and costly; however, in the presence of malfunctioning equipment, it is the definitive option. Monitoring alarms and alarm limits are designed to provide patient safety. Before the commencement of any procedure, the patient monitors should be turned on and the alarm parameters activated. Alarm limits should not be so broad that dangerous clinical situations are undetected. Parameters must not be so narrow that they cause undue stress to the patient or clinician throughout the procedure. Initial alarm limits may be set approximately 20% above or below the patient's presedation baseline vital signs. Effective monitoring of the patient receiving sedation/analgesia includes continuous assessment,

TABLE 6-3

Observer's Assessment of Alertness/Sedation Scale

RESPONSIVENESS	SPEECH	FACIAL EXPRESSION	EYES	COMPOSITE SCORE (LEVEL)
Responds readily to name spoken in normal tone	Normal	Normal	Clear, no ptosis	1 (alert)
Lethargic response to name spoken in normal tone	Mild slowing or thickening	Mild relaxation	Glazed or mild ptosis (less than half the eye)	2
Responds only after name is called loudly and/or repeatedly	Slurring or prominent slowing	Marked relaxation (slacked jaw)	Glazed and mild ptosis (half the eye or more)	3
Responds only after mild prodding or shaking	Few recognizable words			4
Does not respond to mild prodding or shaking				5 (deep sleep)

Assign the composite score corresponding to the highest level at which any statement is checked. Responsiveness should be evaluated first.

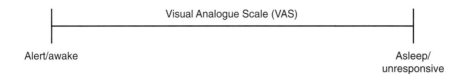

FIGURE 6-18 Sedation visual analogue scale. (From McCaffery M, Pasero C. *Pain: Clinical Manual.* St. Louis: Mosby; 1999:62.)

the use of ECG, noninvasive blood pressure (NIBP), pulse oximetry, ETCO$_2$ analysis (where applicable), and the implementation of critical thinking skills to provide safe, effective quality patient care.

> Disabling of alarms is dangerous and may lead to devastating complications.

BOX 6-7

Differential Diagnosis of Sedation/Postsedation Complications

Restlessness
- Hypoxemia ($\downarrow$ Spo$_2$)
- Pain
- Hypotension
- Bladder distention/urinary retention
- Emotional response
- Shivering/feeling of being cold
- Hypercarbia ($\uparrow$ CO$_2$)
- Emergence delirium
- Gastrointestinal distress/distention
- Psychotropic effects of sedative medications
- $\uparrow$ Intracranial pressure, intracranial event

Hypotension
- Decreased preload
  - Hypovolemia from prolonged fasting or inadequate fasting or inadequate fluid replacement
  - Excessive urinary losses, bleeding
  - Peripheral vasodilation ($\downarrow$ resistance)
- Effects of sedative and narcotic drugs
- Decreased myocardial contractility
- Orthostatic effects of progressive ambulation

Hypertension
- Pain, surgical stimulation
- Hypoxemia ($\downarrow$ Spo$_2$)
- Bladder distention/urinary retention
- Shivering, vasoconstriction due to hypothermia
- Preexisting disease (e.g., hyperthyroidism, essential hypertension, renal disease)
- Emergence delirium, emotional response
- Hypercarbia ($\uparrow$ CO$_2$)
- Retching or vomiting
- Fluid overload
- Effects of medications (e.g., vasopressors, naloxone, ketamine, anticholinergics, cocaine, ephedrine, epinephrine)

Dysrhythmias
- Pain
- Hypoxemia ($\downarrow$ Spo$_2$)
- Procedural myocardial infarction
- Catecholamine release
- Metabolic changes (e.g., acidosis, alkalosis)
- Preexisting disease
- Hypercarbia ($\uparrow$ CO$_2$)
- Failure of artificial pacemaker
- Side effects of sedative/analgesia medications
- Electrolyte imbalance (potassium, calcium)

Tachycardia
- Pain
- Hypovolemia
- Emergence delirium
- Fever (e.g., malignant hyperthermia, sepsis)
- Hyperthyroidism
- Effects of medications (e.g., atropine, glycopyrrolate)

Bradycardia
- Oculocardiac reflex
- Stimulation of baroreceptors
- Hypoventilation, especially in children
- Cardiac effects of heavy athletic activity
- Sedative, analgesic drugs

Respiratory Depression
- Obstructed airway
- Splinting, secondary to pain
- Pulmonary congestion
- Positioning, especially in the obese
- Mechanical failure of equipment (bag/valve/mask)
- Preexisting disease, chronic obstructive pulmonary disease, reactive airway

Modified from Burden N. *Ambulatory Surgical Nursing.* 2nd ed. Philadelphia: WB Saunders; 2000:413.

LEARNER SELF-ASSESSMENT

In order to achieve maximal educational benefit from this chapter, please complete the Learner Self-Assessment below. This self-assessment tool provides the learner with the ability to identify areas requiring additional review. Reference material for each question is provided in Appendix F.

1. Healthcare practitioner considerations associated with **JCAHO Standards** related to physiologic monitoring requirements for sedation/analgesia patients include:

2. **Practice Guidelines for Sedation and Analgesia by Non-Anesthesiologists recommendations** promulgated by the ASA Task Force on Sedation **related to physiologic monitoring** of the patient presenting for sedation/analgesia clinical services include:

3. **The rationale, advantages, and disadvantages associated with ECG, blood pressure, pulse oximetry, and level of consciousness monitoring** utilized during sedation procedures include:

4. **Which ECG lead positions are best utilized in the detection of dysrhythmias versus ischemia?**

5. **Which rhythm disturbances may impact on the patient's physiologic status** during sedation/analgesia procedures?

6. **Recommended treatment protocols for hypertension/hypotension** and their prescribed treatment protocols include:

7. **Advantages associated with use of end-tidal carbon dioxide monitoring** during sedation/analgesia procedures include:

8. Required **components of the sedation/analgesia record** include:

POST-TEST QUESTIONS

Please note: If you are applying for CE credit, you must contact Specialty Health Education, Inc. @ 800-694-8041 for a CE Application Packet.

1. Which ECG monitoring lead is useful in the detection of dysrhythmias secondary to the increased visibility of the P wave in this lead? _____
   A. Lead I
   B. Lead II
   C. Lead III
   D. Lead IV

2. Which of the following ECG monitoring leads is useful in the detection of dysrhythmias because a large portion of the left ventricle is located beneath its position and is a useful lead in the detection of myocardial ischemia? _____
   A. Lead I
   B. Lead II
   C. Lead III
   D. Lead V_5

3. The monitoring lead of choice for a patient with a significant past medical history of severe coronary artery disease and myocardial ischemia is _____.
   A. Lead I
   B. Lead II
   C. Lead III
   D. Lead V_5

4. A cardiac dysrhythmia that is characterized by fluctuations in heart rate influenced by the respiratory pattern and the degree of parasympathetic nervous system control over the SA node and features a heart rate increase during inspiration is identified as _____.
   A. Sinus tachycardia
   B. Sinus bradycardia
   C. Sinus arrhythmia
   D. Premature atrial contraction

5. Cardiac dysrhythmias that are characterized by rapid ectopic atrial discharge at a rate of 250 to 350 beats per minute with inability of the ventricle to respond to each impulse is identified as _____.
   A. Premature atrial contractions
   B. Atrial flutter
   C. Ventricular fibrillation
   D. Ventricular tachycardia

6. A life-threatening dysrhythmia that results in the inability of the ventricle to contract with no recovery phase between ventricular contractions is identified as _____.
   A. Ventricular tachycardia
   B. Ventricular fibrillation

C. Atrial fibrillation
D. Atrial tachycardia

7. Hypotension is identified as a decrease in systemic arterial blood pressure of _____ below the patient's baseline blood pressure.
   A. 5%-10%
   B. 10%-15%
   C. 20%-30%
   D. Less than 30%

8. All of the following are treatment protocols for managing procedural hypotension except _____.
   A. Administration of hydralazine (alpha blocker)
   B. Correction of acidosis or hypoxemia
   C. Administration of oxygen
   D. Administration of ephedrine

9. Hypertension is defined as a systolic blood pressure greater than _____ mm Hg and a diastolic blood pressure greater than _____ mm Hg.
   A. 90 and 60
   B. 130 and 80
   C. 135 and 80
   D. 140 and 90

10. An SaO_2 of 90% correlates with an approximate PO_2 of _____ mm Hg on the oxyhemoglobin dissociation curve.
    A. 30
    B. 40
    C. 50
    D. 60

11. Which of the following monitors introduced into clinical anesthesia practice in 1996 is utilized to assess level of consciousness? _____
    A. Pulse oximeter
    B. Capnography
    C. Bispectral analysis monitor
    D. Peripheral nerve stimulator

12. Which of the following procedural monitoring tool requires patient response to commands? _____
    A. Assessment of vital signs
    B. Level of consciousness monitoring
    C. Pulse oximetry measurement
    D. ECG monitoring

REFERENCES

1. Grauer K. *A Practical Guide to ECG Interpretation.* St. Louis: Mosby; 1992.
2. Cummins R. *Advanced Cardiac Life Support.* Dallas: American Heart Association; 1998.
3. Morgan G, Mikhail M. *Clinical Anesthesiology.* 3rd ed. New York: McGraw-Hill; 2002;87.
4. Morgan G, Mikhail M. *Clinical Anesthesiology.* 2nd ed. Stamford, CT: Appleton & Lange; 1996:800.
5. The sixth report of the Joint National Committee on Prevention, Detection, Evaluation, and Treatment of High Blood Pressure (JNC VI). *Arch Intern Med.* 1997:2413-2420.
6. Gravenstein JS, Paulus DA, Hayes TJ. *Gas Monitoring in Clinical Practice.* 2nd ed. Boston: Butterworth-Heinemann, 1995;202.
7. LaValle TL, Perry AG. Capnography: Assessing end-tidal CO_2 levels. *Dimens Crit Care Nurs.* 1995;14(14):67-68.
8. Trillo G, von Planta M, Kette F. $ETCO_2$ monitoring during low flow states: Clinical aims and limits. *Resuscitation.* 1994;25(6):412.
9. Sanders A. Contemporary in Emergency Medicine. *Ann Emerg Med.* 1989;18:1287-1290.
10. Smart CapnoLine, http//www.oridion.com (accessed June 3, 2003). Oridion Capnography Inc., Needham, MA.
11. Capnography Waveforms: Interpreting the Capnogram, http//www.oridion.com (accessed 3 June 2003). Oridion Capnography Inc., Needham, MA.
12. Capnography Overview: Waveforms, http//www.oridion.com (accessed June 3, 2003). Oridion Capnography Inc., Needham, MA.
13. Bower AL, et al. Bispectral index monitoring of sedation during endoscopy. *Gastrointest Endosc.* 2000;52(2-4).
14. Kaplan L, et al. Bispectral index monitoring: An essential element of conscious sedation. *Crit Care Med.* 29(Suppl 12): 11-15.
15. Aspect Medical Systems, http//www.aspectmedical.com/sec_sedation (accessed June 9, 2003).
16. Glass PSA, Bloom MJ, Kearse L, et al. Bispectral analysis measures sedation and memory effects of propofol, midazolam, isoflurane, and alfentanil in healthy volunteers. *Anesthesiology.* 1997;86:836-847.
17. Kearse L, Rosow C, Glass PSA, et al. Monotonic changes in EEG bispectral index correlate with targeted plasma concentration of propofol and midazolam. *Anesth Analg.* 1996;82:S220.
18. Avramov MN, White PF. Methods for monitoring the level of sedation. *Crit Care Clin.* 1995;11:803.
19. Ramsay MA, Savage TM, Simpson BR, et al. Controlled sedation with alphaxalone-alphadolone. *BMJ.* 1974;2:656.
20. Chernik DA, Gillings D, Laine H, et al. Validity and reliability of the observer's assessment of alertness/sedation scale: Study with intravenous midazolam. *J Clin Psychopharmacol.* 1990; 10:244.
21. White PF, Negus JB: Sedative infusions during local and regional anesthesia. *J Clin Anesth* 3:32, 1991.
22. Ramirez-Ruiz M, Smith I, White PF: Use of analgesics during propofol sedation: A comparison of ketorolac, dezocine, and fentanyl. *J Clin Anesth* 7:481, 1995.
23. Borgeat A, Wilder-Smith OH, Saiah M, et al: Subhypnotic doses of propofol possess direct antiemetic properties. *Anesth Analg* 74:539, 1992.

CHAPTER 7

Airway Management and Management of Respiratory Complications

At the completion of this chapter, the learner shall:

◆ Identify the components of a presedation airway evaluation.

◆ State the clinical signs and symptoms associated with respiratory insufficiency and airway obstruction.

◆ List treatment modalities designed to relieve airway obstruction and restore air flow in the sedated patient.

◆ State the proper technique for nasal and oral airway insertion.

◆ Demonstrate the proper application of a face mask for positive-pressure ventilation.

◆ Identify the components and treatment modalities associated with the "Sedation Airway Algorithm."

Joint Commission on Accreditation of Healthcare Organizations Standards for Operative or Other High-Risk Procedures and/or the Administration of Moderate or Deep Sedation or Anesthesia

Standard PC.13.20
Operative or other procedures and/or the administration of moderate or deep sedation or anesthesia are planned.

Rationale for PC.13.20
Because the response to procedures is not always predictable and sedation-to-anesthesia is a continuum, it is not always possible to predict how an individual patient will respond. Therefore, qualified individuals are trained in professional standards and techniques to manage patients in the case of a potentially harmful event.

Elements of Performance for PC.13.20
1. Sufficient numbers of qualified staff are available* to evaluate the patient, perform the procedure, monitor, and recover the patient.
2. *Individuals administering moderate or deep sedation and anesthesia are qualified*† *and have the appropriate credentials to manage patients at whatever level of sedation or anesthesia is achieved, either intentionally or unintentionally.*
3. *A registered nurse supervises perioperative nursing care.*
4. *Appropriate equipment to monitor the patient's physiologic status is available.*
5. *Appropriate equipment to administer intravenous fluids and drugs, including blood and blood components, is available as needed.*
6. *Resuscitation capabilities are available.*

Before operative and other procedures or the administration of moderate or deep sedation or anesthesia:

7. Patient acuity is assessed to plan for the appropriate level of postprocedure care.

8. Preprocedural education, treatments, and services are provided according to the plan for care, treatment, and services.

9. The site, procedure, and patient are accurately identified and clearly communicated before surgery.

10. A presedation or preanesthesia assessment is conducted.

11. *Before sedating or anesthetizing a patient, a licensed independent practitioner with appropriate clinical privileges plans or concurs with the planned anesthesia.*

12. *The patient is reevaluated immediately before moderate or deep sedation and before anesthesia induction.*

Standard PC.13.30
Patients are monitored during the procedure and/or administration of moderate or deep sedation or anesthesia.

Elements of Performance for PC.13.30

1. *Appropriate methods are used to continuously monitor oxygenation, ventilation, and circulation during procedures that may affect the patient's physiological status.*

2. *The procedure and/or administration of moderate or deep sedation or anesthesia for each patient are documented in the medical record.*

---

*For hospitals providing obstetric or emergency operative services, this means they can provide anesthesia services as required by law and regulation.

†**Qualified** The individuals providing moderate or deep sedation and anesthesia have at a minimum had competency-based education, training, and experience in the following:

1. Evaluating patients before moderate or deep sedation and anesthesia.

2. *Performing the moderate or deep sedation and anesthesia, including rescuing patients who slip into a deeper-than-desired level of sedation or analgesia. This includes the following:*
   a. *Moderate sedation – are qualified to rescue patients from deep sedation and are competent to manage a compromised airway and to provide adequate oxygenation and ventilation.*
   b. *Deep sedation – are qualified to rescue patients from general anesthesia and are competent to manage an unstable cardiovascular system as well as a compromised airway and inadequate oxygenation and ventilation.*

© Joint Commission: Standards for Operative or Other High-Risk Procedures and/or the Administration of Moderate or Deep Sedation or Anesthesia, January, 2004. Reprinted with permission.

Practice Guidelines for Sedation and Analgesia by Non-Anesthesiologists

American Society of Anesthesiologists Task Force on Sedation and Analgesia by Non-Anesthesiologists

Recommendations. Clinicians administering sedation/analgesia should be familiar with sedation-oriented aspects of the patient's medical history and how these might alter the patient's response to sedation/analgesia. These include: (1) abnormalities of the major organ systems; (2) previous adverse experience with sedation/analgesia as well as regional and general anesthesia; (3) drug allergies, current medications, and potential drug interactions; (4) time and nature of last oral intake; and (5) history of tobacco, alcohol, or substance use or abuse. **Patients presenting for sedation/analgesia should undergo a focused physical examination, including vital signs, auscultation of the heart and lungs, and evaluation of the airway (Example I).** Preprocedure laboratory testing should be guided by the patient's underlying medical condition and the likelihood that the results will affect the management of sedation/analgesia. These evaluations should be confirmed immediately before sedation is initiated.

EXAMPLE I: AIRWAY ASSESSMENT PROCEDURES FOR SEDATION AND ANALGESIA

Positive-pressure ventilation, with or without tracheal intubation, may be necessary if respiratory compromise develops during sedation/analgesia. This may be more difficult in patients with atypical airway anatomy. In addition, some airway abnormalities may increase the likelihood of airway obstruction during spontaneous ventilation. Factors that may be associated with difficulty in airway management include:

History

- Previous problems with anesthesia or sedation
- Stridor, snoring, or sleep apnea
- Advanced rheumatoid arthritis
- Chromosomal abnormality (e.g., trisomy 21)

Physical examination

- Habitus: Significant obesity (especially involving the neck and facial structures)
- Head and neck: Short neck, limited neck extension, decreased hyoid-mental distance (<3 cm in an adult), neck mass, cervical spine disease or trauma, tracheal deviation, dysmorphic facial features (e.g., Pierre-Robin syndrome)
- Mouth: Small opening (<3 cm in an adult), edentulous, protruding incisors, loose or capped teeth, dental appliances, high, arched palate, macroglossia, tonsillar hypertrophy, nonvisible uvula
- Jaw: Micrognathia, retrognathia, trismus, significant malocclusion

Recommendations. Equipment to administer supplemental oxygen should be present when sedation/analgesia is administered. Supplemental oxygen should be considered for moderate sedation and should be administered during deep sedation unless specifically contraindicated for a particular patient or procedure. If hypoxemia is anticipated or develops during sedation/analgesia, supplemental oxygen should be administered.

From American Society of Anesthesiologists Task Force on Sedation and Analgesia by Non-Anesthesiologists. Practice guidelines for sedation and analgesia by non-anesthesiologists. *Anesthesiology.* 2002;96(4):1010. Reprinted with permission.

Respiratory insufficiency is a condition characterized by reduced gas exchange, which is inadequate to meet the body's metabolic demands. Use of sedative, hypnotic, and opioid medications in conjunction with pathophysiologic disease processes predisposes patients receiving sedation/analgesia to the development of respiratory compromise. The synergistic respiratory depressant effects of opioids, sedatives, and hypnotics may produce respiratory insufficiency and airway obstruction in all patient populations including the young, healthy patient. Respiratory insufficiency may develop at any time during the procedure or in the postsedation period.

> It is imperative that healthcare providers participating in sedation patient care understand the principles of oxygen delivery and respiratory physiology. Providers must also demonstrate clinical competency in their ability to utilize oxygen delivery and mechanical airway devices.

Attempts to decrease morbidity associated with the administration of sedation/analgesia are enhanced by identification of patients at risk of respiratory complications with optimization of presedation medical therapy (see Chapter 2). The focus of this chapter includes a review of the anatomy of the airway, airway management, positive-pressure ventilation, and use of oxygen-delivery devices.

Before the administration of sedation/analgesia, healthcare providers must be clinically competent with airway management skills and treatment protocols used in the event of airway obstruction or a respiratory event. These objectives may be accomplished by means of a thorough review of this chapter and practical clinical application. Preceptorship by an anesthesiologist, a certified registered nurse anesthetist, or a qualified airway management specialist is strongly recommended to facilitate this learning process.

ANATOMY

To competently master airway management skills, it is important to understand the functional anatomy of the human airway. Air enters the pulmonary system through the nose, which has a bone and cartilage framework. The upper airway is defined as that portion above the vocal cords.

Upper Airway

The oral cavity consists of the tongue and teeth. The pharynx is a 13-cm-long tube that begins at the internal nares and consists of the tonsils, uvula, and epiglottic structure. The pharynx is divided into three parts:

1. *Nasopharynx:* The nasopharynx begins just posterior to the internal nasal cavity and extends to the soft palate. It contains the adenoids located at the posterior pharyngeal wall.

2. *Oropharynx:* The oropharynx begins at the soft palate and extends to the level of the hyoid bone. It contains the paired palatine and lingual tonsils. The oropharynx serves as both a respiratory and a food passageway.

3. *Laryngopharynx:* The laryngopharynx begins at the level of the hyoid bone and diverges posteriorly to connect with the esophagus and anteriorly into the larynx. Like the oropharynx, the laryngopharynx also functions as a respiratory and gastrointestinal passageway.

Anatomy of the upper airway is depicted in Figure 7-1. The glottic aperture (glottis) is the opening to the larynx, which is covered by the epiglottis. The epiglottis is a large, leaflike structure with its stem attached anteriorly to the thyroid cartilage with no posterior attachment. The leaf portion of the epiglottis moves freely to prevent aspiration of gastric contents from the oropharynx into the trachea. During swallowing, the epiglottis covers the glottic opening. To avoid gastric acid aspiration, it is advisable that the gag reflex be maintained during the administration of sedative/analgesic medications.

Lower Airway

The lower airway includes structures below the level of the vocal cords. The adult larynx (voice box) lies below the glottic opening anterior to the fourth through the sixth cervical vertebra. The larynx is composed of three single and three paired cartilages.

The three single cartilages include:

◆ Thyroid
◆ Cricoid
◆ Epiglottis

The three paired cartilages include:

◆ Corniculate
◆ Cuneiform
◆ Arytenoid

Laryngeal cartilages are displayed in Figure 7-2. The thyroid cartilage (Adam's apple) comprises the anterior portion of the larynx. The cricoid cartilage is the single complete cartilaginous ring, which comprises the lower border of the larynx. Of the three paired cartilages, the arytenoid cartilages control vocal cord function through pharyngeal muscle movement.

The trachea (windpipe) is an air passageway, approximately 12 cm in length, which extends from the larynx to the fifth thoracic vertebra.[1] The trachea lies anterior to the esophagus and bifurcates into the right and left mainstem bronchi. The right and left bronchi progressively branch to eventually form the terminal bronchioles. The lungs consist of smooth muscle innervated by the autonomic nervous system. The lungs extend from just above the clavicles to the diaphragm and are housed within the rib cage. The function and purpose of the upper airway, larynx, trachea, lungs, and pulmonary circulation is to provide exchange of oxygen and carbon dioxide at the alveolar level. A primary concern of the healthcare provider participating in the administration of sedation/analgesia is to maintain and protect the integrity of respiratory processes. In the presence of comorbid states, synergistic pharmacologic effects, and individual patient variability, protection of the patient's airway may become tenuous during procedural sedation. The focus of this chapter is to assist in identification or diagnosis of potential airway problems and to offer intervention strategies to alleviate airway obstruction and prevent the development of respiratory insufficiency.

EVALUATION OF THE AIRWAY

Comprehensive presedation patient assessment is complemented by a focused physical examination, which includes:

◆ Oral cavity evaluation
◆ Temporomandibular joint evaluation
◆ Thyromental distance evaluation
◆ Atlanto-occipital movement evaluation
◆ Physical characteristics related to airway management
◆ Assignment of Mallampati Airway Classification

Equally important is the ability to identify patients with subtle physical anomalies that may predispose them to development of respiratory compromise. All patients presenting for sedation/analgesia should undergo a focused physical examination, which includes evaluation of the airway as a key component. The American Society of Anesthesiologists Task Force on Sedation and Analgesia by Non-Anesthesiologists' "Practice Guidelines for Sedation and Analgesia" advocate a **focused physical examination, including vital signs, auscultation of the heart and lungs, and evaluation of the airway.**[2]

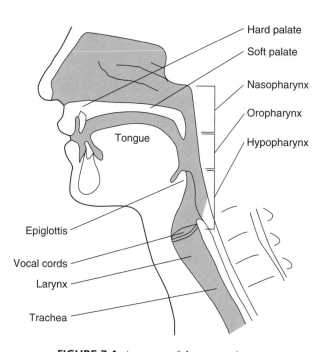

Hard palate
Soft palate
Nasopharynx
Oropharynx
Hypopharynx
Tongue
Epiglottis
Vocal cords
Larynx
Trachea

FIGURE 7-1 Anatomy of the upper airway.

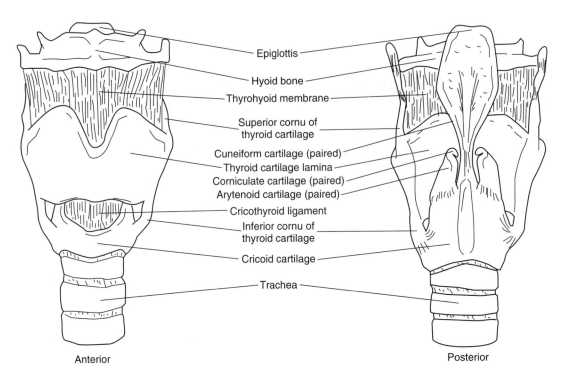

Epiglottis
Hyoid bone
Thyrohyoid membrane
Superior cornu of thyroid cartilage
Cuneiform cartilage (paired)
Thyroid cartilage lamina
Corniculate cartilage (paired)
Arytenoid cartilage (paired)
Cricothyroid ligament
Inferior cornu of thyroid cartilage
Cricoid cartilage
Trachea

Anterior

Posterior

FIGURE 7-2 Laryngeal cartilages.

Oral Cavity Inspection

The oral cavity identified in Figure 7-3 is assessed to identify loose, chipped, or capped teeth. Documentation of the presence of dental anomalies, crowns, bridges, and dentures should be completed before the start of the procedure. The oral cavity should be examined for the presence of tumors or obstruction of air flow.

Temporomandibular Joint Examination

The assessment of the temporomandibular joint (interincisor distance) identified in Figure 7-4 is conducted with the patient's mouth opened as wide as possible. In the adult, the distance between the upper and lower central incisors is normally 4 to 6 cm (2.54 cm = 1 inch).[3,4] An adult should be able to open the mouth at least 40 cm (2 large finger breadths) between the upper and lower incisors. **An interincisor gap of less than 2 finger breadths may be associated with difficult endotracheal intubation.** The presence of a clicking sound, pain associated with opening of the mouth, or a reduced ability to open the mouth indicates reduced temporomandibular joint mobility. Patients with preexisting temporomandibular joint disease may have limited airway mobility if mechanical conduits (oropharyngeal airways, endotracheal tubes, laryngeal mask airways) are required to treat respiratory distress during procedural sedation care.

Thyromental Distance Evaluation

Thyromental distance represents the straight distance, with the neck fully extended and the mouth closed. As demonstrated in Figure 7-5, the distance between the prominence of the thyroid cartilage and the bony point of the lower mandibular border should be more than 7 cm (3 finger breadths). A distance of less than 7 cm may indicate that the patient may be difficult to intubate should the need arise during an airway emergency. The rationale for potential difficult airway management includes inadequate alignment of the pharyngeal and laryngeal axis, which is required for direct visualization and intubation of the larynx.

Atlanto-Occipital Movement

Side to side movement, neck extension, and neck flexion must be assessed before the procedure. Alignment of the three axes required for successful endotracheal intubation (oral, pharyngeal, and laryngeal) requires a combination of flexion and extension with a goal of attainment of the "sniffing" position. Limitations in the ability to achieve the "sniff" position can impair laryngoscopy and endotracheal intubation during emergency airway maneuvers. Therefore, as demonstrated in Figure 7-6, evaluation of the airway includes assessing atlanto-occipital movement through full range of motion.

Physical Characteristics

The following physical characteristics may indicate the potential for difficult airway management:
◆ Hypognathic (recessed) jaw
◆ Hypergnathic (protruding) jaw
◆ Deviated trachea

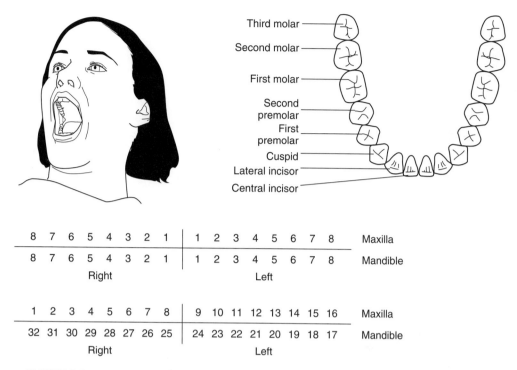

8	7	6	5	4	3	2	1	1	2	3	4	5	6	7	8	Maxilla
8	7	6	5	4	3	2	1	1	2	3	4	5	6	7	8	Mandible
			Right								Left					

1	2	3	4	5	6	7	8	9	10	11	12	13	14	15	16	Maxilla
32	31	30	29	28	27	26	25	24	23	22	21	20	19	18	17	Mandible
			Right								Left					

FIGURE 7-3 Oral cavity assessment. During oral cavity assessment the patient is instructed to open the mouth wide for the healthcare practitioner. The oral cavity is then examined for the presence of anomalies that may obstruct air flow or impede instrumentation of the airway in the event of an airway emergency.

- Large tongue
- Short, thick neck
- Protruding teeth
- High arched palate

Mallampati Airway Classification System

The modified Mallampati Airway Classification System, described in 1983, attempts to grade the degree of difficulty of endotracheal intubation from grade I to IV.[5] The examination is conducted with the patient in a sitting position. The patient's head is maintained in a neutral position, and the mouth is opened as wide as possible (50 to 60 mm).[6] Classification of the patient's airway is based on a description of the anatomic area visualized (Fig. 7-7). **During the examination the patient is encouraged NOT to phonate because this maneuver may elevate the soft palate and interfere with accurate classification.**

The Mallampati Airway Classification System should not be utilized as the only method of airway evaluation and assessment. The system has been criticized secondary to false-positive and false-negative difficult airway identification associated with its use.

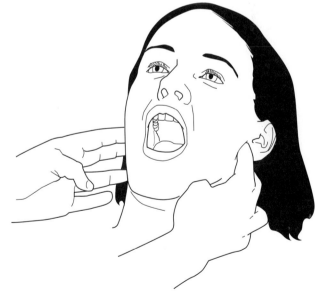

FIGURE 7-4 Temporomandibular joint examination. While the patient's mouth is opened during temporomandibular joint examination, the clinician may assess joint mobility by palpating the temporomandibular joint in an attempt to identify pain or limited range of motion.

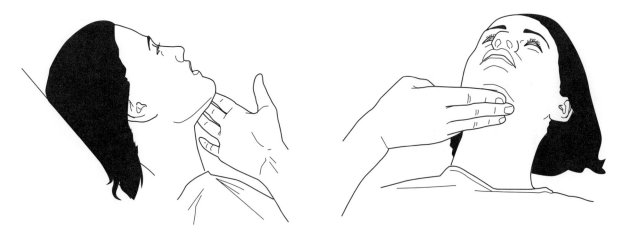

FIGURE 7-5 Thyromental distance evaluation. Presedation patient assessment of the airway should reveal a thyromental distance of more than 7 cm (3 finger breadths).

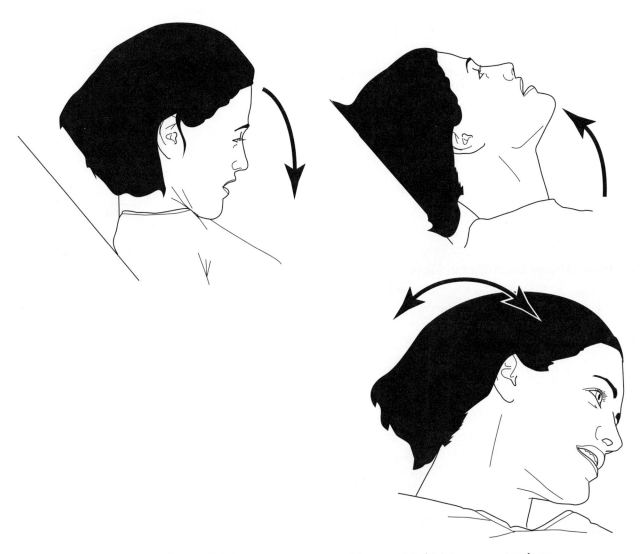

FIGURE 7-6 Atlanto-occipital movement assessment. Atlanto-occipital joint assessment evaluates range of motion through flexion, extension, and side to side movement.

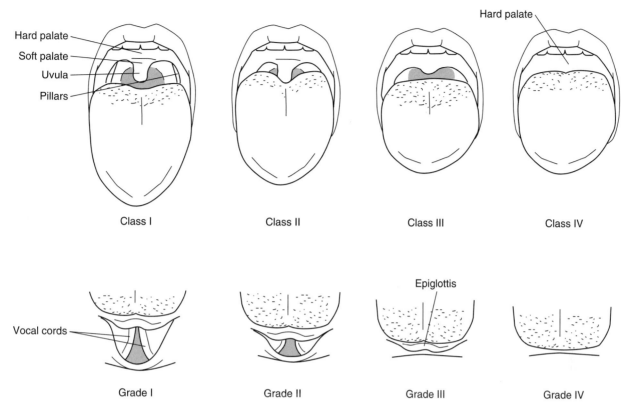

Class I   Class II   Class III   Class IV

Grade I   Grade II   Grade III   Grade IV

FIGURE 7-7 Mallampati Airway Classification System. A difficult intubation (grade III or IV) may be predicted by the inability to visualize certain pharyngeal structures (class III or IV) during the presedation examination of a seated patient.

AIRWAY MANAGEMENT

Skilled clinicians engaged in the administration of sedation/analgesia perform thousands of uneventful procedures annually. When complications do arise, the practitioner must immediately recognize the signs and symptoms of airway compromise and deal with them effectively. **The pharmacologic effect associated with sedative, hypnotic, and analgesic medications in combination is synergistic.** This synergism, or the pharmacologic effects of individual medications, alters airway muscle activity. Alterations in airway muscle activity may lead to airway obstruction. Signs and symptoms of airway obstruction include the following:

- Increased respiratory effort
- Sternal retraction
- Rocking chest motion (not in sync with respiratory effort)
- Inspiratory stridor (harsh, high-pitched inspiratory sounds)
- Hypoxemia
- Hypercarbia
- Absence of breath sounds

Although many clinicians believe that airway obstruction occurs from the base of the tongue occluding the airway, contemporary research reveals that airway obstruction is a more complex phenomenon.[7] **Airway patency is the result of an active mechanism associated with muscles that attach to the hyoid bone and thyroid cartilages.** The tonic nature of muscle activity is responsible for maintaining airway patency by functioning as airway dilators with a resultant increase in air flow and decrease in resistance of breathing. Airway obstruction is a very complex series of architectural changes, which involve changes in pharyngeal and laryngeal muscle support.[8] The epiglottis or posterior movement of the soft palate is often the cause of airway obstruction. Relief of airway obstruction can be demonstrated through displacement of the hyoid bone anteriorly with restoration of a patent airway. Therefore, clinical treatment of airway obstruction is not simply "clearing the tongue" from the posterior pharynx. Figure 7-8 demonstrates forward displacement of the mandible, with resultant stretch of the front of the neck and elevation of the preepiglottic soft tissues anteriorly.[7] **The focus of this chapter is to assist the clinician in rapid diagnosis and intervention in the presence of respiratory complications.** Treatment modalities that may restore effective ventilation include:

- Auditory/tactile stimulation
- Head tilt
- Chin lift
- Jaw thrust
- Nasal/oral airway insertion

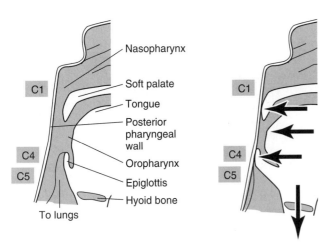

FIGURE 7-8 Restoration of effective ventilation. The upper airway in the sagittal plane. **A,** Nasopharynx and oropharynx are patent due to proper tone and position of airway architectural structures. **B,** Significant posterior displacements of the soft palate and base of the tongue occur. Note also the downward displacement of the hyoid bone. Even with insertion of an oral airway the soft palate and epiglottic obstructions would likely not resolve. Patient inspiratory effort in **B** could easily provoke even more soft tissue derangement, further exacerbating the airway distress.

◆ Pharmacologic reversal of sedative/analgesic (Romazicon/Narcan)

> The goal of these interventions is to restore air flow. The "Sedation Airway Management Algorithm" featured in Figure 7-9 should be used in the event of airway obstruction and respiratory compromise encountered during procedural sedation.

Lateral Head Tilt

If verbal and tactile stimulation fail to relieve airway obstruction, the lateral head tilt depicted in Figure 7-10 is a mechanical maneuver that moves the head from the neutral position to the lateral (side) position. This maneuver may result in tongue displacement from the posterior pharyngeal wall to the side of the oropharynx. Complete or partial relief of upper airway obstruction may occur after use of this maneuver.

Chin Lift

When the head tilt is unsuccessful, a chin lift may be utilized. The chin lift depicted in Figure 7-11 permits anterior movement of the mandible through superior displacement of the chin. This maneuver combined with hyperextension of the head and neck and forward displacement of the mandible will elevate the soft tissue anteriorly.

Jaw Thrust

If verbal or tactile stimulation, head tilt, and chin lift do not produce relief of airway obstruction, the patient has entered a

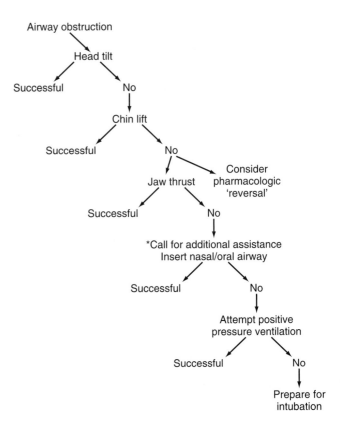

FIGURE 7-9 The sedation airway management algorithm.

state of deep sedation or general anesthesia. Unless the obstruction is relieved and air flow restored, oxygen desaturation and hypoxemia will ensue. The jaw thrust maneuver depicted in Figure 7-12 requires the use of both hands. A jaw thrust provides significant anterior displacement of the mandible, stretches the anterior aspects of the neck, and elevates the preepiglottic soft tissues anteriorly. Great care must be taken not to exert excessive pressure for a prolonged period of time when performing a jaw thrust to prevent damage to the facial nerve. As depicted in Figure 7-13, the facial nerve runs behind the ramus of the mandible and fans out across the face. Damage to the facial nerve or its central pathway may result in facial palsy.[9] In the event that these maneuvers do not relieve airway obstruction, pharmacologic reversal should be considered. Nonreversible medications may require the use of an oral or nasal airway to relieve obstruction.

> Airway obstruction not relieved by head tilt, chin lift, and jaw thrust may require immediate consultation by a certified registered nurse anesthetist or anesthesiologist for additional airway support.

Nasal Airway

If airway obstruction continues after the previous maneuvers, an airway conduit may be needed to physically displace

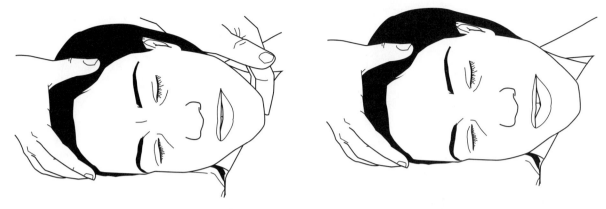

FIGURE 7-10 Lateral head tilt. Lateral head tilt allows the healthcare practitioner the ability to move the head from the neutral to the "side" position, which may result in relief of airway obstruction.

the tongue from the posterior pharyngeal wall. In the sedated patient, nasal airways are generally better tolerated than oral airways. Oral airways frequently stimulate the gag reflex, with resultant vomiting or laryngospasm. However, nasal airways are not without risks. Inherent risks associated with nasopharyngeal airway use include epistaxis, hypertension, and difficult placement in patients with nasal deformity. Epistaxis in the presence of respiratory distress results in blood in the oropharynx, which may stimulate laryngospasm or bronchospasm. Nasopharyngeal airways are not recommended in the presence of anticoagulants, cerebrospinal fluid rhinorrhea, septal deformity, or nasal polyps. They should not be forced in the presence of obstruction. Insertion of nasopharyngeal airways requires assessment of nare size. Nasopharyngeal airways come in an assortment of adult sizes:

- 6.0 mm
- 6.5 mm
- 7.0 mm
- 7.5 mm
- 8.0 mm

These sizes for nasopharyngeal airways indicate the internal diameter in millimeters. The larger the internal diameter, the longer the airway.[10] As demonstrated in Figures 7-14 and 7-16, the nasopharyngeal airway must be long enough to physically displace the base of the tongue from the posterior pharyngeal wall. Approximate length of the nasopharyngeal airway is measured from the tip of the nares to the lobe of the ear. Before insertion, the nasopharyngeal airway should be lubricated well. This can be accomplished with water-soluble lubricant, 2% lidocaine (Xylocaine) jelly, or 5% lidocaine ointment. Lubrication also helps to decrease the incidence of epistaxis. During insertion (Fig. 7-15), gentle pressure may be used after initial insertion into the nare. **However, one should never force a nasopharyngeal airway that is impeded in the posterior nasopharynx.** The nasal airway

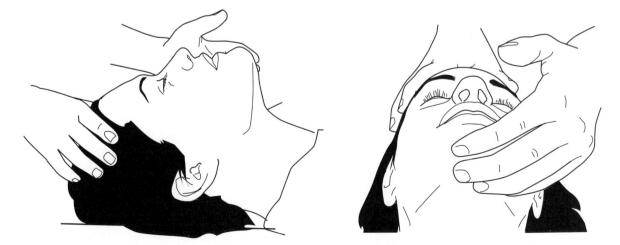

FIGURE 7-11 Chin lift. The chin lift maneuver places traction on the mentum of the chin providing forward displacement of the mandible in an attempt to restore air flow.

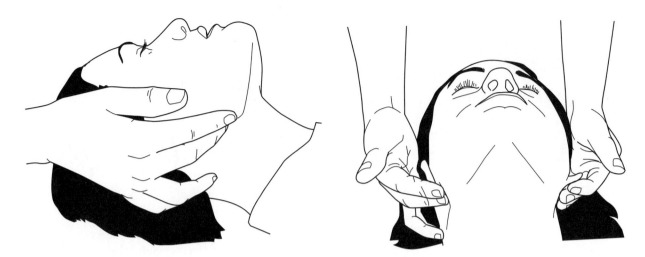

FIGURE 7-12 Jaw thrust. The jaw thrust maneuver places significant anterior forward displacement on the jaw in an attempt to relieve obstruction and restore air flow.

must be inserted perpendicular to the face. Figure 7-16 demonstrates a properly positioned nasal airway, which provides a physical conduit for air passage.

Oral Airway

Just as a nasopharyngeal airway provides a mechanical passage for air flow, the oropharyngeal airway physically

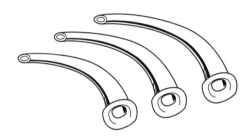

FIGURE 7-14 Nasal airway.

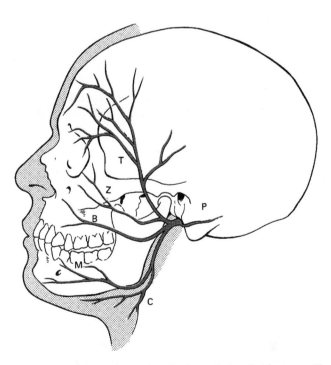

FIGURE 7-13 Anatomic distribution of the facial nerve. *T,* temporal; *Z,* zygomatic; *B,* buccal; *M,* mandibular; *C,* cervical; *P,* posterior auricular branch. (From Ellis H, Feldman S. *Anatomy for Anaesthetists.* 6th ed. Cambridge, MA: Blackwell Scientific Publications; 1993:284.)

displaces the tongue off of the posterior pharyngeal wall. The oropharyngeal airway may stimulate vomiting if the gag reflex remains intact. Additional complications associated with insertion of an oropharyngeal airway include the following:

- Bradycardia secondary to vagal stimulation
- Retching with resultant hypertension and tachycardia
- Laryngospasm
- Dental damage
- Pharyngeal or lip lacerations

When indicated, insertion of an oropharyngeal airway must be performed carefully to avoid complications noted previously. Proper placement of an oropharyngeal airway, depicted in Figure 7-17, is outlined in Box 7-1.

> Patients who require and tolerate the insertion of nasal/oral airways have entered into a state of deep sedation or general anesthesia.

Pharmacologic Antagonists

Consideration should be given to the administration of pharmacologic antagonists to "reverse" the respiratory depressant effects associated with benzodiazepines and narcotic medications. A complete pharmacokinetic/

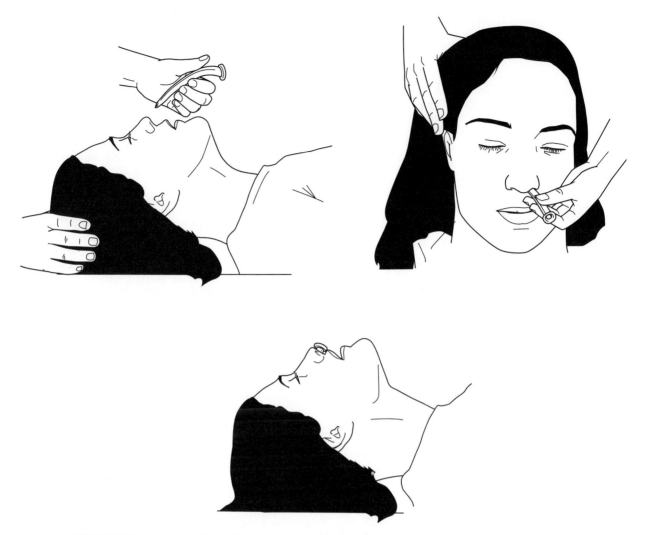

FIGURE 7-15 Insertion of nasopharyngeal airway. Gentle pressure is used to advance a well-lubricated nasopharyngeal airway into place. Excessive force must be avoided to prevent epistaxis. If excessive pressure is encountered on placement of the airway, one should withdraw and attempt placement on the opposite side.

pharmacodynamic profile of these medications is provided in Chapters 4 and 5.

Laryngospasm

Laryngospasm is a spasm of the laryngeal musculature. Often initiated by mucus, blood, or saliva irritating the vocal cords, laryngospasm results in complete or partial closure of the cords with inability of the patient to ventilate. Patients with total airway obstruction will often display "rocky" abdominal respirations with no air exchange. Initial treatment for laryngospasm is positive-pressure ventilation with 100% oxygen. A secure mask fit is required to generate positive pressure to break the spasm. If this maneuver is unsuccessful, an anesthesia provider or airway management expert should

be summoned immediately. A nonparalyzing dose (approximately one tenth of the full intubating dose) of succinylcholine is administered. Because of the need for advanced airway support associated with the utilization of muscle relaxants, this treatment modality should only be attempted by airway management experts. Coupled with ventilatory support, relaxation of the skeletal muscles of the larynx generally ensues. If necessary, endotracheal intubation is employed as a last resort to break a laryngospasm.

EMERGENCY AIRWAY MANAGEMENT
Mask Management

Upper airway obstruction and respiratory insufficiency must be recognized promptly and treated effectively.

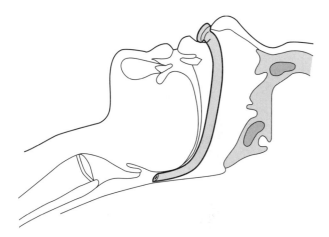

FIGURE 7-16 The nasopharyngeal airway in place. The airway passes through the nose and extends to just above the epiglottis.

Mechanisms to relieve upper airway obstruction must be provided in a systematic manner as outlined in Figure 7-9. In the presence of respiratory depression, apnea, or airway obstruction, the healthcare provider must be prepared to ventilate the patient with a positive-pressure breathing device. If all maneuvers previously outlined fail to relieve upper airway obstruction and do not restore effective ventilation, an airway management expert should be summoned emergently to correct the airway obstruction and administer positive-pressure ventilation.

Commercially available bag-valve-mask devices are disposable systems for single patient use. Generally, packaged with this system is one disposable mask for use with the bag-valve device. It is important to note that many of the masks packaged with these units are large adult sizes. However, the facial anatomy of each individual patient may be markedly

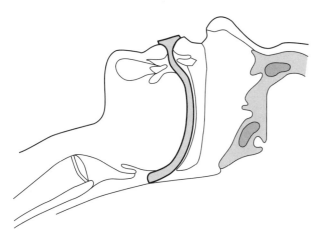

FIGURE 7-17 The oropharyngeal airway in place. The airway follows the curvature of the tongue, pulling it and the epiglottis away from the posterior pharyngeal wall and providing a channel for air passage.

BOX 7-1

Proper Placement of an Oropharyngeal Airway

1. Carefully open the patient's mouth, exercising caution to prevent finger injury to the clinician or dental damage to the patient.
2. Once the mouth is open, insert the tongue blade into the posterior pharynx.
3. Insert the tongue blade toward the base of the tongue. Apply pressure with the tongue blade to displace the base of the tongue anteriorly.
4. Insert the oropharyngeal airway into the oropharynx. The oropharyngeal airway is designed to follow the natural curvature of the oropharynx. The tongue blade should expose a clear view of the posterior oropharynx. Do not force or blindly position the oropharyngeal airway. Malpositioning of the oropharyngeal airway can force the base of the tongue against the posterior pharyngeal wall, completely obstructing the airway.
5. After insertion, verify that the tongue and lips have not been inadvertently positioned between the teeth.
6. A patient who tolerates the insertion of an oropharyngeal airway is deeply sedated and at this point the practitioner is advised to consult an anesthesia practitioner to provide additional airway management assistance.

---

different on the basis of patient weight, mandibular size, age, nutritional status, presence of facial hair, and dentition. Therefore, it is important to select a proper size mask based on these individualized patient factors. To account for patient variability, a variety of disposable mask sizes must be available in each sedation area. **It is critical to have an assortment of these masks available before the commencement of any sedation procedure.** As identified in Figure 7-18, a properly fitting mask should fit snugly between the bridge of the patient's nose, the mentum or the chin, and the medial aspects of the face. Masks that extend above the bridge of the nose, below the level of the mandible, or past the lateral aspects of the face are inappropriately sized. This results in ineffective positive-pressure ventilation.

To secure an appropriate mask fit for positive-pressure ventilation, the mask must form an effective seal between the skin of the face and the mask. Once the mask has been properly positioned (Fig. 7-19), the third and fourth or fourth and fifth fingers (depending on the clinician's hand size) are placed on the mandible. This maneuver elevates the jaw and the base of the tongue off the posterior pharyngeal wall. On delivery of the first positive-pressure ventilation, there should be chest rise and fall, breath sounds, and no air escape around the mask. If the patient remains apneic, positive-pressure ventilation should ensue at a rate of 16 to 20 breaths per minute until additional assistance arrives. **Preparation for a respiratory emergency is required**

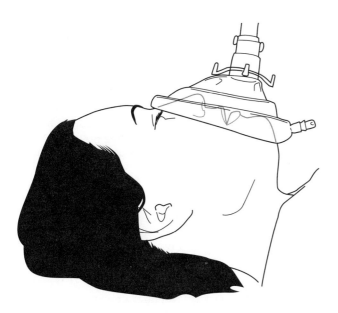

FIGURE 7-18 Properly fitting mask.

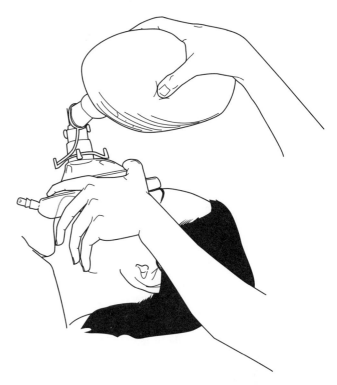

FIGURE 7-19 Positive-pressure ventilation. An effective seal is formed by placing the third, fourth, and fifth fingers below the mandible and exerting gentle pressure on the bridge of the nose. A proper mask fit does not allow oxygen to escape between the patient's face and the mask seal. Notice how the hands produce an effective mask seal and also extend the head to produce a patent airway. (Redrawn from Butterworth J. *Atlas of Procedures in Anesthesia and Critical Care.* Philadelphia: WB Saunders; 1991:23.)

wherever the administration of sedation/analgesia is performed. When summoned, anesthesia personnel or the attending physician will need specific equipment and supplies to secure the airway and establish effective ventilation. Therefore, it is important to maintain specific emergency airway equipment at each designated sedation location.

Endotracheal Tubes

An assortment of endotracheal tubes must be kept on hand at all times for the variety of age groups receiving procedural sedation. Endotracheal tube sizes are designated in millimeters of internal diameter. Box 7-2 lists recommended endotracheal tube sizes on the basis of patient age.

Stylet

An endotracheal stylet (Fig. 7-20) is a polyvinylchloride or aluminum instrument that provides rigidity to the endotracheal tube. It enhances the clinician's ability to place the endotracheal tube in a variety of positions to aid in the intubation process. Stylets allow direction of the endotracheal tube through the glottic opening and are frequently utilized for difficult intubations. Stylets are available in malleable aluminum or metal with or without a rubberized cover. Adult and pediatric sizes are available, and the stylet should not extend past the tip of the endotracheal tube or into the Murphy eye. To facilitate the insertion and easy removal of stylets from endotracheal tubes, a water-soluble lubricant should be applied along its axis before insertion.

Laryngoscope Handle and Blade

The laryngoscope handle and blade are used to manipulate the oropharyngeal tissue and epiglottis. The blade provides the ability to visualize the glottic aperture and facilitate insertion

of the endotracheal tube into the trachea. The laryngoscope handle serves a dual function. First, it acts as a power supply that is powered by nicad or alkaline batteries. Its second function is to act as a receptacle for the blade. A variety of blades are available for use with the handle.

BOX 7-2	
Recommended Sizes for Endotracheal Tubes	
Age	**Endotracheal Tube Size (Internal Diameter, mm)**
Newborn	3.0
6 mo	3.5
18 mo	4.0
36 mo	4.5
5 yr	5.0
6 yr	5.5
8 yr	6.0
12 yr	6.5
16 yr	6.5-7.0
Adult female	7.0
Adult male	8.0

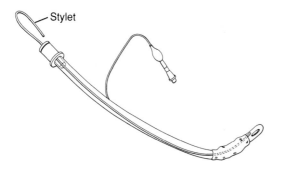

FIGURE 7-20 Endotracheal tube stylet. Stylets should be well lubricated before insertion in the endotracheal tube. The stylet must be bent to prevent the proximal end from extending past the tip of the endotracheal tube. (From Morgan G, Mikhail M. *Clinical Anesthesiology.* 2nd ed. Stamford, CT: Appleton & Lange; 1996:62.)

Selection of a blade depends on patient age, anatomic variabilities of the patient, and clinician preference. Age-appropriate selection of blades listed in Figure 7-21 should be maintained in each practice setting. In most adults, intubation can be done successfully with a Macintosh No. 3 blade or a Miller No. 2 blade. Having both readily available significantly enhances the clinician's ability to secure endotracheal tube placement and a patent airway in emergent situations.

Magill Forceps

Magill forceps are ancillary airway tools used to direct an endotracheal tube during nasotracheal intubation. Endotracheal tubes inserted for nasotracheal intubation hug the posterior pharyngeal wall and may require use of the Magill forceps to distally direct the tube anteriorly and through the glottic opening.

Suction Equipment

A variety of suction equipment is available. An ample supply of suction liners, filters, tubing, and suction tips must be readily accessible in each sedation location. In areas where sedation procedures are performed concurrently, one suction unit must be available for each patient. Yankauer suction tips aspirate large volumes of material from the oropharynx. They also offer the advantage of aspiration of larger particulate matter. Disadvantages associated with Yankauer suction tips include lip laceration, oropharyngeal damage, and dental trauma. No. 16 French suction catheters must be available to suction the oropharynx in the event of patients biting or clenching down. Advantages of No. 16 French suction catheters include insertion into small areas

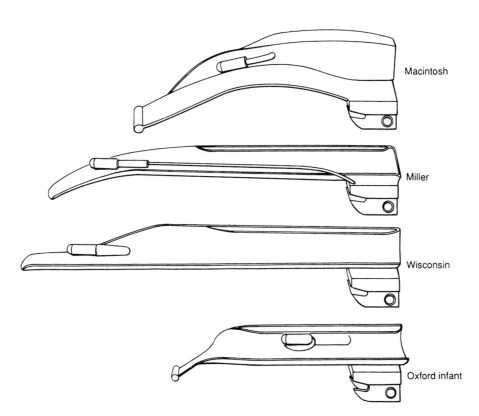

FIGURE 7-21 Laryngoscope blades. (From Morgan G, Mikhail M. *Clinical Anesthesiology.* 2nd ed. Stamford, CT: Appleton & Lange; 1996:61.)

Minimum Recommended Emergency Airway Setup

- Nasopharyngeal airways (age-appropriate sizes)
- Oropharyngeal airways (age-appropriate sizes)
- Tongue blades
- Lidocaine (Xylocaine) ointment or jelly and water-soluble lubricant
- Two laryngoscope handles
- Two MacIntosh blades (age-appropriate sizes)
- Two Miller blades (age-appropriate sizes)
- Spare blade light bulbs
- Endotracheal tubes (age-appropriate sizes)
- Two stylets (adult and pediatric)
- Magill forceps (adult and pediatric)
- Suction units
- Yankauer suction tips
- No. 16 French suction catheters
- Supplemental oxygen E cylinders
- Oxygen
- Bag valve mask device
- Face mask (age-appropriate size)

and the nasopharynx. Use of emergency airway equipment for respiratory resuscitation is dependent on clinician preference, the degree of respiratory distress, and the patient's anatomy. Box 7-3 outlines minimum recommended emergency airway setup.

An ample supply of respiratory equipment must be immediately available in all sedation locations.

OXYGEN DELIVERY DEVICES

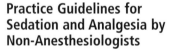

Practice Guidelines for Sedation and Analgesia by Non-Anesthesiologists

American Society of Anesthesiologists Task Force on Sedation and Analgesia by Non-Anesthesiologists

Recommendations. Equipment to administer supplemental oxygen should be present when sedation/analgesia is administered. Supplemental oxygen should be considered for moderate sedation and should be administered during deep sedation unless specifically contraindicated for a particular patient or procedure. If hypoxemia is anticipated or develops during sedation/analgesia, supplemental oxygen should be administered.

From American Society of Anesthesiologists Task Force on Sedation and Analgesia by Non-Anesthesiologists. Practice guidelines for sedation and analgesia by non-anesthesiologists. *Anesthesiology.* 2002;96:1010. Reprinted with permission.

Supplemental oxygen may be administered by a variety of methods. The primary goal of oxygen therapy is the prevention of hypoxia, hypoventilation, and respiratory depression. Table 7-1 presents oxygen systems available to deliver an enriched oxygen environment to the patient.

Because of the respiratory depressant effects associated with all sedatives, hypnotics, and analgesics, serious consideration should be given to the administration of supplemental oxygen to all patients receiving sedation/analgesia unless specifically contraindicated.

Nasal Cannula

Nasal cannulas are low-flow oxygen-administration systems that increase the patient's inspired oxygen concentration. Comfortable and inexpensive, they increase inspired oxygen concentration and allow the nasopharynx to serve as an oxygen reservoir. Inspired oxygen concentration increases 3% to 4% for each liter delivered through the nasal cannula.[11] Nasal cannulas are not recommended for flow rates exceeding 4 to 5 L/min. Flow rates greater than 4 L/min may lead to drying of mucous membranes, irritation, and bleeding.

Oxygen Face Mask

Simple oxygen face masks permit delivery of inspired oxygen of 40% to 60%. This increase in F_{IO_2} occurs secondary to increased reservoir space and oxygen flow. An F_{IO_2} of 40% to 60% depends on oxygen flow rate, the patient's inspiratory flow, and mask fit.

Nonrebreathing Masks

A distinct advantage of a reservoir bag to the oxygen face mask is that it allows delivery of up to 100% oxygen when a tight face seal is assured. Rebreathing is diminished through a combination of unidirectional valves and high inspiratory flow rates.

Humidified Oxygen

Humidified oxygen is indicated in the presence of increased pulmonary secretions, increased viscosity, and mobilization of secretions. The goal of humidification is to decrease viscosity and mobilize secretions by increasing water content in the alveoli. Humidification requires high flow rates to convert water to a vapor state.

Manual Resuscitative Devices: Bag-Valve Device (AMBU Bag)

It is important for the clinician participating in the administration of sedation to ventilate patients both efficiently and effectively. As outlined earlier, the provider must be cognizant of airway obstruction and take definitive action when necessary. In the presence of apnea, hypoxemia, or respiratory distress, positive-pressure ventilation must be used. In emergent situations the bag-valve mask is the ventilation

TABLE 7-1

Methods of Oxygen Administration

METHOD	F_{IO_2}	FLOW (L/min)	COMMENTS
Low-Flow Methods			
Nasal cannula (prongs)	0.24-0.4	5-6	Comfortable to wear; patient can breathe orally or nasally and still raise F_{IO_2}; humidification unnecessary
Simple face mask	0.4-0.6	5-8	Adjustable to fit face; may be hot and uncomfortable for patients. Poorly tolerated; potential for skin irritation from tight fit and oxygen contact.
Face tent	0.3-0.55	4-10	Less confining; useful when extra humidity needed.
Partial rebreathing mask	0.35-0.6	6-10	Mask with attached reservoir bag; no valves on mask (exhalation ports open).
High-Flow Methods			
Nonrebreathing mask	0.4-1	6-15	Mask with reservoir bag; one-way valves on exhalation side ports of mask, one-way valve between mask and bag for inhalation.
"Venturi" mask	0.24-0.55	2-14	Believed accurate delivery of desired F_{IO_2}; may be less if patient is hyperpneic or unable to keep mask in position on face.
T-piece or Brigg's	0.21-1	2-10	Used with endotracheal or tracheostomy tube; provides accurate delivery of desired F_{IO_2} and humidification; most often used when weaning patients from ventilator assistance before endotracheal tube removal.
Mechanical ventilator	0.21-1	Direct from supply	Pressure, volume, flow, and oxygen percentage all adjustable.

F_{IO_2}, Fraction of inspired oxygen concentration.
From Drain C. *The Post Anesthesia Care Unit.* 4th ed. Philadelphia: WB Saunders; 2003:401.

system of choice to deliver oxygen-enriched positive-pressure ventilation to the patient. Manual resuscitative devices are known by a variety of names, including the following:

◆ Bag valve masks
◆ Bag valve resuscitative device
◆ Respiratory bags
◆ Self-inflating resuscitators
◆ Ambu bag

During the past several years, manual resuscitators have evolved from a multiple patient use device to a disposable resuscitator for single patient use. Advantages of bag-valve masks include the following:

◆ Inexpensive
◆ Permit an enriched oxygen environment
◆ Portable
◆ Lightweight

The bag of the resuscitator is self-inflating and is coupled with a nonrebreathing valve to prevent rebreathing of exhaled gases. The American Society for Testing and Materials requires manual resuscitators to be equipped with a mechanism to increase inspired oxygen concentration.[12] When oxygen is delivered into the self-inflating bag, the inspired oxygen concentration increases. Some bags also have an additional reservoir, which allows an opportunity for oxygen to accumulate. Oxygen flows directly into the self-inflating bag when the refill valve opens. During a respiratory crisis, the oxygen flow rate should be 10 to 15 L in the adult patient.[13] Positive-pressure ventilation requires the clinician to grasp the self-inflating bag in the middle with firm pressure and depress the bag to deliver an effective ventilation. If the patient is not completely apneic, the delivery of the manual ventilation should be synchronized with the inspiratory phase of the patient. Complications associated with use of the bag valve mask devices are generally related to valve failure, with resultant rebreathing of expired gases and decreased F_{IO_2}. Additional complications include gastric insufflation secondary to attempted ventilation through a nonpatent airway. Since the advent of disposable single-use units, these complications occur with less frequency. **A bag-valve-mask device that is self-inflating must be present with a backup source of oxygen available in each sedation practice setting. The presence of a backup oxygen source (E cylinders) should be reserved in the event that the regular tank system or hospital pipeline system fails.**

SUMMARY

Clinicians engaged in caring for patients receiving any degree of sedation must be prepared to manage airway compromise. Airway obstruction, arterial desaturation, and respiratory insufficiency may develop secondary to the synergistic effects of the medication or untoward patient response. **Healthcare providers who assume the responsibility of administering sedative and opioid medications must be clinically competent to respond to airway emergencies.** A self-inflating bag-valve-mask device must be present with a backup source of oxygen in each sedation practice setting.

In order to achieve maximal educational benefit from this chapter, please complete the Learner Self-Assessment below. This self-assessment tool provides the ability to identify areas requiring additional review. Reference material for each question is provided in Appendix F.

1. Healthcare practitioner considerations associated with **JCAHO Standards** related to airway management, oxygenation, and ventilation associated with sedation/analgesia include:

2. **Practice Guidelines for Sedation and Analgesia by Non-Anesthesiologists** promulgated by the ASA Task Force on Sedation **related to airway management, oxygenation, ventilation, focused physical examination, and oxygen delivery devices** associated with the administration of sedation/analgesia include:

3. **Components of the presedation airway evaluation** include:
   a.

   b.

   c.

   d.

   e.

4. **Clinical signs and symptoms associated with respiratory insufficiency and airway obstruction** include:

5. **Treatment modalities designed to relieve airway obstruction and restore air flow** include:
   a.

   b.

   c.

   d.

   e.

6. The **proper technique for nasal and oral airway insertion** includes:
   a. Nasal insertion

   b. Oral insertion

7. Considerations for **proper application of a face mask for positive-pressure ventilation** include:

8. Components of the **"Sedation Airway Algorithm"** include:

POST-TEST QUESTIONS

Please note: If you are applying for CE credit, you must contact Specialty Health Education, Inc. @ 800-694-8041 for a CE Application Packet.

1. A pulmonary condition characterized by reduced gas exchange that is inadequate to meet the body's metabolic demand is identified as _____.
   A. Pulmonary embolus
   B. Pulmonary obstruction
   C. Respiratory arrest
   D. Respiratory insufficiency

2. Identification of loose, chipped, or capped teeth and observation of tumors or physical anomalies that may interfere with procedural airway management is identified during which of the following presedation examinations? _____
   A. Temporomandibular joint examination
   B. Atlanto-occipital movement examination
   C. Assignment of Mallampati airway classification
   D. Oral cavity inspection

3. During assessment of the temporomandibular joint (interincisor distance), the distance between the upper and lower central incisors is normally _____.
   A. 1 to 2 cm
   B. 3 to 4 cm
   C. 4 to 6 cm
   D. 15 to 18 cm

4. A normal thyromental distance during physical examination would reveal a distance _____.
   A. Less than 2 cm
   B. Less than 4 cm
   C. Greater than 7 cm
   D. Greater than 28 cm

5. A mechanical maneuver used initially to restore air flow during airway obstruction, which moves the head from the neutral position to the "side" position is identified as _____.
   A. Chin lift
   B. Lateral head tilt
   C. Jaw thrust
   D. Finger sweep

6. Epistaxis (nasal bleeding) may be associated with which of the following airway maneuvers? _____
   A. Oral airway insertion
   B. Nasal airway insertion
   C. Chin lift
   D. Jaw thrust

7. Positive airway pressure may be delivered to the sedated patient in respiratory distress by which of the following devices? _____
   A. Nasal airway
   B. Oxygen cylinder
   C. Self-inflating Ambu bag
   D. Oral airway

8. One of the primary goals of oxygen therapy is _____.
   A. Prevention of anoxia
   B. Treatment of airway obstruction
   C. Prevention of hypoxia, hypoventilation, and respiratory depression
   D. Elimination of carbon dioxide

9. Which of the following airway devices provides an increase in oxygen concentration of 3% to 4% for each liter delivered? _____
   A. Nasal airway
   B. Oral airway
   C. Endotracheal tube
   D. Nasal cannula

10. Which of the following is not a sign of airway obstruction? _____
    A. Inspiratory stridor
    B. Hypercarbia
    C. Hypoxemia
    D. Hypocarbia

REFERENCES

1. Barash P, Cullen B, Stoelting R. *Clinical Anesthesia.* 4th ed. Philadelphia: Lippincott Williams & Wilkins; 2001;595.
2. American Society of Anesthesiologists Task Force on Sedation and Analgesia by Non-Anesthesiologists. Practice guidelines for sedation and analgesia by non-anesthesiologists. *Anesthesiology.* 2002;96(4).
3. Rose DK, Cohen MM. The airway: problems and predictions in 18,500 patients. *Can J Anaesth.* 1994;41:372-383.
4. Block C, Brechnew VL. Unusual problems in airway management: II. The influence of the temporomandibular joint, the mandible, and associated structures on endotracheal intubation. *Anesth Analg.* 1971;50:114-123.
5. Faust R, Danielson D. Management of the difficult airway. In *Anesthesiology Review.* 3rd ed. New York: Churchill Livingstone; 2002;482.
6. Stoelting R, Miller R. *Basics of Anesthesia.* 4th ed. New York: Churchill Livingstone; 2000;148.
7. Biddle C. Reflections on "Maintaining an Airway." *Curr Rev Perianesth Nurs.* 1993;15(21):169-176.
8. Boidin MP. Airway patency in the unconscious patient. *Br J Anaesth.* 1985;57:306-310.
9. Ellis H, Feldman S. *Anatomy for Anaesthetists.* 6th ed. Cambridge, MA: Blackwell Scientific Publications; 1993:285.
10. Cummins R. *American Heart Association Advanced Life Support.* Dallas: The Association; 1994:2.
11. Morgan G, Mikhail M, Muray M. *Clinical Anesthesiology.* 3rd ed. New York: Lange Medical Books/McGraw-Hill, 2002.
12. Dorsch J, Dorsch S. *Understanding Anesthesia Equipment.* 4th ed. Baltimore: Williams & Wilkins, 2001:231.
13. Dorsch J, Dorsch S. *Understanding Anesthesia Equipment.* 4th ed. Baltimore: Williams & Wilkins, 2001:234.

Intravenous Insertion Techniques/Intravenous Solutions

At the completion of this chapter, the learner shall:

◆ State the principles of intravenous therapy.

◆ List the methods of intravenous cannula insertion required for moderate sedation patients.

◆ Identify systemic complications associated with intravenous catheter placement.

◆ State common intravenous solutions utilized during the administration of moderate sedation/analgesia.

◆ State the presedation, procedural, and postprocedural care associated with intravenous therapy.

Joint Commission on Accreditation of Healthcare Organizations Standards for Operative or Other High-Risk Procedures and/or the Administration of Moderate or Deep Sedation or Anesthesia

Standard PC.13.20
Operative or other procedures and/or the administration of moderate or deep sedation or anesthesia are planned.

Rationale for PC.13.20
Because the response to procedures is not always predictable and sedation-to-anesthesia is a continuum, it is not always possible to predict how an individual patient will respond. Therefore, qualified individuals are trained in professional standards and techniques to manage patients in the case of a potentially harmful event.

Elements of Performance for PC.13.20
1. Sufficient numbers of qualified staff are available* to evaluate the patient, perform the procedure, monitor, and recover the patient.
2. Individuals administering moderate or deep sedation and anesthesia are qualified† and have the appropriate credentials to manage patients at whatever level of sedation or anesthesia is achieved, either intentionally or unintentionally.
3. A registered nurse supervises perioperative nursing care.
4. Appropriate equipment to monitor the patient's physiologic status is available.
5. ***Appropriate equipment to administer intravenous fluids and drugs, including blood and blood components, is available as needed.***
6. Resuscitation capabilities are available.

Before operative and other procedures or the administration of moderate or deep sedation or anesthesia:
7. Patient acuity is assessed to plan for the appropriate level of postprocedure care.

8. Preprocedural education, treatments, and services are provided according to the plan for care, treatment, and services.

9. The site, procedure, and patient are accurately identified and clearly communicated before surgery.

10. A presedation or preanesthesia assessment is conducted.

11. Before sedating or anesthetizing a patient, a licensed independent practitioner with appropriate clinical privileges plans or concurs with the planned anesthesia.

12. The patient is reevaluated immediately before moderate or deep sedation and before anesthesia induction.

---

*For hospitals providing obstetric or emergency operative services, this means they can provide anesthesia services as required by law and regulation.

†**Qualified** The individuals providing moderate or deep sedation and anesthesia have at a minimum had competency-based education, training, and experience in the following:

1. Evaluating patients before moderate or deep sedation and anesthesia.
2. Performing the moderate or deep sedation and anesthesia, including rescuing patients who slip into a deeper-than-desired level of sedation or analgesia. This includes the following:
   a. *Moderate* sedation – are qualified to rescue patients from deep sedation and are competent to manage a compromised airway and to provide adequate oxygenation and ventilation.
   b. *Deep* sedation – are qualified to rescue patients from general anesthesia and are competent to manage an unstable cardiovascular system as well as a compromised airway and inadequate oxygenation and ventilation.

© Joint Commission: Standards for Operative or Other High-Risk Procedures and/or the Administration of Moderate or Deep Sedation or Anesthesia, January, 2004. Reprinted with permission.

Practice Guidelines for Sedation and Analgesia by Non-Anesthesiologists
American Society of Anesthesiologists Task Force on Sedation and Analgesia by Non-Anesthesiologists

Recommendations. In patients receiving intravenous medications for sedation/analgesia, vascular access should be maintained throughout the procedure and until the patient is no longer at risk for cardiorespiratory depression. In patients who have sedation/analgesia by nonintravenous routes, or whose intravenous line has become dislodged or blocked, practitioners should determine the advisability of establishing or reestablishing intravenous access on a case-by-case basis. In all instances, an individual with the skills to establish intravenous access should be immediately available.

From American Society of Anesthesiologists Task Force on Sedation and Analgesia by Non-Anesthesiologists. Practice guidelines for sedation and analgesia by non-anesthesiologists. *Anesthesiology.* 2002;96(4):1011. Reprinted with permission.

PRINCIPLES OF INTRAVENOUS THERAPY

The purpose of intravenous cannulation is to provide direct vascular access for administration of medications and supplemental fluid during sedation/analgesia procedures. **Intravenous access provides immediate uptake and distribution of sedation medications and serves as a lifeline in the event of patient decompensation or crisis.** Placement of the intravenous cannula is critical to the success of the planned procedure.

Whenever there is doubt regarding successful cannulation or possible infiltration, the clinician should err on the side of caution and replace the catheter.

INTRAVENOUS INSERTION TECHNIQUES

Supplies and equipment are assembled before the application of a tourniquet and selection of a vein. Supplies and equipment required for intravenous insertion are listed in Box 8-1. Intravenous solutions have been available in plastic containers since 1971.[1] Plastic containers displayed in Figure 8-1 offer the following advantages when compared with glass containers:

- They do not require that air be admitted to the system for fluid to flow.
- They do not require vented intravenous administration sets.
- They use atmospheric pressure to collapse the container as the intravenous solution flows into the patient.
- They do not break or rupture during routine use.

BOX 8-1

Intravenous Insertion Supplies

- Disposable gloves
- Alcohol swabs/antiseptic solution
- Tourniquet
- Selection of IV catheters:
  16 gauge
  18 gauge
  20 gauge
  22 gauge
- 1% lidocaine
- Local anesthesia (EMLA) cream for pediatric patients
- Adhesive/paper tape
- Tuberculin syringe with 25- or 30-gauge needle for local anesthetic injection
- Assortment of syringes: 3 mL, 5 mL, 10 mL
- Intravenous tubing (Venoset, minidrip, macrodrip)
- Extension tubing
- Intravenous solutions (lactated Ringer's, normal saline, dextrose)
- Sterile, transparent, semipermeable dressings

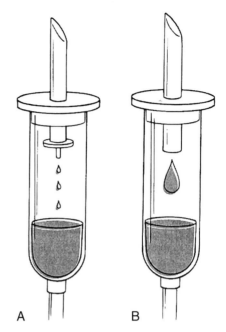

FIGURE 8-2 Administration Venoset drip chambers. **A,** Minidrip. **B,** Macrodrip. (From Booker MF, Ignatavicius DD. *Infusion Therapy: Techniques and Medications.* Philadelphia: WB Saunders; 1996:51.)

A variety of administration sets are available for use. Administration sets are selected on the basis of the following criteria:

- Length
- Location of access ports
- Size of drip chamber: microdrip vs. macrodrip (Fig. 8-2)
- Type of flow regulator (Fig. 8-3)
- Connectors

Once supplies and equipment are prepared, the patient is assessed for identification of a vascular access site. Veins generally used for peripheral cannulation are depicted in Figure 8-4. Selection of a vein for vascular access depends on a number of variables, which include surgical site, patient

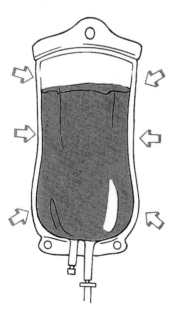

FIGURE 8-1 Plastic intravenous solution containers. Outside atmospheric pressure collapses plastic intravenous containers, which have been commercially available since 1971. (From Booker MF, Ignatavicius DD. *Infusion Therapy: Techniques and Medications.* Philadelphia: WB Saunders; 1996:46.)

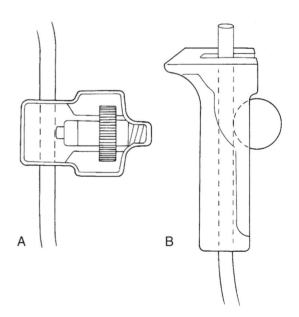

FIGURE 8-3 Administration set fluid regulating clamps. **A,** Screw clamp. **B,** Roller clamp. (From Booker MF, Ignatavicius DD. *Infusion Therapy: Techniques and Medications.* Philadelphia: WB Saunders; 1996:51.)

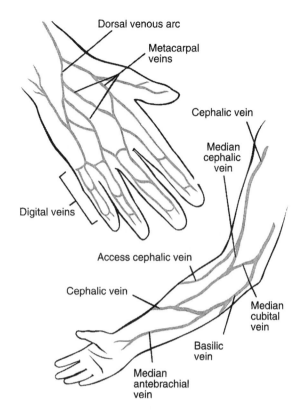

FIGURE 8-4 Peripheral vein cannulation sites. Peripheral veins appropriate for vascular access in older children and adults. (From Booker MF, Ignatavicius DD. *Infusion Therapy: Techniques and Medications.* Philadelphia: WB Saunders; 1996:91.)

positioning, diagnostic procedure, patient status (inpatient vs. outpatient), anticipated postsedation activity level, and length of time that intravenous access is required. Previous mastectomy, lymph node dissection, and the presence of renal access grafts are contraindications for vascular access in the affected extremity.

Inpatients receiving prolonged intravenous fluid therapy benefit from intravenous insertion at the most distal portion of the upper extremity. Advantages and disadvantages of peripheral vein selection are listed in Table 8-1. The catheter selected for intravenous cannulation for short-term care should be ¾ to 1 inch (2 to 2.5 cm) in length with a 20- or 22-gauge diameter.[2] However, larger-gauge catheters may be required to facilitate hydration or for specific diagnostic or therapeutic procedures. Application of a tourniquet approximately 6 inches above the insertion site (Fig. 8-5) distends the peripheral blood vessels. Periodic clenching of the patient's hand distends the vessel more fully. Warm cloths and rubbing of the extremity provide vasodilation and venous filling in patients who are peripherally vasoconstricted. Before insertion, the area should be cleansed in a circular fashion (Fig. 8-6) with a 2- to 2.5-inch radius from the intended insertion site. The cleansing agent (iodine, alcohol) is allowed to air dry to provide antibacterial action.

When a local anesthetic is used to anesthetize the skin, it should be injected superficially. A small intradermal skin wheal (0.1 mL of plain lidocaine, 30-gauge needle)

TABLE 8-1

Advantages and Disadvantages of Peripheral Vein Selection

SITE	ADVANTAGES	DISADVANTAGES
Basilic	Largest vein; straight pathway in upper arm and thorax	May be located too far to the posterior side for sterile procedure and routine care; may only be able to palpate a short segment
Median	Communicates with larger basilic; easily accessible for insertion and routine care	
Median cubital		
Median basilic	Joins with larger basilic; easily accessible for insertion and routine care	Valve may be located at junction with basilic, causing obstruction to cannula advancement
Median cephalic	Easily accessible	Valve may be located at junction with basilic, causing obstruction to cannula advancement; terminates in smaller cephalic; may not be present in some patients
Accessory cephalic	Easily accessible for insertion and routine care	Valve may be located at junction with cephalic, causing obstruction to cannula advancement; terminates in smaller cephalic; may not be present in some patients
Cephalic	Easily accessible for insertion and routine care; easy palpation and visualization above and below antecubital fossa	Smaller than basilic; pathway in upper arm and thorax is variable and unknown

From INS (Intravenous Nurses Society). *Intravenous Therapy: Clinical Principles and Practice.* Philadelphia: WB Saunders; 1995:101.

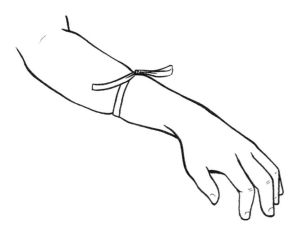

FIGURE 8-5 Application of venous tourniquet provides venous engorgement before intravenous cannulation. (From Booker MF, Ignatavicius DD. *Infusion Therapy: Techniques and Medications.* Philadelphia: WB Saunders; 1996:115.)

anesthetizes the local tissue. Care must be taken not to insert the local needle deeply into the skin or venous perforation and hematoma formation may occur. Once the area has been localized, traction on the vein is applied by the nondominant hand to secure or anchor the vein. This prevents the vein from "rolling" and from excessive movement when one is preparing to insert the intravenous catheter.

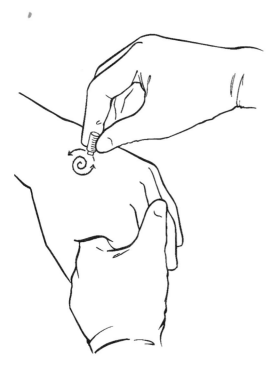

FIGURE 8-6 Preparation of intravenous cannulation site. Prior to vascular access, cleansing agent is applied in a circular fashion within a 2 to 2.5 inch radius and permitted to dry. (From Booker MF, Ignatavicius DD. *Infusion Therapy: Techniques and Medications.* Philadelphia: WB Saunders; 1996:116.)

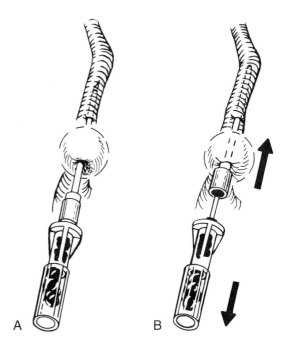

FIGURE 8-7 Presence of venous flash with advancement of catheter. **A,** Venous access is ascertained with the presence of a flash followed by (**B**) advancement of the catheter into the peripheral blood vessel. (From Butterworth J. *Atlas of Procedures in Anesthesia and Critical Care.* Philadelphia: WB Saunders; 1991:72.)

When the appropriately sized intravenous catheter is selected, it should be inserted through the small skin wheal of local anesthesia. The needle is then advanced at a 30- to 40-degree angle in the direction of the vein to be cannulated. Once a "flash" of blood is noted in the catheter chamber (Fig. 8-7), the needle should be advanced slightly (several millimeters). This maneuver ensures that the plastic catheter is situated in the vein and not positioned superficially over the vein. At this point, extreme care must be taken not to advance the needle through the back wall of the vein. Malpositioning of the catheter may result in local tissue trauma, hematoma formation, and a nonfunctional intravenous site. If the attempt to secure an intravenous line is unsuccessful, it is beneficial to leave the original plastic catheter in place while an attempt is made at another intravenous access to avoid hematoma formation. After venous access is established, the unsuccessful intravenous catheter may then be removed. Pressure is then applied until hemostasis is achieved.

Once the intravenous line is established, the caregiver advances the catheter over the trocar with the index finger of his or her dominant hand or opposite hand. Either technique is acceptable for positioning the intravenous catheter into the vein. The Venoset is then connected with pressure applied between the male Venoset connector and the female catheter connector. Firm pressure should be applied at this junction to avoid unintentional disconnect. It is important to secure the catheter and tubing with a sterile dressing, tape, or transparent dressing. Transparent dressings afford direct visualization of the intravenous site. Redness, swelling, edema, or leakage around the site may be evaluated directly through the presence of the clear Tegaderm dressing.

> New systems for intravenous access are incorporating "needleless" technology. Self-retracting trocars on systems that "cover" the sharp tip of the needle must now be available to all providers.

COMPLICATIONS OF INTRAVENOUS CATHETER INSERTION

Local complications associated with intravenous catheter insertion include infiltration, extravasation, phlebitis, hematoma formation, catheter embolism, local infection, and venous irritation. Local and systemic complications associated with intravenous therapy are listed in Table 8-2.

INTRAVENOUS FLUIDS

Intravenous fluid replacement is typically accomplished with crystalloid solutions during the administration of sedation/analgesia. Intravenous solutions maintain fluid and

TABLE 8-2

Intravenous Therapy Complications

COMPLICATION	ETIOLOGY	SIGNS/SYMPTOMS	TREATMENT	PREVENTION
Local Complications				
Infiltration	Infusion of seepage of intravenous fluid into extravascular tissue caused by partial or complete venous access dislodgment	Decreased infusion rate Localized edema Complaints of burning, pain, and tenderness at IV site	Remove catheter Application of warm, moist heat to enhance fluid absorption	Stabilize catheter insertion site Avoid catheter insertion at points of flexion Frequent assessment of catheter site
Extravasation	Accidental administration of medication or solution, which results in tissue destruction (dopamine, diazepam)	Patient complaint of: • Stinging or localized burning at the catheter insertion site • Swelling • Localized tissue destruction (blister formation)	Stop the infusion Related to the amount of concentration of the medication or solution Physician notification Catheter remains in place	Monitor insertion site frequently Stabilize catheter insertion site Administer IV push medications via a free-flowing intravenous insertion site
Phlebitis	Inflammation along the course of the vein. Contributing factors in the development of phlebitis include: • Insertion technique • Type of medication • Catheter size and length	Pain at the catheter site Red, inflamed "knotty" cord-like vein Temperature	Catheter removal Warm compresses	Change catheter site every 48-72 hours Use of large veins when irritating solutions (highly osmolar) are used Strict aseptic handling of catheter during insertion

Continued

TABLE 8-2

Intravenous Therapy Complications—cont'd

COMPLICATION	ETIOLOGY	SIGNS/SYMPTOMS	TREATMENT	PREVENTION
Local Complications—cont'd				
Hematoma formation	Leakage of blood into the surrounding tissue	Bruising around the intravenous insertion site. Pain at the site	Removal of catheter. Application of direct pressure at insertion site. Warm soaks applied if hematoma site is stable	Selection of small-gauge catheter. Careful advancement of catheter parallel to patient's skin
Local infection	Contamination at the intravenous insertion site secondary to a break in aseptic technique	Red, swollen, warm area or presence of purulent exudate at the insertion site	Catheter removal. Catheter tip may be sent for culture. Site is cleansed with antibacterial solution and covered with a sterile dressing	Strict aseptic technique. Change of infusion containers after a minimum of 24 hours. Venoset change every 48-72 hours
Catheter embolization	A piece of the intravenous catheter breaks off and floats freely in the blood vessel. Embolization can occur when the needle is reinserted into the catheter and advanced once a flash has been obtained.	Cardiovascular compromise: • Hypotension • Tachycardia • Cyanosis Pain along the vein	Catheter removal. Tourniquet placement proximal to the insertion site. Radiograph to locate catheter tip. Surgical excision of catheter tip	Never reinsert the needle into the catheter during Jelco catheter insertion. During medication administration, use the shortest needle to puncture the injection port (1 inch)
Systemic Complications				
Systemic infection/ sepsis	Pathogenic organism entrance into the systemic circulation. Results from poor aseptic technique, contaminated solution, or catheter insertion.	Early: • Fever • Chills • Headache • Malaise Late: • Cardiovascular collapse • Death	Change entire infusion system. Notify physician. Obtain cultures as ordered	Strict adherence to aseptic technique. Change of infusion containers at a minimum of every 24 hours. Venoset change every 48-72 hours
Air embolism	Air entrains into the systemic circulation. Entrainment may occur secondary to empty solution container, air in Venoset tubing, and loose intravenous connections.	Chest/shoulder pain. Back pain. Dyspnea. Hypotension. Cyanosis	Position patient on left side in the Trendelenburg position to contain air in right atrium. Notify physician. Administer oxygen. Cardiovascular support as ordered	Use of Luer-Lok connectors. Careful monitoring of IV volume infused. Use of electronic control device to detect presence of air

Continued

TABLE 8-2

Intravenous Therapy Complications—cont'd

COMPLICATION	ETIOLOGY	SIGNS/SYMPTOMS	TREATMENT	PREVENTION
Systemic Complications—cont'd				
Circulatory overload	Excess fluid within the circulatory system at a rate greater than the patient's cardiovascular system can accommodate	Shortness of breath Rales on auscultation Engorged neck veins Dependent edema	Reduce IV flow rate Administer oxygen, monitor vital signs as ordered Administration of diuretics as ordered	Monitor intake and output
Allergic reaction	A localized or systemic reaction to an allergen	Skin wheal Redness, edema Hypotension, tachycardia Bronchospasm Wheezing Cardiovascular collapse	Remove allergen Redress with hypoallergenic tape If medication is suspected allergen, discontinue medication Systemic treatment is dependent on presenting symptoms and includes administration of: • Oxygen • Antihistamines • Epinephrine • Steroids	Careful preprocedure assessment to elicit allergy status Assessment for medication cross-reaction

electrolyte balance. Body fluids are divided into intracellular and extracellular fluids. Intracellular fluids are contained within the cells of the body. Extracellular fluid is divided into three compartments:

♦ Interstitial
♦ Intravascular
♦ Transcellular

Interstitial fluid is located between cells, whereas intravascular fluid lies within blood vessels or plasma. Transcellular fluid is secreted by epithelial cells and constitutes cerebrospinal fluid, intraocular fluid, and digestive fluids. Factors that have an impact on intravascular fluid replacement include the presence of concomitant disease states (hypertension, dehydration), intraprocedure fluid losses, and the patient's cardiovascular status. In emergency situations, restoration of intravascular volume restores plasma volume and optimizes cardiac output to ensure adequate tissue oxygen delivery.

Crystalloid solutions can be differentiated according to their osmolality. *Osmolality* **is a term used to identify the number of particles in a liter of solution.** Measured in milliosmoles per liter (m)Osm/L, the osmolality of the extracellular fluid is determined by measuring solute concentration of the blood (normal serum osmolality equals 280 to 300 (m)Osm). Electrolyte solutions (crystalloid) are capable of conducting an electrical charge. Cations (potassium, sodium) maintain a positive charge, and anions (chloride) produce a negative charge. Anions and cations of intracellular, interstitial, and intravascular fluids are identified in Figure 8-8.

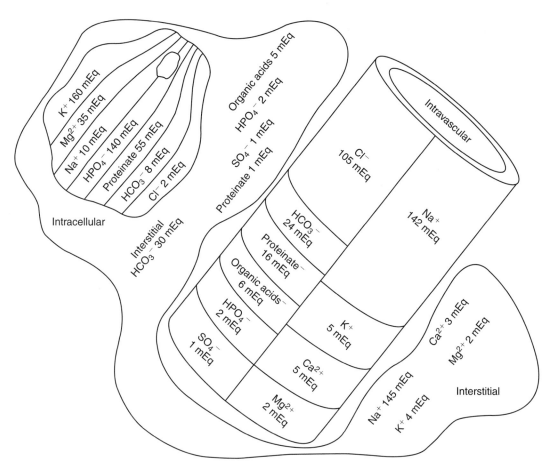

FIGURE 8-8 Anions and cations of intracellular, interstitial, and intravascular fluids. (From Hankins J, et al. *Infusion Therapy,* 2nd ed. Philadelphia: WB Saunders; 2001:103.)

The tonicity of crystalloids is also a major factor in the selection of intravenous fluids. Crystalloid solutions are therefore divided into the following classifications:

♦ **Hypotonic:** Lower osmotic pressure than plasma
♦ **Isotonic:** Same osmotic pressure as plasma
♦ **Hypertonic:** Greater osmotic pressure than that of plasma

With the administration of hypotonic solution (0.45% saline), cells begin to swell. As hypotonic solution is added to the extracellular fluid, the osmolality decreases, forcing water to enter the cells in an area of higher osmolality. **Hypertonic solution (3% saline) increases osmolality of the surrounding extracellular fluid and forces water to leave the cell and enter the extracellular fluid with resultant cellular shrinkage.** In comparison, isotonic solutions (0.9% normal saline, lactated Ringer's) produce no change in osmolality of body fluids. The infusion of isotonic solutions results in equal distribution throughout the extracellular compartment since the tonicity is similar to plasma (300 (m)Osm). The characteristics of commonly utilized intravenous solutions are provided in Table 8-3.

> Isotonic solutions are generally the crystalloid of choice for intravenous maintenance during the administration of sedation/analgesia.

Before discharge, ambulatory care patients should have the intravenous catheter removed. Firm, consistent pressure is applied until hemostasis is achieved. A 4 × 4- or 2 × 2-inch reinforcement dressing applied with tape provides additional pressure after discharge. Patients should be instructed to remove the gauze once they are at home and replace it with a Band-Aid. This additional reinforcement

TABLE 8-3

Common Intravenous Solutions

MANUFACTURER(S)/IV SOLUTIONS*	TONICITY	OSMOLARITY (mOsm/L)			APPROXIMATE pH			Na+	K+	Ca+	Mg²⁺	Cl⁻	HCO₃⁻	LACTATE	ACETATE	CITRATE
		A	B	M	A	B	M									
DEXTROSE/SALINE SOLUTIONS																
A, B, M/dextrose 2.5% and 0.45% sodium chloride	Isotonic	280	280	280	4.3	4.5	4.6	77				77				
M/dextrose 5% and 0.11% sodium chloride	Isotonic			290			4.3	19				19				
A, B, M/dextrose 5% and 0.2% sodium chloride	Hypertonic	329	321	320	4.3	4.0	4.4	34 38.5*				34 38.5*				
A, B, M/dextrose 5% and 0.3% sodium chloride	Hypertonic	355	365	365	4.3	4.0	4.4	56 51*				56 51*				
A, B, M/dextrose 5% and 0.45% sodium chloride	Hypertonic	406	406	405	4.3	4.0	4.3	77				77				
A, B, M/dextrose 5% and 0.9% sodium chloride	Hypertonic	560	560	560	4.3	4.0	4.4	154				154				
M/dextrose 10% and 0.2% sodium chloride	Hypertonic			575			4.3	34				34				
M/dextrose 10% and 0.45% sodium chloride	Hypertonic			660			4.3	77				77				
A, B, M/dextrose 10% and 0.9% sodium chloride	Hypertonic	813	813	815	4.4	4.0	4.3	154				154				

SALINE SOLUTIONS															
A, B, M/0.45% sodium chloride	Hypotonic	154	154	155	5.6	5.0	5.6	77				77			
A, B, M/0.9% sodium chloride	Isotonic	308	308	310	5.6	5.5	5.6	154				154			
B, M/3% sodium chloride	Hypertonic		1027	1030		5.0	5.8	513				513			
A, B, M/5% sodium chloride	Hypertonic	1711	1711	1710	5.6	5.0	5.8	855				855			
								856§†				856§†			
DEXTROSE SOLUTIONS															
A, B, M/5% dextrose and water	Isotonic	253	252	253	5.0	5.0	4.5								
A, B/10% dextrose and water	Hypertonic	505	505		4.6	4.0									
A, B/50% dextrose and water	Hypertonic	2526	2520		4.9	4.5									
ELECTROLYTE SOLUTIONS															
A/Normosol R	Isotonic	294			6.6			140	5		3	98	23‡		27	
B/Plasmalyte A	Isotonic		294			7.4		140	5		3	98	23‡		27	
B/Plasmalyte R	Isotonic		312			5.5		140	10	5	3	103		8	47	
M/Isolyte E	Isotonic			310			6.0	140	10	5	3	103			49	8
A, B, M/Ringer's	Isotonic	309	309	310	5.4	5.5	5.8	147		4		155				
								147.5†	4	4.5§†		156§†				
A, B, M/lactated Ringer's	Isotonic	273	273	275	6.6	6.5	6.2	130	4	2.7†		109†				
										3		110§		28		
DEXTROSE/ELECTROLYTE SOLUTIONS															
A, B, M/dextrose 5% in Ringer's	Hypertonic	561	561	560		4.3		147		4.5†		156†				
						4†		147.5†	4	4*§		155*§				
A, B, M/dextrose 5% in lactated Ringer's	Hypertonic	525	525	527	4.9	5.0	4.6	130	4	2.7†		109†				
										3.0		112§		28		
A, B, M/dextrose 2.5% in half-strength lactated Ringer's	Isotonic		263	263		5.0	5.0	65	2	1.4		54				
										1.5§		55†		14		

From Hankins J, et al: *Infusion Therapy,* 2nd ed. Philadelphia: WB Saunders; 147–148.

A, Abbott; *B,* Baxter; M, B, Braun/McGaw.

*Abbott.

†Baxter.

‡Gluconate.

§*B,* Braun/McGaw.

Continued

TABLE 8-3
Common Intravenous Solutions—cont'd

MANUFACTURER(S)/IV SOLUTIONS*	TONICITY	OSMOLARITY (mOsm/L)			APPROXIMATE pH			Na+	K+	Ca2+	Mg2+	Cl−	HCO3−	LACTATE	ACETATE	CITRATE
		A	B	M	A	B	M									
MISCELLANEOUS SOLUTIONS																
A, B/5% sodium bicarbonate injection	Hypertonic	1203	1190		7.8	8.0		595					595			
A, B/sodium lactate injection (1/6 M sodium lactate)	Hypertonic	334	334		6.7	6.5		167						167		
B/10% mannitol injection	Hypertonic		549			5.0										
B/15% mannitol injection	Hypertonic		823			5.0										
A, B/20% mannitol injection	Hypertonic		1098			5.0										
A, B/6% dextran and 0.9% sodium chloride	Isotonic	309	309		4.5	5.0		154				154				
A, B/10% dextran and 0.9% sodium chloride	Isotonic	310	311		4.7	5.0		154				154				
A, B/10% dextran and 5% dextrose injection	Slightly hypotonic	255	255		4.4	4.0										

DX

IV PROFILE CARD

ALLERGIES

ADDRESSOGRAPH

MD ORDERS

7175-50-1086 (12/91)

SITE 1								2nd SITE		REASON For 2nd Site
Date	Size	Date	Size	Date	Size	Date	Size	Date	Size	

COMMENTS:

RESTRICTIONS

NRSC	CODE	
	Y	N
Date Requested	PALL	
Date Obtained	Y	N

FIGURE 8-9 Intravenous profile card for peripheral catheter care.

may decrease the incidence of hematoma formation. Inpatients or patients who require prolonged intravenous therapy require peripheral catheter care. Nursing documentation of patients with peripheral catheters is summarized in Figure 8-9. Documentation of intravenous cannulation required on the sedation flowsheet or medical record includes the following:

◆ Identification of intravenous insertion site
◆ Catheter gauge
◆ Number of attempts
◆ Intravenous volume infused

SUMMARY

It is imperative that patients presenting for sedation services have adequate intravenous access. Intravenous access provides a convenient mode of administration for intravenous medications while serving as a lifeline to the patient in the event of cardiopulmonary distress. Sedation providers must demonstrate competence in their ability to establish intravenous access. Complications associated with intravenous cannulation should be dealt with in a timely manner. Isotonic solutions are generally selected as the intravenous solution of choice for sedation procedures.

LEARNER SELF-ASSESSMENT

In order to achieve maximal educational benefit from this chapter, please complete the Learner Self-Assessment below. This self-assessment tool provides the ability to identify areas requiring additional review. Reference material for each question is provided in Appendix F.

1. The **principles of intravenous therapy** include:

2. **List methods of intravenous cannula insertion** required for moderate sedation patients.

3. **Identify systemic complications** associated with intravenous catheter placement.

4. **State common intravenous solutions** utilized during the administration of moderate sedation/analgesia.

5. **State the presedation, procedural, and postsedation care associated with intravenous therapy.**

POST-TEST QUESTIONS

Please note: If you are applying for CE credit, you must contact Specialty Health Education, Inc. @ 800-694-8041 for a CE Application Packet.

1. Intravenous cannulation for administration of fluids/medications provides _____.
   A. Delayed uptake of sedative and analgesic medications
   B. Delayed distribution of sedative and analgesic medications
   C. Immediate uptake of sedative and analgesic medications
   D. Random distribution of sedative and analgesic medications

2. Contraindications for vascular access in an affected extremity include all of the following except _____.
   A. Previous mastectomy
   B. Lymphoid dissection
   C. Presence of renal access graphs
   D. Minimal adipose tissue in the affected side

3. The largest vein with the straightest pathway in the upper arm is the _____.
   A. Basilic
   B. Median
   C. Accessory
   D. Median cubital

4. Warm cloths and rubbing of the extremity provides _____ for ease of intravenous cannula insertion.
   A. Vasoconstriction
   B. Vasodilation
   C. Reduced venous filling
   D. Peripheral edema

5. After appropriate localization via a small skin wheal of local anesthesia, the intravenous needle is advanced at a _____ degree angle in the direction of the vein to be cannulated.
   A. 10-20
   B. 21-30
   C. 31-40
   D. Greater than 50

6. Inflammation along the course of a vein that may occur in response to specific intravenous insertion techniques, types of medications infused, and catheter size is termed _____.
   A. Infiltration
   B. Extravasation
   C. Phlebitis
   D. Hematoma formation

7. Infusion or seepage of intravenous fluid into extra-vascular tissue that is caused by partial or complete venous access dislodgement is termed _____.
   A. Infiltration
   B. Extravasation
   C. Phlebitis
   D. Hematoma formation

8. The presence of concomitant disease states (hypertension, dehydration, procedural fluid losses) and the patient's cardiovascular status are factors that have an impact on _____.
   A. Transcellular fluid replacement
   B. Intravascular fluid replacement
   C. Interstitial fluid replacement
   D. Iso-osmolar fluid replacement

9. Crystalloid solutions that have a greater osmotic pressure than plasma include _____.
   A. Hypotonic solutions
   B. Isotonic solutions
   C. Hypertonic solutions
   D. Iso-osmolar solutions

10. Which of the following intravenous solutions is considered the crystalloid of choice for intravenous maintenance during the administration of sedation? _____
   A. Hypotonic solutions
   B. Isotonic solutions
   C. Hypertonic solutions
   D. Iso-osmolar solutions

REFERENCES

1. Booker M, Ignatavicius D. *Infusion Therapy: Techniques and Medications.* Philadelphia: WB Saunders; 1996:46.
2. Booker M, Ignatavicius D. *Infusion Therapy: Techniques and Medications.* Philadelphia: WB Saunders; 1996:103.

ADDITIONAL RESOURCES

Hankins J, Lonsway R, Hedrick C, Perdue M. *Infusion Therapy in Clinical Practice,* 2nd ed. Philadelphia: WB Saunders; 2001.

CHAPTER 9

Geriatric Patient Care

At the completion of this chapter, the learner shall:

◆ Identify Practice Guidelines for Sedation and Analgesia by Non-Anesthesiologists related to the geriatric patient presenting for sedation.

◆ Define the term *geriatric*.

◆ Identify the cardiorespiratory, renal, hepatic, and central nervous system physiologic alterations that impact geriatric patient care.

◆ List pharmacodynamic/pharmacokinetic considerations associated with the aging process.

◆ State specific procedural considerations associated with administering benzodiazepines, opioids, and sedative/hypnotics to the geriatric patient population.

◆ State airway management issues associated with caring for the "aged" patient.

Practice Guidelines for Sedation and Analgesia by Non-Anesthesiologists
American Society of Anesthesiologists Task Force on Sedation and Analgesia by Non-Anesthesiologists

Recommendations. Whenever possible, appropriate medical specialists should be consulted before administration of sedation to patients with significant underlying conditions. The choice of specialists depends on the nature of the underlying condition and the urgency of the situation. For severely compromised or medically unstable patients (e.g., anticipated difficult airway, severe obstructive pulmonary disease, coronary artery disease, or congestive heart failure), or if it is likely that sedation to the point of unresponsiveness will be necessary to obtain adequate conditions, practitioners who are not trained in the administration of general anesthesia should consult an anesthesiologist.

From American Society of Anesthesiologists Task Force on Sedation and Analgesia by Non-Anesthesiologists. Practice guidelines for sedation and analgesia by non-anesthesiologists. *Anesthesiology.* 2002;96(4):1013. Reprinted with permission.

All patients scheduled for procedural sedation require judicious titration of medications and vigilant care. The "geriatric" patient population requires particular attention when presenting for sedation services. Their altered response to pharmacologic compounds occurs secondary to the physiologic alterations and pharmacokinetic and pharmacodynamic changes associated with the aging process. This chapter will focus on the specific needs of the geriatric patient presenting for sedation services.

Gerontology is the study of the effects of time on human development, specifically the study of the aged.[1] Increased life expectancy and decreased mortality associated with the aging process in the United States has led to an explosion in the geriatric patient population. The aged population currently composes approximately 12% to 15% of the United States population. Because the baby boomer population (those born between 1940 through the 1960s) contributes more than 75 million people to the population, this figure is expected to rise to 20% by the year 2020.[2] Additionally, the 2000 U.S. Census estimates 31 million people older than 80 years of age by the year 2050.[3] **As healthcare continues to evolve and organizations prepare to provide medical care in the future, the impact of the aging population and their specific clinical needs must be considered.**

> It is apparent that a considerable percentage of sedation clinical practice will involve the geriatric patient population.

The aged population is arbitrarily defined as those patients who have reached the age of 65. In 1907, the "aged" population was defined as 50 years or older. The definition of the term *aged* or *geriatric* is continually changing. A currently accepted definition of the beginning of old age (geriatrics) is 65 years. **However, an appreciation of the patient's functional age is far more important than the individual's chronologic age.** The aging process affects all individuals and is accompanied by a decline in organ system function. This progressive decline in organ function is responsible for the **physiologic** aging process. Aging is associated with progressive decreases (1% to 1.5% per year) in function of major organ systems after the age of 30.[4] Organ function eventually cannot compensate to restore the body to a homeostatic state. This reduction in functional capacity predisposes the body to additional stressors. Box 9-1 identifies the physiologic aspects associated with the aging process.

> It is important that the sedation practitioner appreciate the specific needs of the geriatric patient and their impact on procedural care.

CARDIOVASCULAR SYSTEM

A variety of anatomic and physiologic changes occur in the cardiovascular and autonomic nervous system as the patient ages. Diminished parasympathetic nervous system tone, a decline in beta-receptor responsiveness, and stiffening of the vascular tree have serious consequences for the geriatric patient. Table 9-1 features specific cardiovascular changes, clinical features, and sedation considerations associated with the geriatric patient.

PULMONARY SYSTEM

Geriatric patients requiring sedation present with respiratory changes associated with the normal aging process. In addition, some patients may present with age-related respiratory disease that includes features of chronic obstructive pulmonary disease:

◆ Asthma
◆ Emphysema

Clinical considerations associated with these disease entities are presented in Chapter 2, Presedation Assessment and Patient Selection.

BOX 9-1

Physiologic Effects of the Aging Process

Body Composition
- ↑ Proportion of body fat
- ↓ Skeletal muscle mass
- ↓ Intracellular fluid

Cardiovascular System
- ↓ Tissue elasticity, which results in increased blood pressure
- ↑ Systolic blood pressure secondary to ventricular hypertrophy and decreased arterial wall compliance
- ↓ Cardiac output by 1% for each year after age 30
- Cardiac dysrhythmias secondary to degenerative changes of the cardiac conduction system
- ↓ Baroreceptor activity

Pulmonary System
- ↓ Total lung capacity
- ↓ Vital capacity
- ↓ FEV_1
- ↑ Residual volume
- ↑ Dead space
- ↓ Pao_2
- Altered ventilation response to hypercapnia and hypoxia

Neurologic System
- ↓ Cerebral blood flow
- ↓ Cerebral oxygen uptake
- ↑ Sensitivity to central nervous system depressant drug

Renal System
- ↓ Glomerular filtration rate (1% to 1.5% per year)
- ↓ Creatinine clearance
- ↓ Tubular function (excretion)

Hepatic System
- ↓ Hepatic blood flow
- ↓ Microsomal enzyme activity
- ↓ Albumin leads to decreased plasma protein binding with resultant increased available free drug

Endocrine System
- ↓ Basal metabolic rate, 1% per year after age 30
- Glucose intolerance

Airway
- Laryngeal and pharyngeal reflexes are diminished
- Inadequate mask fit for positive-pressure ventilation
- ↓ Neuronal function

The aging process reduces elasticity in the geriatric pulmonary system. This decreased elastic recoil coupled with calcific changes decreases lung compliance. As evidenced by loss of body height, the intervertebral spaces are diminished, causing reduction in the thoracic curvature. This leads to changes in chest wall compliance. There is also an increase in anatomic and physiologic dead space secondary to loss of gas exchanging units. The normal aging process is associated with progressive loss and destruction of the alveolar septa,

TABLE 9-1

Geriatric Cardiovascular Alterations

ANATOMIC/PHYSIOLOGIC ALTERATION	CLINICAL FEATURE	SEDATION CONSIDERATIONS
Increased arterial rigidity Increased sympathetic nervous system activity	Left ventricle has to work harder to eject blood into a rigid aorta. Elevates systemic vascular resistance. Increased left ventricular strain may lead to the development of left ventricular hypertrophy.	Alterations in cardiovascular response to sedative, analgesic, and hypnotic medications. Vital signs may be labile secondary to left ventricular hypertrophy, increased afterload, and increased myocardial oxygen consumption associated with increased sympathetic nervous system activity and "stiff" vessels
Vein stiffening	Decreased compliance of capacitance vessels	Reduces the body's ability to "buffer" hemodynamic changes in intravascular tone Exaggerated hypotension
Left ventricular hypertrophy	Impaired diastolic filling	Reduction in end-diastolic function and coronary artery filling
Decreased peripheral nervous system tone	Tonic peripheral nervous system outflow declines	Inability to adjust cardiac output and blood pressure during sedation challenges (pain, anxiety, alterations in preload or afterload)
Decreased response to beta-adrenergic stimulation	Decreased inotropic and chronotropic response to beta stimulant medications	Decreased response to sympathetic nervous system stimulant medications. May result in profound bradycardia and hypotension, which is refractory to pharmacologic treatment
Impaired chronotropic and inotropic responsiveness of the heart	Inability to respond to metabolic demands	Heart rate and ejection fraction may not be capable of maintaining cardiac output during periods of stress and anxiety
Altered baroreceptor response	Aortic arch and carotid sinus stretch receptor effectiveness is reduced secondary to arterial stiffening with resultant decrease in baroreflex	Increased susceptibility in geriatric patients to orthostatic hypotension and heart rate compensatory mechanisms
Decreased cardiac output	Reduced blood flow to major organ systems	Intravenously administered sedative, analgesic, and hypnotic medications take longer to reach their target receptor sites. Full pharmacologic effect may be delayed in excess of 6 to 10 minutes depending on the patient's cardiac output, which frequently results in excessive doses of medication administration. *To avoid oversedation, hypercarbia, hypoxia, and airway obstruction, allow ample time for the full pharmacologic effect of the medication to be appreciated before administering additional medication.*
Fibrotic changes in conduction system	Sinoatrial node and pacemaker cells are accompanied by atrophy of conducting tissue	Conduction system anomalies may manifest as dysrhythmias, decreased conduction through the atrioventricular node, fascicular blocks, and sick sinus syndrome

which leads to this increase in physiologic dead space. These changes eventually lead to reduction in tidal volume, increased air trapping, atelectasis, and shunting. A reduction in respiratory ciliary activity, in airway reactivity, and in protective reflexes predisposes the geriatric patient to the development of gastric acid aspiration and pulmonary dysfunction.

These pulmonary anatomic and physiologic alterations reveal that the geriatric sedation patient has a limited pulmonary reserve coupled with an inability to increase respiratory rate and volume in the presence of hypoventilation and hypoxia. Ventilatory muscles fatigue early secondary to anatomic structural changes outlined. In addition, the clinician providing sedation services to this sensitive patient population must recognize that procedural ventilatory inadequacy may occur.

> The mechanical, anatomic, and physiologic pulmonary changes associated with the aging process predisposes the geriatric patient to pharmacologic sensitivity that can lead to potential respiratory distress.

RENAL SYSTEM

Loss of kidney mass, vascular changes, decreased renal blood flow, and decreased glomerular filtration rate in the geriatric patient require decreased dosage requirements and use of drugs with short half-lives and no active metabolites. This diminished renal reserve may increase the risk of renal insufficiency and also affects the duration of action of many anesthetic medications and adjuvant drugs.[5] Presedation patient assessment requires careful review of fluid and electrolyte status secondary to the geriatric patient's inability to conserve sodium, which may predispose to the development of hemodynamic instability.

HEPATIC SYSTEM

Liver blood flow at the age of 65 is reduced to approximately 40% of the liver blood flow in patients at the age of 30. **Hepatic microsomal enzymes, important in oxidizing drugs, are less active in older patients.** The conversion by the liver of lipid-soluble drugs to water-soluble metabolites by conjugation is also reduced. This may also lead to increased duration of action for many lipid-soluble drugs, including some anesthetics and sedatives.

CENTRAL NERVOUS SYSTEM

Among the important age-related changes in the geriatric patient is a consistent loss of neuronal density of approximately 50,000 neurons per day.[6] Biochemical changes associated with the aging process include a decrease in the neurotransmitters identified in Box 9-2. It is generally agreed that the geriatric patient has a higher incidence of central nervous system–related complications.[7] **The effects of aging on the central nervous system frequently results**

> **BOX 9-2**
>
> **Reduced Biochemical Transmitters**
>
> Acetylcholine   Serotonin
> Dopamine   Norepinephrine
> Tyrosine

in an increased incidence of confusion, delirium, and sensitivity to pharmacologic agents.

> To avoid adverse central nervous system effects, geriatric patients require dosage reduction of 30% to 50%, use of small incremental doses of sedative and analgesic agents, and longer time between doses to assess full pharmacologic effect.

THERMOREGULATION

Although patients presenting for sedation are not exposed to the wide temperature fluctuations or environmental extremes of the general operating room population, geriatric patients do not regulate their body temperature as efficiently as young adults. Geriatric patients in the sedation setting should be kept warm during all procedures to prevent the development of shivering. Shivering has been shown to increase oxygen consumption as much as 100% to 200%.[8] This increase in oxygen consumption increases myocardial strain and may result in the development of tissue hypoxia. **Pharmacologic considerations associated with hypothermia include decreased clearance of medications with resultant pronounced and prolonged pharmacologic effect.**

PHARMACOKINETICS AND PHARMACODYNAMICS IN THE ELDERLY

The physiologic changes outlined impact on the geriatric patient's response to pharmacologic compounds. Additional considerations associated with the aged population include:
- Decreased plasma protein binding
- Body composition changes

Plasma protein binding is often decreased in the geriatric patient population owing to a reduced amount of circulating protein. Plasma proteins "bind" pharmacologic compounds with the "bound" portion of the drug inactive secondary to its inability to penetrate cell membranes and exert pharmacologic effect. The remaining "free" fraction of the drug exerts pharmacologic effect. **This decrease in plasma protein binding is one of the important reasons that geriatric patients frequently exhibit an exaggerated clinical effect to sedatives, hypnotics, and opioid medications.**

Additionally, age-related changes in body composition include a loss of skeletal muscle (lean body mass) and an increase in the percentage of body fat. This increased adipose content coupled with a 20% to 30% reduction in blood volume occurs with the aging process. Therefore, injection

TABLE 9-2
Elimination Half-Life

DRUG	YOUNG ADULT	OLDER ADULT
Morphine	2.9 hr	4.5 hr
Fentanyl	250 min	925 min
Diazepam	24 hr	72 hr
Midazolam	2.8 hr	4.3 hr

of anesthetic drugs will initially be dispersed into a contracted blood volume in the elderly patient, producing a higher than expected initial plasma drug concentration.[9] Furthermore, many anesthetic drugs are then redistributed to the fat tissue, leading to prolonged somnolence in the geriatric patient. Table 9-2 features the impact of many of these changes on the half-lives of commonly utilized sedation medications.

Pharmacologic Profile

A complete profile of each pharmacologic classification and reversal agent is presented in Chapter 5, Sedation/Analgesia Pharmacologic Profile.

Benzodiazepines

Geriatric patients are particularly vulnerable to the sedative effects associated with the administration of benzodiazepines.[10,11] Dosage reduction of 30% to 50% may be required when benzodiazepines are administered to the geriatric patient. The sedative effects of benzodiazepines are enhanced by decreased hepatic microsomal enzyme activity and renal clearance. Considerations with the administration of benzodiazepines include careful titration, decreased total dose, and the use of benzodiazepines with inactive metabolites (midazolam).

Opioids

Decreased protein binding and reduced pharmacologic clearance, coupled with an increased volume of distribution, may result in a prolonged duration of action and an enhanced pharmacologic effect. These variations also result in significant respiratory and cardiovascular depression in the geriatric patient population. The addition of opioids in the presence of benzodiazepines produces a pronounced synergistic effect. Respiratory depression is a common complication associated with the combination of benzodiazepines and opioids.

Sedatives

Decreased total dosage of all central nervous system depressant medications is required in the geriatric patient population. Reduced clearance coupled with altered pharmacokinetics requires careful titration of all sedative and opioid medications. Specific gerontologic considerations include reduced total dose (30% to 50%), titrated slowly to clinical effect. **Reduced cardiac output in the geriatric**

patient population requires the sedation practitioner to wait several minutes after the administration of each medication dose to allow sufficient circulation time to fully assess pharmacologic effect.

Airway Evaluation

During sedation procedures, management of the geriatric patient's airway may prove particularly challenging. Redundant oropharyngeal tissue in the edentulous patient may result in premature airway collapse and upper airway obstruction. Arthritis in this patient population frequently results in limited range of motion and the potential for a difficult airway. Limited range of motion must be appreciated by sedation clinicians to avoid deep sedative states. The limited range of motion of arthritic patients predisposes them to potential difficult airway management if an emergency situation occurs. Loss of bony jaw structure in the aged patient distorts the face, which may make it difficult to resuscitate the patient or deliver positive-pressure ventilation. An oropharyngeal or nasopharyngeal airway may be required to function as a mechanical conduit to maintain air flow.

Psychologic Well-Being

It is important to consider the psychologic well-being of the geriatric patient when providing sedation services. Many geriatric patients are acclimated to a specific daily routine. Administration of sedation for diagnostic, therapeutic, or minor surgical procedure removes the patient from his or her specific pattern of daily behavior. Physical limitations (hearing, vision loss) and lack of autonomy may lead to increased levels of frustration and feelings of confusion. The practitioner engaged in the care of this patient population should use slow diction, assess specific patient needs, and provide information as needed.

> Geriatric patients do not respond well to fast-paced, disorganized practice settings. A controlled environment is required for the geriatric patient that is sensitive to the individual's social and clinical needs.

SUMMARY

Administration of sedation to the geriatric patient must focus on proper presedation and preparation strategies (see Chapter 2) to identify the presence of concomitant disease, prescribed treatment protocol, and effectiveness of therapy. A careful review of the cardiopulmonary system is required to identify the presence of coronary artery disease, hypertension, prior myocardial infarction, or chronic obstructive pulmonary disease. Careful titration with reduced doses of medications is required to avoid the development of deep sedation states, prolonged recovery time, and cardiovascular depression. Decreased gastroesophageal sphincter tone, decreased laryngeal reflexes, and the physiologic changes associated with the aging process listed in Box 9-1 increase the potential for morbidity and mortality in the geriatric patient.

LEARNER SELF-ASSESSMENT

In order to achieve maximal educational benefit from this chapter, please complete the Learner Self-Assessment below. This self-assessment tool provides the learner with the ability to identify areas requiring additional review. Reference material for each question is provided in Appendix F.

1. **Practice Guidelines for Sedation and Analgesia by Non-Anesthesiologists** promulgated by the ASA Task Force on Sedation **related to geriatric patient** care include:

2. The term *geriatric* is defined as:

3. **Cardiorespiratory, renal, hepatic, and central nervous system physiologic alterations** that impact on geriatric patient care include:

4. **Pharmacodynamic and pharmacokinetic considerations** associated with the aging process include:

5. Specific **procedural considerations** associated with administering benzodiazepines, opioids, and sedative hypnotics to the geriatric patient include:

6. Airway **management issues** associated with caring for the geriatric sedation patient include:

POST-TEST QUESTIONS

Please note: If you are applying for CE credit, you must contact Specialty Health Education, Inc. @ 800-694-8041 for a CE Application Packet.

1. The study of the effects of time on human development and study of aging is termed _____.
   A. Internal medicine
   B. Radiology
   C. Pediatrics
   D. Gerontology

2. The "geriatric" population is defined as those patients older than _____ years of age.
   A. 50
   B. 55
   C. 60
   D. 65

3. After the age of 30, aging is associated with progressive decreases in major organ system function of approximately _____ percent per year.
   A. 1-1.5
   B. 2-2.5
   C. 3-3.5
   D. 4-4.5

4. Cardiovascular system changes associated with the geriatric patient include _____.
   A. Enhanced parasympathetic nervous system tone
   B. Diminished parasympathetic nervous system tone
   C. Enhanced beta-receptor responsiveness
   D. Relaxation of the vascular tree

5. Hepatic microsomal enzyme activity is _____ in the geriatric patient.
   A. Decreased
   B. Not affected
   C. Increased
   D. Nonexistent

6. Among the important age-related changes in the geriatric patient is a consistent loss of neuronal density of approximately _____ neurons per day.
   A. 20,000
   B. 30,000

   C. 40,000
   D. 50,000

7. To avoid adverse central nervous system effects, geriatric patients generally require drug dosage reduction of _____.
   A. 10% to 20%
   B. 30% to 50%
   C. 60% to 70%
   D. 80%

8. Plasma protein binding is decreased in the geriatric patient, resulting in excess _____ portion of sedative medications with resultant exaggerated pharmacologic effect.
   A. Bound
   B. Unbound
   C. Nonreactive
   D. Reactive

9. Injection of anesthetic drugs will initially be dispersed into a _____ blood volume in the elderly patient, producing a higher than expected initial plasma drug concentration.
   A. Diluted
   B. Contracted
   C. Hyperthermic
   D. Hypothermic

10. Which of the following conditions predisposes the geriatric patient to the possibility of difficult airway management if an emergency situation occurs? _____
   A. Stiffening of peripheral blood vessels
   B. Increased beta-receptor responsiveness
   C. Polycythemia
   D. Arthritis

REFERENCES

1. Schneider EL, Rowe JW (eds). *Handbook of the Biology of Aging.* 3rd ed. San Diego: Academic Press; 1990:439.
2. US Department of Commerce, Bureau of the Census, 1994.
3. US Department of Commerce, Bureau of the Census, 2000.
4. Evans TI. The physiological basis of geriatric anesthesia. *Anesth Intensive Care.* 1973;1:319-328.
5. Barlow I. Perioperative renal insufficiency and failure in elderly patients. In *Syllabus on Geriatric Anesthesiology.* Park Ridge, IL, American Society of Anesthesiologists; 2002.
6. Schejeide OA. Relation of development and aging; pre-and postnatal differentiation of the brain as related to aging. *Adv Behavioral Biol.* 1975;16:37-83.
7. Bosek V. Anesthesia for the elderly. *Curr Rev Nurs Anesth.* 1999;21(17):153-160.
8. Morgan G, Mikhail M, Murray M. *Clinical Anesthesiology.* 3rd ed. New York: Lange Medical Books/McGraw-Hill; 2002.
9. McLeskey C. Pharmacokinetic and pharmacodynamic differences in the elderly. In *Syllabus on Geriatric Anesthesiology.* Park Ridge, IL, American Society of Anesthesiologists; 2002.
10. Schoeler S, Schafer D, Potter J. The effect of age on the relative potency of midazolam and diazepam sedation in upper gastrointestinal endoscopy. *J Clin Gastroenterol.* 1990;12:145.
11. McLeskey C. *Geriatric Anesthesiology.* Baltimore: Williams & Wilkins; 1997;134.

CHAPTER 10

Pediatric Patient Care*

Krista Bragg

CORE COMPETENCIES

At the completion of this chapter, the learner shall:

◆ State the goals of pediatric procedural sedation.

◆ Define the developmental subsets of pediatrics and state examples of developmentally appropriate rapport.

◆ State the role of the parents or primary caregivers of children receiving procedural sedation.

◆ List the infant's physiologic response to pain.

◆ List three characteristics of the infant central nervous system.

◆ State the relationship of the parasympathetic vs. sympathetic nervous system in children younger than 1 year of age.

◆ List significant differences between the cardiovascular system of a small child vs. an adult.

◆ State the primary cause of bradycardia in infants.

◆ Identify at least three methods to avoid air administration via pediatric intravenous catheters.

◆ List five distinct features of the infant upper airway.

◆ List three distinct features of the infant's lower airway.

◆ Explain the significance of subglottic edema in children.

◆ State one method to determine the appropriate-sized pediatric endotracheal tube.

◆ List five airway maneuvers that may improve ventilation in a sedated pediatric patient.

◆ Describe the natural breathing pattern of infants.

◆ List the physiologic response of infants and young children to hypothermia.

◆ Describe methods to decrease heat loss in sedated pediatric patients.

◆ State the relationship between infant and adult total body water.

◆ State the method of determining hourly fluid requirements in pediatric patients.

◆ List the current recommended NPO guidelines for pediatric patients before sedation:
  • Clear liquids
  • Solid food

◆ List at least three anatomic features that may predict a difficult pediatric airway.

◆ List at least two pediatric-specific anatomic features that may require further consultation with a pediatric anesthesiologist before the administration of sedation.

◆ List at least five pediatric medical problems that may require cancellation of the planned procedure.

*A special thanks to Peter Davis, MD; Chief Anesthesiologist at Children's Hospital at Pittsburgh.

◆ Describe a pediatric-friendly environment as defined by the American Academy of Pediatrics (AAP).

◆ List three methods of monitoring the sedated pediatric patient.

◆ Name one sedation scale that is useful in pediatrics.

◆ State the relationship between the administration of three or more sedating medications and pediatric outcomes.

◆ Describe the importance of titration in pediatric patients.

◆ Identify sedation drugs with long half-lives and the consequential effects on infants and small children.

◆ Describe the features of the pediatric patient during a "failed sedation."

◆ List six criteria that should be met before pediatric patient discharge after procedural sedation.

◆ Describe one possible mechanism of infant desaturation in car seats after procedural sedation.

Guidelines for Monitoring and Management of Pediatric Patients During and After Sedation for Diagnostic and Therapeutic Procedures: American Academy of Pediatrics (AAP), Committee on Drugs (COD): October 2002 Addendum

"Regardless of the intended level of sedation or route of administration of sedative, sedation of a patient represents a continuum and may result in loss of the patient's protective reflexes; a pediatric patient may move easily from a level of light sedation to obtundation."

The COD continues to emphasize that sedation of children is different from sedation of adults. Sedatives are generally administered to gain the cooperation of the child. The ability of the child to cooperate depends on chronologic and developmental age. Often, children younger than 6 years and those with developmental delays require deep levels of sedation to gain their cooperation. Children in this age group are particularly vulnerable to the adverse effects of sedatives on respiratory drive, patency of airway, and protective reflexes. Because deep sedation may occur after administration of sedatives in any child, the practitioner must have the skills and equipment necessary to safely manage patients who are sedated.

Recommendations. The "Guidelines for Monitoring and Management of Pediatric Patients During and After Sedation for Diagnostic and Therapeutic Procedures" apply regardless of the settings in which sedatives are administered or the specific training or profession of the practitioners involved.

Recommendations. Sedative or anxiolytic medications should not be administered at home or as part of a preprocedural sedation plan.

Recommendations. Sedative or anxiolytic medications should not be administered by anyone who is not medically skilled or supervised by skilled medical personnel.

Recommendations. When children are deeply sedated, at least one individual must be present who is trained in, and capable of, providing pediatric basic life support, and who is skilled in airway management and cardiopulmonary resuscitation; training in pediatric advanced life support is strongly encouraged.

Recommendations. It is crucial that age-appropriate resuscitation equipment and medications be immediately available.

Recommendations. Children who receive sedative medications with a long half-life may require extended observation.

Recommendations. On occasion, on the basis of careful, documented review of the medical history, physical examination, and proposed procedure, a practitioner may determine that a hospital is the only appropriate venue for administering sedatives.[1]

The goals of pediatric procedural sedation include:

◆ To provide analgesia
◆ To decrease patient movement
◆ To enhance patient cooperation

Children younger than 6 years of age and those with developmental delays often require deep levels of sedation to perform the intended procedure.[1] The more invasive the procedure, the more likely it is that the child's required level of sedation will border on general anesthesia. **It is extremely important for practitioners engaged in pediatric sedation not to treat the child as a small adult.** This chapter will address the emotional needs of children, the physiological variations among children, assessment and monitoring parameters, and pharmacologic techniques to provide safe procedural sedation.

> Treating a child as a small adult will inevitably lead to errors in drug dosage, fluid administration, and airway management. These errors may ultimately compromise patient safety.

The indications for pediatric procedural sedation cover a broad spectrum. Procedural sedation is used for diagnostic studies (CT scans), minor surgical procedures (suturing skin lacerations), and invasive procedures (endoscopies and drainage of abscesses) for the pediatric patient population. Some sedation techniques are necessary to keep the child motionless, whereas other techniques require a substantial amount of analgesia. Many children receive procedural sedation therapy in non-hospital facilities. It is in the non-hospital environment that skilled pediatric rescue teams may be least accessible. Adverse events that occur during office-based sedation are more likely to be fatal than events that occur in a hospital or hospital-like setting.[2] Because the indications for procedural sedation are broad, sedative regimens are also wide ranging, and no one technique fits all children and their needs.

Pediatrics is defined by the American Academy of Pediatrics as the medical care of patients younger than the age of 21.[3] The pediatric population is diverse with age-related physical, intellectual, and psychological differences. Information available on anesthesia adverse outcomes suggests neonates are at higher risk than older infants and, in turn, older infants are at greater risk than pediatric patients older than 2 years of age.[4-11] Because of the anatomic, physiologic, and psychological differences that occur among children, additional differentiation of pediatric age groups for patients older than 2 years is recommended.[12]

The pediatric practitioner administering sedation must be knowledgeable about various subset groups within pediatrics and the specific relative physiologic and anatomic differences. Airway management and pharmacologic administration must be age and procedure specific. The pediatric population is identified as:

◆ Newborn (<1 day old)
◆ Neonate (<30 days)
◆ Infants (1 to 12 months)
◆ Children (1 to 12 years of age)
◆ Adolescent (13 to 19 years of age)
◆ Young Adult (20 to 21 years of age)

> It is imperative that the pediatric sedation provider is competent and comfortable in providing sedation to the pediatric patient.

PSYCHOLOGICAL NEEDS

Medical procedures can be psychologically distressing.[13] Children must cope with separation from caregivers, introduction of strangers, an unfamiliar environment, and invasive, painful procedures. Practitioners can ease some of the child's anxiety by creating a child-friendly environment and communicating at an age-appropriate level. The developmental mechanisms of pediatric patient rapport include[14]:

◆ Trust vs. Mistrust (birth to 1 year)
  ● Familiarity and trust with the primary caregiver(s) is essential.
  ● Separation (especially after 6 months of age) may result in a screaming, clinging infant.
◆ Autonomy vs. Shame and Doubt (1 to 3 years)
  ● Children are striving to maintain control of themselves and their environment.
  ● Fears of abandonment and separation anxiety are characteristic.
  ● Parental presence during the initial sedation can be very valuable in encouraging cooperation from the child.
  ● Allow objects of security (stuffed animal, blanket).
  ● Clearly delineate end of procedure ("all done," "no more").
◆ Initiative vs. Guilt (3 to 5 years)
  ● Children are working for a sense of independence.
  ● Fears of bodily harm and mutilation can be concerns.
  ● Simple, concise information and directions should be relayed to the child.
  ● Positive reinforcement is valuable.
◆ Industry vs. Inferiority (6 to 12 years)
  ● School is a good topic for conversation.
  ● Making choices is crucial to this age group.
  ● Participation and completion of tasks can decrease stress.
  ● Example: patient helping push stretcher to procedure room.
◆ Identity vs. Role Confusion (12 to 18 years)
  ● Self consciousness and modesty are hallmarks of this age group.
  ● Providing privacy is important.
  ● Peer relationships are valued.
  ● Conversing in friendly, relaxed, informational manner can be helpful.
  ● Music may be useful.

Parents are becoming increasingly involved in their children's medical care and may expect to be present during the initiation of procedural sedation. Other family or surrogate caregivers may participate in lieu of biologic parents. Parental presence during the induction of general anesthesia has been shown particularly beneficial to children older than 4 years of age, especially if both parent and child are relatively calm before the procedure.[15] Before the procedure, parental anxiety should be addressed in a caring, considerate manner by the practitioner. Parental anxiety may be transmitted to the patient, further upsetting the child. Open, honest communication with the parent along with a clear concise description of the sedation process is often helpful.[13]

CENTRAL NERVOUS SYSTEM

The infant central nervous system (CNS) is underdeveloped relative to older children and adults until 1 year of age.[16] **It is well established that newborns and infants experience pain similar to adults, with resultant tachycardia, increased blood pressure, and increased intracranial pressure.**[17,18] The CNS's immaturity predisposes newborns to dangers such as seizures, increased intracranial pressure, and subsequent intraventricular hemorrhages.[19] The infant skull is less rigid than that of adults, with expandable fontanelles making it more yielding to pressure. This compliance provides accommodation to increases in cerebral volume and pressure. Palpation of the fontanelles can provide information regarding infant intracranial pressure.[20]

Infants born with baseline hydrocephalus have increased cerebral pressure and because of the large occiput may become difficult airway management patients.[19] In these patients, sedation is often contraindicated secondary to the risk of hypoventilation, hypercapnia, and possible brain herniation.[18] Procedures for patients with known elevated intracranial pressure should be performed in a hospital setting with appropriate personnel, equipment, and medications necessary to treat a neurologic medical or surgical emergency.

Newborns are prone to intraventricular hemorrhages (IVH) related to increased intracranial pressure associated with the fragile cerebral capillary network.[18] IVH is a leading cause of mortality and morbidity in this patient population.[16] Box 10-1 identifies factors that contribute to IVH in newborns. Stress factors such as intubation in awake patients with inadequate analgesia are notable contributors to increased intracranial pressure.[16] Pharmacologic management should attempt to limit increases in intracranial pressure and maintain adequate cerebral perfusion.

Little is known about newborn cerebral blood flow. Global cerebral blood flow is 65-85 mL/100 gm/min in older infants and children, whereas the adult value is 50 mL/100 gm brain tissue/minute.[19] The cerebral metabolic rate for oxygen is also higher in children (5 mL/min) as opposed to adults (3 to 4 mL/min). Oxygen metabolic rates are further increased with seizures and fever. Oxygen metabolic rates are decreased with barbiturate administration and hypothermia.

The neuroendocrine response exhibited by infants in reaction to painful procedures may surpass that of adults.

> **BOX 10-1**
>
> ### Potential Sources of Infant Increased Intracranial Pressure During Procedural Sedation
>
> - Hypoxia
> - Hypercarbia
> - Fluctuations in blood pressure
> - Low hematocrit
> - Hypertonic fluid administration
> - Intubation in the awake patient

From Hamid RK, Newfield P. Pediatric neuroanesthesia. In *Handbook of Neuroanesthesia*. Philadelphia: Lippincott Williams & Wilkins; 1994:270-284.

Behavior and short term development have been shown to be adversely affected immediately after procedures in infants without adequate analgesia.[20] Analgesia should be administered to infants with same care and compassion that would be provided a verbalizing adult.

> Studies suggest infants exposed to painful procedures may develop an increased sensitivity to pain later in life.[21]

CARDIOVASCULAR SYSTEM

When caring for the pediatric patient, knowledge of age appropriate vital signs cannot be overly emphasized. Table 10-1 identifies pediatric cardiovascular parameters. The adage "one size fits all" is not true with pediatric patients. Care must be taken to use proper sized equipment to obtain accurate vital signs.[22]

The infant myocardium is significantly less compliant than the adult heart.[23] Increased preload does little to improve stroke volume in the less compliant ventricle. Heart rate is the primary factor responsible for changes in pediatric cardiac output.[24] Bradycardia is poorly tolerated in the infant population and is generally accompanied by hypotension. The heart rate during pediatric sedation should be monitored with an electrocardiogram (ECG) or precordial stethoscope (see monitoring section). Table 10-2 summarizes cardiovascular variations between the infant and adult heart.

> Hypoxia is a primary cause of bradycardia in infants.[25]

Hypoxemia and bradycardia decrease cardiac output and increase systemic acidosis and pulmonary vasoconstriction.[24] Airway obstruction is a major cause of hypoxemia in children. The child's airway should be reassessed frequently for signs of obstruction and 100% oxygen administered when the heart rate decreases. Proactive intervention is necessary to prevent a rapid physiologic spiral toward cardiac arrest. Atropine must be available for all pediatric

TABLE 10-1

Pediatric Cardiovascular Parameters

AGE AND WEIGHT (kg)	RESPIRATIONS (BREATHS PER MINUTE: MIN-MAX)	HEART RATE (BEATS PER MINUTE: MIN-MAX)	SYSTOLIC BLOOD PRESSURE (mm Hg: MIN-MAX)
Preemie (1-2)	30-60	90-180	50-70
Newborn (3.5)	30-60	90-180	50-70
6 mo (7)	24-40	85-170	65-106
1 yr (10)	20-40	80-140	72-110
3 yr (15)	20-30	80-130	78-114
6 yr (20)	18-25	70-120	80-116
8 yr (25)	18-25	70-110	84-122
10 yr (30)	16-20	65-110	90-130
12 yr (40)	14-20	60-110	94-136
15 yr (50)	12-20	55-100	100-142
18 yr (65)	12-18	50-90	104-148

From Pediatric Field Reference Card, Children's Hospital of Pittsburgh Publication.

patients presenting for sedation. Table 10-3 identifies Pediatric Advanced Life Support (PALS) emergency drug dosages. Additional pediatric medications which should be included in the sedation setting are listed in the equipment/drug preparation section.

The parasympathetic nervous system is particularly active in pediatric patients. Hypoxia, deep sedation, and painful events can produce bradycardia which left untreated leads to cardiovascular decompensation conversely. The sympathetic nervous system is underdeveloped in children less than one year of age.[26] Adrenergic receptors are decreased along with circulating catecholamines. Additionally, a diminished response to exogenous catecholamines can be expected.

Constriction of the ductus arteriosus, the fetal connection between the pulmonary artery and aorta, occurs soon after birth in response to increased PaO_2 with ventilation. Hypoxemia may contribute to the reopening of the ductus and shunting of deoxygenated blood from the pulmonary system to the systemic system.[24]

TABLE 10-2

Cardiovascular Variations: Infants vs. Adults

	NEONATE	ADULT
Cardiac output	Rate dependent	Increased by stroke volume/hr
Contractility	Reduced	Normal
Starling response	Limited	Normal
Catecholamine response	Reduced	Normal
Compliance	Reduced	Normal

Modified from Lake CL. *Pediatric Cardiac Anesthesia*. 2nd ed. Norwalk, CT, Appleton; 1993:37.

Functional closure of the foramen ovale, the fetal connection between the atria, typically occurs shortly after birth with anatomic closure following in 4 to 6 weeks.[27] However, anatomic closure may be delayed up to one year.[28] Probe-patent foramen ovale can be found in up to 20% to 30% of adults.[29] Atrial septal defects and ventricular septal defects provide direct access to the cerebral circulation bypassing the lungs. Normally the pulmonary vascular bed functions as a safety reservoir such that small air emboli can be absorbed prior to systemic or cerebral circulation. Intravenous stopcocks and injection ports tend to entrain air and should be manually expunged. Box 10-2 identifies safety measures to prevent inadvertent air administration via intravenous lines.

> It is particularly important to remove all air bubbles from intravenous lines used in small children and infants.

Patients with congenital heart defects or anomalies can be particularly challenging to manage medically. These patients should be referred to a hospital setting with a pediatric anesthesia team prepared to thoroughly assess and treat the hemodynamic consequences of sedation in patients with congenital heart defects. In order to make the appropriate referral, practitioners should be aware of some pediatric syndromes associated with cardiac anomalies which are identified in Box 10-3.

PEDIATRIC RESPIRATORY SYSTEM AND AIRWAY MANAGEMENT

The intent of pediatric procedural sedation is for the child to maintain his/her own airway with minimal support from the practitioner. Concerted effort and care with drug administration frequently prevents procedural sedation from obtunding most patients. However, the continuum of

TABLE 10-3

Emergency Pediatric Advanced Life Support (PALS) Drug Dosages

AGE AND WEIGHT (kg)	EPINEPHRINE 1:10,000 (10 mcg/kg)	ATROPINE 400 mcg/cc (20 mcg/kg)	BICARBONATE (8.4%) (1 mEq/kg)	GLUCOSE	LIDOCAINE 1% 1 mg/kg	CRYSTALLOID BOLUS 10 cc/kg
Preemie (1-2)	20 mcg or 0.2 mL	Minimum dose 100 mcg	4 mL (4.2%)	5 mL (D$_{10}$)	2 mg or 0.2 mL	20 mL
Newborn (3-5)	40 mcg or 0.4 mL	Minimum dose 100 mcg	8 mL (4.2%)	10 mL (D$_{10}$)	4 mg or 0.4 mL	40 mL
6 months (7)	70 mcg or 0.7 mL	140 mcg or 0.35 mL	7 mL (8.4%)	14 mL (D$_{25}$)	7 mg or 0.7 mL	140 mL
1 yr (10)	100 mcg or 1 mL	200 mcg or 0.5 mL	10 mL (8.4%)	20 mL (D$_{25}$)	10 mg or 1 mL	200 mL
3 yr (15)	150 mcg or 1.5 mL	300 mcg or 0.75 mL	15 mL (8.4%)	30 mL (D$_{25}$)	15 mg or 1.5 mL	300 mL
6 yr (20)	200 mcg or 2 mL	400 mcg or 1 mL	20 mL (8.4%)	40 mL (D$_{25}$)	20 mg or 2 mL	400 mL
8 yr (25)	250 mcg or 2.5 mL	500 mcg or 1.25 mL	25 mL (8.4%)	50 mL (D$_{25}$)	25 mg or 2.5 mL	500 mL
10 yr (30)	300 mcg or 3 mL	600 mcg or 1.5 mL	30 mL (8.4%)	30 mL (D$_{50}$)	30 mg or 3 mL	600 mL
12 yr (40)	400 mcg or 4 mL	800 mcg or 2 mL	40 mL (8.4%)	40 mL (D$_{50}$)	40 mg or 4 mL	800 mL
15 yr (50)	500 mcg or 5 mL	1000 mcg (1mg) or 2.5 mL	50 mL (8.4%)	50 cc (D$_{50}$)	50 mg or 5 mL	1000 mL
18 yr (65+)	650 mcg - 1000 mcg (1 mg) or 6.5-10 mL	1000 mcg (1mg) or 2.5 mL	50 mL (8.4%)	50 cc (D$_{50}$)	65-100 mg or 6.5-10 mL	1300 mL

Adapted from Children's Hospital of Pittsburgh publication: Pediatric Field Reference 2001.
Bircher N. Cardiopulmonary resuscitation of infants and children. In Motoyama EK, Davis PJ (eds). *Smith's anesthesia for Infants and Children.* 6th ed. St. Louis: Mosby; 1996:889.

sedation, analgesia, and patient pharmacokinetics does not support this goal in all cases. Practitioners engaged in pediatric sedation must be comfortable with pediatric airway assessment and management. Airway skills must include bag and mask management as well as tracheal intubation if needed.[1]

The infant upper airway is characterized by distinct anatomical features, which vary from adults[30]:

◆ Relatively larger tongue
◆ Short neck
◆ Small mandible
◆ Large occiput
◆ Narrow nasal passages

BOX 10-2

Prevention of Intravascular Air Bubbles

1. Thoroughly remove all air from intravenous line before the child enters the sedation suite or procedure room.
2. Just prior to the child entering the room, inspect the tubing again.
3. When connecting fluid-filled tubing to IV cannulas, have a free flow of both tubing and cannula (blood).
4. Before injecting a drug from a syringe intravenously, eject a small amount of drug from syringe to clear air from the syringe and needle hub.
5. Do not inject the last millimeter of syringe contents because of microbubbles on the plunger.
6. Use air traps on intravenous lines if they are available.
7. Never leave central lines open to air.

Adapted from Lake CL. *Pediatric Cardiac Anesthesia.* 2nd ed. Norwalk, CT: Appleton; 1993:216.

BOX 10-3

Pediatric Syndromes Associated with Cardiac Anomalies

• DiGeorge syndrome
• Down syndrome (trisomy 21)
• Goldenhar's syndrome
• Marfan's syndrome
• Noonan's syndrome
• Polysplenia
• Sebaceous nevi syndrome
• VATER syndrome
• Williams' syndrome

Syndromes Associated with Cardiomyopathy

• Duchenne muscular dystrophy
• Hunter's syndrome
• Hurler's syndrome
• Stevens-Johnson syndrome

Adapted from Krane JK, Davis PJ, Smith RM. Preoperative preparation. In Motoyama EK, Davis PJ (eds). *Smith's Anesthesia for Infants and Children.* 6th ed. St. Louis: Mosby; 1996:219.

TABLE 10-4

Age-Appropriate Oral Airways

AGE	SIZE	SIZE (cm)	SIZE (mm)
Preterm	000 or 00	3.5 or 4.5	35 or 45
Neonate to 3 mo	0	5.5	55
3-12 mo	1	6.0	60
1-5 yr	2	7.0	70
>5 yr	3	8.0	80

Modified: mm length added because mm length is a common identifier and label.

From Bell C. *The Pediatric Anesthesia Handbook.* 2nd ed. St. Louis: Mosby; 1997:42.

Size 0, **infant,** 50 mm
Size 1, **small child,** 60 mm
Size 2, **child,** 70 mm
Size 3, **small adult,** 80 mm
Size 4, **medium adult,** 90 mm
Size 5, **large adult,** 100 mm

Traditional

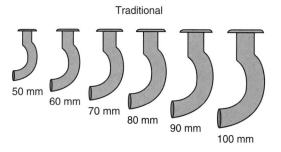

Color coded

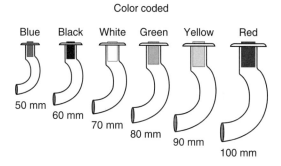

FIGURE 10-1 Oral airway sizing.

This combination of anatomical features can make the infant difficult to bag and mask ventilate when deep sedation or general anesthesia inadvertently occurs. The large tongue easily falls toward the roof of the mouth in a sedated infant or small child and obstructs ventilation.[31-33] This may necessitate the need for an appropriate-sized oral airway. A guide for selecting an age appropriate-sized oral airway is identified in Table 10-4. The appropriate length of the oral airway can be predicted by choosing an airway that is the same length as the distance from the mouth to the angle of the mandible. This can be estimated by holding the airway next to the side of the face and comparing the mouth to mandibular distance with the length of the plastic oral airway. An oral airway that is too long will push the epiglottis down; an airway that is too small will push the tongue toward the oropharynx roof.[33] Properly placed oral airways significantly decrease airway resistance, thus the work of breathing in spontaneously breathing sedated patients is decreased.[34] As identified in Figure 10-1, oral airways may elicit a gag response that can generate vomiting and vagal nerve-mediated bradycardia in mildly sedated or awake patients, therefore they should only be placed in deeply sedated patients requiring bag and mask ventilation. As depicted in Figure 10-2, oral airways should always be placed with a tongue blade to avoid folding the tongue back on itself and exacerbating the obstruction.

In patients requiring bag and mask ventilation, the practitioner's fingers should remain on the bony mandible and off the soft tissue beneath the mandible (Fig. 10-3). Incorrect positioning exerts pressure on the soft tissue beneath the bony mandible, pushing the tongue forward, and further obstructing the airway.

Soft nasal airways (nasal trumpets) are more appropriate for the mild or moderately sedated patient. Narrow nasal passages are easily obstructed with secretions. Nasal obstruction can create respiratory problems because infants cannot easily convert to mouth breathing.[31-33] Placement of an appropriate-sized nasal trumpet will ease ventilation by physically displacing the tongue obstruction and decrease the resistance of breathing. To avoid trauma to the adenoidal tissue, nasal airways must be lubricated.[33] Nasal trumpets are more comfortable than oral airways and generally elicit less gagging, vomiting, and vagally mediated bradycardia.

Alignment of the oral, pharyngeal, and laryngeal axis is necessary for adequate view of the vocal cords during laryngoscopy.[35] The characteristic short neck, small mandible, and large occiput may prevent the oral-pharyngeal-laryngeal axis from aligning, thereby creating airway obstruction in the sedated child. Extreme flexion of the neck is shown to increase airway obstruction in obstructive apneic patients.[31,32] A neck or shoulder roll, depicted in Figure 10-4 may be necessary to ensure neutral head placement for alignment of the airway axes. The infant's lower airway is characterized by the following considerations[31-33]:

- The infant's larynx is higher (cephalad) in the neck (C3-4) than in adults (C4-5).
- The infant's epiglottis is omega or "U" shaped and stiff.
- The narrowest part of the infant's larynx is the cricoid cartilage *below* the level of the vocal cords.

These characteristics can affect the intubation of the infant in several ways. Head elevation to achieve the "sniffing position" in adults may inhibit vocal cord visualization in infants. Keeping the head neutral or slightly flexed is recommended.[31,32,35,36] During laryngoscopy the stiff epiglottis may totally obscure visualization of the glottic opening.

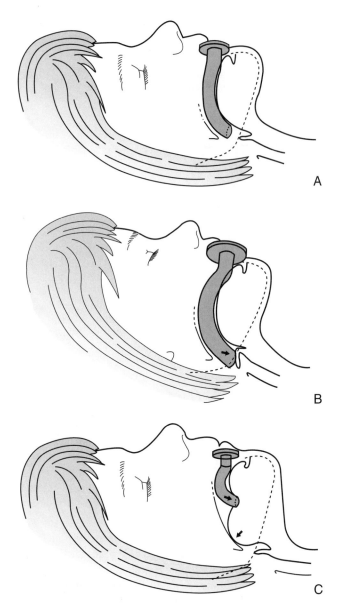

FIGURE 10-2 Correct vs. incorrect oral airway placement during mask ventilation of the obstructed pediatric sedation patient. An artificial airway of proper size should relieve airway obstruction secondary to the tongue without damaging laryngeal structures. The appropriate size can be estimated by holding the airway against the child's face. **A,** The tip of the oral airway should end just cephalad to the angle of the mandible, resulting in proper alignment with the glottic opening. **B,** If too large of an oral airway is inserted, the tip lines up posterior to the angle of the mandible and mechanically obstructs the glottic opening with the epiglottis. **C,** If too small of an oral airway is inserted, the tip lines up well above the angle of the mandible and exacerbates airway obstruction by kinking the tongue against the roof of the mouth. (Redrawn from Coté CJ. *A Practice of Anesthesia for Infants and Children.* 3rd ed. Philadelphia: WB Saunders; 2000:90.)

Pediatric straight blades are used to manually lift the epiglottis to expose the vocal cords for laryngoscopy (Fig. 10-5).

The narrow cricoid cartilage is lined with pseudostratified, ciliated epithelium that is very sensitive to manipulation and readily forms edema.[32] The pediatric tracheal lumen is cone shaped with the narrowest portion at the cricoid ring just *below* the vocal cords. If an endotracheal tube with an excessively large external diameter is placed in a child, edema in this subglottic space may occur.

> Because the resistance to air flow is proportional to the 4th power of the radius,[31] even slight edema can significantly increase airway resistance. One millimeter of edema or retained secretions will decrease the cross-sectional area of a 4-mm airway by 75%. The same airway will be subjected to a 16-fold increase in airway resistance.

Symptoms of stridor and respiratory distress can develop easily in patients with subglottic edema. For this reason, care must be taken to deliberately choose appropriate-sized endotracheal tubes in children. Box 10-4 identifies endotracheal tube (ETT) sizes for the pediatric patient. The following equation can be used when choosing the appropriate-sized uncuffed endotracheal tube for children younger than 10 years.[37]

$$\frac{16 + age}{4} = ETT\ size$$

Infants who were born premature and require prolonged mechanical ventilation during the neonatal period may be at risk for subglottic stenosis. For these children smaller endotracheal tubes than the age-identified recommendation should also be available. Uncuffed tubes are generally used in children younger than 10 years of age due to the narrow cricoid cartilage. A leak at 20 to 25 cm H_2O pressure indicates an appropriate-sized endotracheal tube. A leak heard at less than 10 cm H_2O pressure may inhibit the ability to generate adequate positive-pressure ventilation. A leak not heard until 30 cm H_2O pressure or greater signals an endotracheal tube that is too large and may contribute to subglottic edema and resulting stridor.[37]

The traditional pediatric airway algorithm has suggested uncuffed tubes in children younger than 10 years of age. However, evidence suggests the use of cuffed tubes in children may be beneficial.[38] The inflatable cuff allows easy manipulation of an airway seal and decreases the repeat intubations needed to establish appropriate endotracheal tube size. If a cuffed endotracheal tube is used in a pediatric patient, the appropriate-sized cuffed tube is at least one size smaller than the appropriate sized uncuffed endotracheal tube.[37]

If the sedated pediatric patient should lose the ability to spontaneously ventilate, or develops airway obstruction, several maneuvers must be considered before intubation (in general order):

◆ Maintenance of the head in neutral position to align the oral-pharyngeal-tracheal axis (removing extreme flexion)[35]

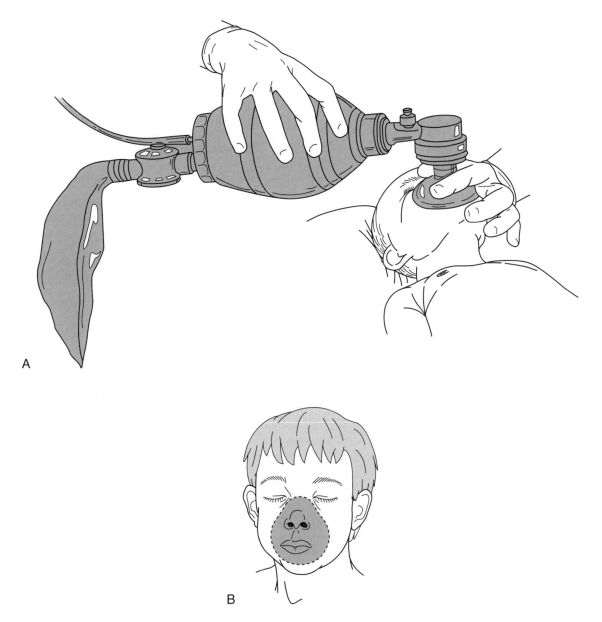

FIGURE 10-3 Proper pediatric mask management technique. **A,** One-handed face mask application technique. Note that the fingers remain on the bony mandible. Incorrect placement of the fingers on the soft tissues beneath the chin pushes the tongue toward the roof of the oropharynx and further obstructs the airway. Note the fingers avoid pressure on the soft tissues of the neck, which could cause laryngeal or tracheal compression. **B,** Proper area of the face for face mask application. Note that no pressure is applied to the eyes. (Redrawn from American Heart Association. Dallas, TX. *Pediatric Advanced Life Support.* American Academy of Pediatrics.)

◆ Gentle jaw lift
◆ Nasopharyngeal airway placement (lubricated nasal trumpet)
◆ Oral airway if patient deeply sedated (placed with tongue blade)
◆ Positive-pressure ventilation with Ambu bag and 100% oxygen

If effective, these measures along with reversal of the sedation/narcotic agent may eliminate the need to intubate.

If the practitioner is unable to effectively oxygenate and ventilate via positive-pressure and a bag-mask-valve, then intubation should be considered.

PEDIATRIC RESPIRATORY PHYSIOLOGY

Full-term newborns breathe irregularly; periods of regular breathing are interposed with 5 to 10 seconds of apnea.[39] This respiratory pattern occurs mostly during quiet sleep. Periodic breathing diminishes with age. Episodic breathing

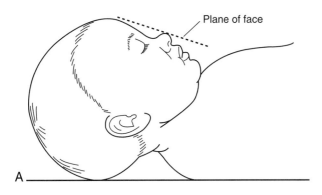

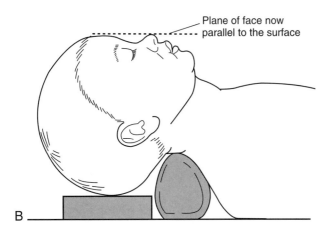

FIGURE 10-4 Proper head position/axis alignment for pediatric endotracheal intubation. **A,** Flexion of the neck producing airway obstruction. This position interrupts the alignment of the oral, pharyngeal, and laryngeal axis necessary for adequate view of the vocal cords during laryngoscopy. **B,** Proper positioning of infant neck/shoulder roll demonstrates proper alignment for endotracheal intubation.

is rarely present at 12 months of age. Central apnea of infancy is defined as a breathing pause greater than 15 to 20 seconds that is associated with bradycardia, cyanosis, or pallor. The immature respiratory center is considered the cause for this phenomenon.[39] Young infants who have received sedation or general anesthesia are at greater risk for apnea and subsequent bradycardia in the first 12 hours after the procedure. Infants most at risk are those younger than 45 weeks postconceptual age.[39-42] Infants younger than this age generally require overnight hospitalization for observation after general anesthesia, even for minor procedures.

Healthcare practitioners sedating infants younger than 45 weeks postconceptual age or a full-term infant younger than 5 to 9 weeks old must be aware of the postsedation risk of apnea and bradycardia. Extended monitoring, prolonged recovery care, and parent education are required for this patient population, and an overnight monitored stay is considered safest.

The muscles associated with ventilation in the newborn are subject to quick fatigue, owing to decreased type I muscle fiber (slow-twitch, fatigue-resistant) distribution.[32,43] The work of breathing is higher overall in the infant than the adult; however, it is compensated for by a higher respiratory rate and minute volume.

Children have an increased metabolic rate, resulting in higher oxygen consumption when compared with adults (6 to 8 mL/kg/min relative to 3 to 4 mL/kg/min in the adult).[31,43] Alveolar ventilation is increased to meet the increase in oxygen demand.[31,39,43] Because of increased oxygen consumption and ventilation, apneic infants can become hypoxic within 30 seconds.[43] Hypoxemia quickly leads to bradycardia in the parasympathetic-predominant child.

If desaturation, cyanosis, or bradycardia occurs, intubation attempts should cease immediately and mask ventilation with 100% oxygen should be administered until the oxygen saturation returns to baseline.[43]

TEMPERATURE REGULATION

The primary types of heat loss experienced by children include conduction, evaporation, radiation, and convection.[44,45] **Conduction** is the heat transfer between two touching objects such as cold irrigation and cold intravenous fluids. **Evaporation** is defined as the difference between the vapor pressure of surface and vapor pressure of environment. Evaporation results in 10% to 20% of all temperature loss in operating room environments. This includes sweating, water loss from open surgical wounds, and evaporation of liquids applied to the skin such as antibiotic solution. Procedural sedation cases would generally have less evaporative losses than open surgical procedures. **Convection** occurs with the transfer of heat from the patient to moving air. The temperature gradient in the room, breezy hallways, and uncovered patients contribute to convective heat losses. **Radiation** is the transfer of heat between two objects not in contact but of different temperatures. This is the main form of heat loss in operating rooms. At 22° C (room temperature), 70% of all heat loss is from radiation.[44]

Hypothermia causes multiple physiologic alterations, which include[44,46]:

◆ Peripheral vasoconstriction
◆ Decreased myocardial function
◆ Unpredictable changes in drug dose-response curves
◆ Alterations in the ability of hemoglobin to release oxygen at the tissue level

Infants are **homeothermic**[44] (having the ability to maintain a constant internal body temperature) similar to adults; however, they possess a significantly decreased thermoregulatory range. The lower environmental temperature limit for autoregulation in adults is 0° C (32° F). Infants require 22° C (72° F) for adequate autoregulation.

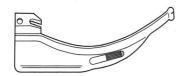

The **MacIntosh** Blade provides the widely preferred curve along its entire length, permitting ease of intubation. The unique reverse Z blade configuration facilitates elevation of the epiglottis without contact on its dorsal surface.

The **Miller** Blade provides a straight design with a gently curved distal tip encompassing approximately two inches from the beak. The flattened flange and gentle curve provide a more direct approach to intubation.

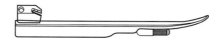

The **Phillips** Blade integrates the straight blade design with the curved distal tip Miller design providing greater visibility and an almost direct line approach to the trachea during intubation. Unique lamp mounting provides deep illumination downward and inward, while the low profile flange reduces the risk of oral damage.

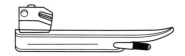

The **Wisconsin** Blade features the straight spatula design with a two-thirds circle flange and blunt tip for elevation of the epiglottis.

Laryngoscope Blade	Age
Miller 0	Preterm, neonate
Miller 1	Neonate to age 2 years
Phillips 1	13 months to 4 years
Whis-Hippel 1.5	Age 2 to 5 years
Miller 2	Age 5 years and older
Macintosh 2	Age 3 to 6 years
Macintosh 3/Phillips 2	Teenagers

FIGURE 10-5 Pediatric laryngoscope blades. (Adapted from Bell C, Kain ZN, Hughes C [eds]. *The Pediatric Anesthesia Handbook.* 2nd ed. St. Louis: Mosby; 1997:43; and Gronert BJ, Motoyama EK. Induction of anesthesia and endotracheal intubation. In Motoyama EK, Davis PJ [eds]. *Smith's Anesthesia for Infants and Children.* 6th ed. St. Louis: Mosby; 1997:292-293.)

Infants have a limited thermoregulatory range secondary to[44,46]:

◆ Small body size
◆ Increased surface-to-volume ratio
◆ Increased thermal conductance

BOX 10-4

Endotracheal Tube Sizes

Age	Size (mm Internal Diameter)
Preterm	
1000 g	2.5
1000-2500 g	3.0
Neonate-6 mo	3.0-3.5
6 mo-1 yr	3.5-4.0
1-2 yr	4.0-5.0
Beyond 2 yr	(age in yr + 16)/4

Nonshivering thermogenesis is an important heat-generating mechanism in infants. This occurs through the metabolism of brown fat. Brown fat composes up to 6% of an infant's total body weight and is composed primarily of mitochondria.[44] Cold stress–induced norepinephrine is the primary impetus for brown fat metabolism. Glucocorticoids and thyroxine have also been implicated in nonshivering thermogenesis.[44]

Methods to decrease temperature loss should be used in the pediatric sedation environment. The simplest maneuver is to simply warm the procedure room to 75° to 80° F. The use of blankets and hats can significantly reduce heat loss. Warming lamps (at an appropriate distance from the infant to avoid burns) are very effective.[46] If warming lamps are used, the area being exposed should not be covered with blankets that would obstruct heat from the lamps.[33] Bair Hugger blankets (forced warm air insufflation) devices must be utilized for longer cases.[47] **It is imperative to utilize blankets with Bair Hugger technology, because case reports of severe burns have been reported in the literature.**[48]

Temperature monitoring for short cases may be unnecessary.[49] Although skin temperature probes are not wholly reliable owing to changes in cutaneous blood flow, they provide information on trends.[33,44] Tympanic membrane temperature probes are easy to use and noninvasive if used properly.[33]

FLUID REPLACEMENT

Infant total body water (75%) is greater than adults (55%).[43,50] The relative percentage of body compartment water featured in Table 10-5 also varies with the pediatric patient population. As much as 80% of the pediatric patient's total blood volume is contained in the venous system.[51] Sedation in a baseline dehydrated child with a long fasting time decreases cardiac output and perpetuates hypovolemia.[51]

Renal function as measured by glomerular filtration rate and tubular function is immature until 6 to 12 months of age.[52] The underdeveloped premature and newborn kidney loses sodium in the urine. For this reason, all intravenous solutions given to infants should contain sodium.[52]

Convenient calculations have been devised to aid the practitioner in fluid maintenance requirements for children. Hourly fluid maintenance should be administered with a balanced salt solution such as lactated Ringers, normal saline (0.9%), or (0.45%). Dextrose 5% to 10% may also be included for intravenous supplementation.

The use of a Buretrol, Venoset, or burette measuring device (Fig. 10-6) allows a predetermined amount of fluid to enter the patient and decreases the chance of inadvertent excess fluid delivery. The use of an infusion pump with free flow protection for accurate fluid volume administration is recommended for pediatric patients.[53] An infusion pump provides an accurate infusion rate, information on volumes administered, and warning if infusion patency becomes obstructed.[32] The following method calculates hourly pediatric fluid requirements.[43,50,52]

WEIGHT	HOURLY FLUID RATE	EXAMPLE
0-10 kg	4 mL/kg/hr	7 kg × 4 = 28 mL/hr
10-20 kg	4 mL/kg/hr for the first 10 kg	10 kg × 4 = 40 mL/hr
	2 mL/kg/hr for remaining kg	5 kg × 2 = 10 mL/hr
		15 kg maintenance = 50 mL/hr
>20 kg	4 mL/kg/hr for first 10 kg	10 kg × 4 = 40 mL/hr
	2 mL/kg/hr for next 20 kg	10 kg × 2 = 20 kg/hr
	1 mL/kg/hr for remaining kg	6 kg × 1 = 6 kg/hr
		26 kg maintenance = 66 mL/hr

TABLE 10-5

Body Composition of Pediatric Patients

	INFANT	CHILD	ADULT
Total body water	75%	70%	55%-60%
Extracellular fluid	40%	30%	20%
Intracellular fluid	35%	40%	40%

GLUCOSE REPLACEMENT

Pediatric patients have a decreased tolerance to starvation when compared with adults; even healthy children with long fasting periods have become hypoglycemic.[54] Severe hypoglycemia has been shown to cause cerebral ischemia and acidosis, leading to brain damage.[55] However, replacement with 5% dextrose solutions is associated with hyperglycemia, which leads to osmolar diuresis and dehydration.[54] Current recommendations suggest maintenance fluids that contain 2.5% dextrose rather than 5% dextrose solutions.[56] The 2.5% dextrose and lactated Ringer's or 2.5% dextrose and half-normal saline are appropriate maintenance fluids for pediatric patients. If 2.5% dextrose is not available, 5% dextrose with sodium at an infusion rate of 4 to 6 mg/kg/min is recommended to maintain glucose concentrations of 50 to 90 mg/dL in newborns.[52] Glucose monitoring is recommended for infants who are not receiving glucose supplementation or who have experienced a prolonged fast.[54]

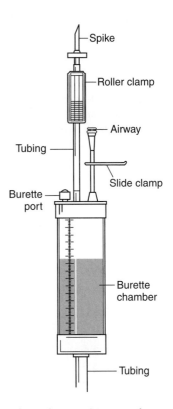

FIGURE 10-6 Pediatric burette. (From Booker M, Ignatavicius D. *Infusion Therapy*. Philadelphia: WB Saunders; 1996:57.)

TABLE 10-6

Current EMLA Dosing Guidelines

AGE AND BODY WEIGHT REQUIREMENTS	MAXIMUM EMLA TOTAL DOSE	MAXIMUM APPLICATION AREA	MAXIMUM APPLICATION TIME
Birth up to 3 mo or <5 kg	1 g	10 cm^2	1 hr
3 mo up to 12 mo and >5 kg	2 g	20 cm^2	4 hr
1 to 6 yr and >10 kg	10 g	100 cm^2	4 hr
7 to 12 yr and >20 kg	20 g	200 cm^2	4 hr

From EMLA Cream. In *Physicians Desk Reference (PDR)*. Montvale, NJ: Thompson PDR; 2003:600.

The AAP Committee on Drugs states "there should be an appropriate interval of fasting before sedation."[1] NPO guidelines established by the American Society of Anesthesiologists were identified in Box 2-7. NPO guidelines were created to decrease the incidence of potential aspiration while at the same time attempting to maintain the child's presedation hydration status. Prior to the administration of sedation, parents should be instructed to continue feeding and liquids to infants as outlined in Box 2-7. This will minimize significant hypovolemia or hypoglycemia in the healthy child. Small children and infants who arrive for sedation with extended NPO times (>12 hours) may need to be rescheduled.

If an intravenous catheter is required, EMLA (Astra Pharmaceuticals) local anesthetic cream may be applied at least 1 hour before the intravenous attempt. EMLA cream is a eutectic (melts into oil below room temperature) mixture of lidocaine 2.5% and prilocaine 2.5% that provides dermal analgesia up to 5 mm deep.[57,58] EMLA is applied to dry intact skin surrounding a potential IV site, covered with an occlusive dressing, and left for 1 hour. EMLA should not be used on open, traumatized, or inflamed skin. EMLA should be used with caution (in appropriate doses) in infants because of methemeglobinemia reports.[57] Table 10-6 categorizes the current guidelines for EMLA administration for avoiding toxicity in patients with normal intact skin and normal hepatic and renal function.

Transient paleness, redness, and edema may occur at the site of EMLA placement, which is thought to be related to vasoconstriction. Maximal local vasoconstriction occurs at 1.5 hours, followed by vasodilatation after 2 to 3 hours.[59] The EMLA cream should be wiped off and appropriate skin preparation applied before intravenous insertions attempts. All other areas with EMLA cream should be cleaned once the intravenous line is placed.

Intravenous placement may be particularly challenging in young children and infants. Intravenous catheters of 22 or 24 gauge are generally adequate in small infants.[60] The dorsum of the hand, the lateral aspect of the foot, and the medial aspect of the ankle are usually the best insertion sites in small children and infants.[32]

PATIENT SELECTION

A thorough presedation patient assessment and focused review of systems is critical to promote safe, appropriate pediatric sedation. The need for the particular procedure requiring sedation should be clear and understood by the practitioners and the parents. The child may have coexisting health issues that affect the sedation plan of care. A proper presedation assessment may impact the type of sedation and the timing of the procedure. This is emphasized in the AAP recommendation.[1]

> On the basis of careful, documented review of the medical history, physical examination, and the proposed procedure, a practitioner may determine that a hospital is the only appropriate choice for administering sedatives.

The American Society of Anesthesiologists (ASA) Physical Status (PS) Classification System identified in Box 10-5 was developed by anesthesia personnel to systematically categorize patient physical status.[61] The JCAHO recommends procedural sedation for ASA PS 1 and ASA PS 2 patients only. Practitioners caring for patients who are ASA PS 3 or higher should consider consultation with an anesthesiologist.[62]

BOX 10-5

American Society of Anesthesiologists Physical Status

PS 1 — a normal, healthy patient

PS 2 — a patient with mild systemic disease that does not limit activities, such as controlled asthma or controlled diabetes, without target organ damage

PS 3 — a patient with severe systemic disease that limits activities, such as severe heart failure or poorly controlled asthma

PS 4 — a patient with severe systemic disease that is a constant threat to life, such as severe heart failure or end-stage renal disease

PS 5 — a moribund patient who is not expected to survive without the operation or other intervention

PS 6 — a patient declared brain dead whose organs are being removed for donation

If the procedure is an emergency, the physical status classification is followed by an E (PS 2 E).

Patients with complex multisystem pathophysiologic disease states require the care from personnel specially educated and prepared to manage the sedation plan of care in this compromised patient population.[60,61]

MEDICAL HISTORY

The medical history should focus on identifying conditions involving major organ systems, previous problems with sedation/analgesia, or regional/general anesthesia. Current medication history (including herbal preparations and over-the-counter products), allergies, and NPO times must also be obtained from the parents. The child's medications should be evaluated carefully. A current pediatric drug reference book should be available in all pediatric settings without exception. The cytochrome P-450 enzyme network within the liver is a primary site for drug metabolism. Prescription and recreational drugs that induce these enzymes may affect the pharmacokinetics and dynamics of the sedative agents. Teenagers should be asked about alcohol, tobacco, and drug use. A urine pregnancy test should be administered to pubescent girls to avoid inadvertent drugs to the fetus. Administration of benzodiazepines in utero has been associated with cleft lip and palate malformations.[64,65]

> Most sedation and analgesia agents have high lipid solubility and low molecular weight and consequently cross the placenta easily.[63]

PHYSICAL EXAMINATION
Airway

The AAP "Guidelines for Monitoring and Management of Pediatric Patients During and After Sedation for Diagnostic and Therapeutic Procedures: Addendum" states that the patient must undergo a documented presedation medical evaluation, including a focused airway examination.[1] Airway evaluation should be performed by someone with expertise in pediatric tracheal intubation.[66] Proper airway evaluation is particularly important if a deep level of sedation is inadvertently reached and respiratory or airway support is required. Most airway disasters are associated with failure to anticipate difficult airway management.[67-69] Many objective measures have been evaluated in the attempt to define particular features associated with difficult bag and mask ventilation and/or tracheal intubation. The Mallampati classification method of airway assessment evaluates the extent the base of the tongue obscures the view of pharyngeal structures.[70] Correlation has been established in adult patients between the Mallampati classification and degree of difficulty exposing vocal cords during direct laryngoscopy (see Fig. 7-7, Chapter 7, Airway Management and Management of Respiratory Complications).

Class I: Uvula, faucial pillars, soft palate visible
Class II: Faucial pillars, soft palate visible
Class III: Only the soft palate visible

The large tongue structure in the pediatric airway frequently leads to poor correlation with the use of the Mallampati Airway Classification System. However, this system can be very useful in evaluating children older than 10 years of age.

Micrognathia (small submandibular space) may indicate the potential for difficult airway management secondary to the mandibular anatomic proportion. In addition, the compactness of the space that it encapsulates may prohibit proper placement of an oral airway and inhibit visibility of the vocal cords during laryngoscopy.[35]

Maxillary-mandibular joint stiffness may inhibit the ability of maximal mouth opening. Patients with temporomandibular joint problems may experience variations in this examination.[35] If there are no limitations during this examination, the atlanto-occipital joint should be assessed. This joint also should be assessed if there are no contraindications such as trisomy 21 or other known patient factors associated with laxity or fusion. The ability to place an older child in the sniffing position will also assist with vocal cord visualization if tracheal intubation is indicated. A complete review of each airway evaluation maneuver is featured in Chapter 7, Airway Management and Management of Respiratory Complications.

Some pediatric patients presenting for sedation have coexisting disease that will affect airway management. Patients with trisomy 21 have large tongues, short mandibles, small oral and nasal passages, and pharyngeal hypotonia.[71] These patients easily experience obstruction when sedated. Twenty percent of Down syndrome patients have ligamentous laxity of the atlantoaxial joint that predisposes to C1-C2 subluxation. This subluxation can lead to spinal cord injury. Care must be taken with these patients while managing the airway.[71]

A systematic approach to pediatric airway evaluation is important. One method of focused evaluation includes stepwise evaluation of[35]:

◆ Mouth and tongue
◆ Extent of mouth opening
◆ Thyromental distance relative to associated structures
◆ Degree of neck extension
◆ Mallampati classification (more valuable in older children and teenagers)

Pediatric syndromes associated with airway management difficulty are identified in Box 10-6. **The management of sedation for these patients must be individualized to the patient's needs and an anesthesia consultation is frequently indicated.**

Children age 6 through adolescence lose deciduous teeth.[43] This age group should be questioned and examined for loose teeth before any sedation procedure. Manipulations such as oral airway and emergency intubation can dislodge a loose tooth and further jeopardize airway management. Orthodontia generally does not interfere with airway manipulation or management. However, metal palate expanders may make intubation slightly more difficult

Pediatric Syndromes Associated with Difficult Airway Management

- Encephalocele
- Cleft palate
- Micronathia or Pierre Robin syndrome
- Craniofacial deformity (Crouzon's syndrome, Apert's syndrome)
- Mandibular hypoplasia (Treacher Collins syndrome, Goldenhar's syndrome)
- Hurler's syndrome

From Motoyama EK, Davis PJ. *Smith's Anesthesia for Infants and Children.* 6th ed. St. Louis: Mosby; 1996:305.

because of pharyngeal spatial restrictions. Patients with wired jaws are not able to open their mouths, and wire clippers must be in the procedural area if these patients are sedated.[72] Patients presenting with fractured jaws that are in the process of healing would benefit from the expertise of an anesthesia provider if sedation services are required in this patient population.

Cardiac

Careful auscultation of the pediatric patient's heart may reveal a murmur not detected previously by other healthcare practitioners. Signs of cardiac disease in children include symptoms of failure to thrive, tachypnea, cyanosis, and diaphoresis. Presedation evaluation of patients with known or suspected cardiac disease should include cardiac consultation and meticulous testing, including an ECG and other specific cardiac diagnostic tests. Pediatric patients with cardiac anomalies should be treated individually and referred to a pediatric cardiac anesthesia team if appropriate.

Central Nervous System

Patients with developmental delay or mental retardation frequently have a less predictable response to the effects of sedation/analgesic medications. Patients with mental retardation or cerebral palsy often have difficulty managing oral secretions and gastroesophageal reflux is common. The increased secretions and the gastroesophageal reflux increase the risk of aspiration, particularly with mentally handicapped patients or those with cerebral palsy. Cerebral palsy is a common disorder (approximately 3 per 10,000 live births) associated with prematurity that is defined as a nonprogressive disorder of movement.[73] Children with cerebral palsy range in intellect: some patients have normal intelligence but are limited in their ability to communicate whereas others have significant developmental delay. This developmental delay can create great difficulty when the patient is separated from daily caregivers. These children often have a seizure disorder treated with one or more seizure medications. It is important to note that any patient's decreased ability to communicate should not be regarded as decreased pain sensation. Parameters other than speech must be monitored closely, such as patient posturing, crying, and vital signs to ensure appropriate analgesia during painful procedures.

PEDIATRIC MEDICAL PROBLEMS

The average child has an average of three to eight colds or upper respiratory tract infections a year.[71] Symptoms of a cold generally manifest as nasal congestion, fever, cough, and general malaise. **Presenting symptoms must be evaluated during the presedation assessment and before administering any sedative agent that may further obstruct breathing in an already compromised patient airway.** A child with significant nasal congestion may be difficult to sedate without simultaneously affecting spontaneous ventilation. Elective sedation cases should be postponed and rescheduled if any of the following are present[71]:

- "Croupy cough"
- Rectal temperature above 38° C (100° F) (+ any other significant sign of an upper respiratory tract infection)
- Malaise or decreased appetite
- Evidence of recent lower respiratory tract infection (rales, wheezing, or productive cough)

Children with hypertrophied tonsils or adenoids tend to have airway obstruction while sleeping, which is manifested as snoring. These patients tend to become hypoxic even during procedures not involving the airway.[74] Patients with baseline airway obstruction may experience increased ventilation difficulty once sedated.[75]

CONSENT

Parents must provide informed consent for the procedure and for procedural sedation. Patients 18 years and older may sign their own consent forms. It is equally important that children are informed about the procedure in a manner consistent with their developmental stage. The intravenous catheter should only be placed after the initial assessment, physical examination, and consent forms are completed.

EQUIPMENT/ENVIRONMENT

The AAP recommendations regarding emergency drug and equipment availability for pediatric sedation facilities are featured in Boxes 10-7 and 10-8.[3] Airway management and sedation equipment in various age-suitable sizes must be immediately available. An emergency cart must be accessible and contain age- and weight-appropriate drugs and equipment to rescue a sedation patient in respiratory distress. The contents of the cart must give the provider the ability to administer continuous life support while the patient is being transported to another area within the medical facility or another medical facility altogether. The specific AAP statement addressing pediatric sedation and magnetic resonance imaging states:

The special technologic problems associated with monitoring patients in a magnetic resonance imaging scanner—specifically,

BOX 10-7

American Academy of Pediatrics: Suggested Resuscitation Drugs for Pediatric Sedation

- Oxygen
- Glucose (50%)
- Atropine
- Epinephrine (1:1,000; 1:10,000)
- Phenylephrine
- Dopamine
- Diazepam
- Diphenhydramine hydrochloride
- Hydrocortisone
- Isoproterenol
- Calcium chloride or calcium gluconate
- Sodium bicarbonate
- Lidocaine (cardiac lidocaine, local infiltration)
- Methylprednisolone
- Succinylcholine
- Aminophylline
- Racemic epinephrine
- Albuterol by inhalation
- Ammonia spirits
- Naloxone hydrochloride
- Hydrocortisone

Note: The choice of emergency drugs may vary according to individual need.

BOX 10-8

Suggested Emergency Equipment for Pediatric Sedation

Intravenous Equipment
Intravenous catheters: 24, 22, 20, 18, and 16 gauge
Tourniquets
Alcohol wipes
Adhesive tape
Assorted syringes: 1 mL, 3 mL, 6 mL, and 12 mL
Intravenous tubing
    Pediatric drip (60 drops/mL)
    Pediatric burette type
    Adult drip (10 drops/mL)
    Extension tubing
Intravenous fluid
    Lactated Ringer's solution
    Normal saline
Three-way stopcocks
Pediatric intravenous (IV) boards
Assorted IV needles: 22, 20, and 18 gauge
Intraosseous bone marrow needle
Sterile gauze pads

Airway Management Equipment
Face masks: infant, child, small adult, medium adult, large adult
Breathing bag and valve set
Oral airways: infant, child, small adult, medium adult, large adult
Nasal airways: small, medium, large
Laryngoscope handles
Laryngoscope blades
    Straight (Miller) No. 1, 2, 3
    Curved (Macintosh) No. 2, 3
Endotracheal tubes
    2.5, 3.0, 3.5, 4.0, 4.5, 5.0, 5.5, 6.0 uncuffed
    6.0, 7.0, 8.0 cuffed

the powerful magnetic field and the generation of radiofrequency— necessitates the use of special equipment to provide continuous patient monitoring throughout the scanning procedure. Pulse oximeters capable of continuous function even during scanning are now available and should be used in any sedated or restrained pediatric patient. Thermal injuries can result if appropriate precautions are not taken; avoid coiling the oximeter wire and place the probe as far from the magnetic coil as possible to diminish the possibility of injury. Electrocardiogram monitoring during magnetic resonance imaging has been associated with thermal injury, and it should be used with caution in this setting.

Age and size appropriate equipment and medications to sustain life must be checked before every sedation case.[3] An appropriate pediatric environment is composed of a child-friendly facility, proper equipment selection, and competent personnel with experience working with children.[76]

Clinical competence is required of all healthcare practitioners participating in the sedation care of young children and infants.

Training and experience in pediatric airway management and basic resuscitation techniques, as well as the ability to recognize a child in distress and provide immediate assistance while calling for support staff/resuscitation team, are necessary. Pediatric Advanced Life Support Course certification should be required.[76]

MONITORING MECHANISMS

Monitoring requirements for pediatric patients undergoing procedural sedation closely parallel the requirements for monitoring a patient receiving general anesthesia. Constant objective and subjective patient assessment as promulgated by the AAP include: **An individual must be specifically assigned to monitor the patient's cardiorespiratory status during and after the procedure; for deeply sedated patients that individual should have no other responsibilities and should record vital signs at least every 5 minutes.**[1]

Precordial stethoscopes are used in pediatric anesthesia and are a useful adjunct for the pediatric sedation provider. The precordial stethoscope (Fig. 10-7) is positioned over the child's left sternal border at the second to fourth intercostals space.[56] This placement allows the practitioner to clearly hear breath sounds, heart rate, and heart tones indicating changes in cardiac output. Double stick adhesive (3M Company, St. Paul, MN) maintains contact of the bell of the stethoscope to the skin. The opposite end of the stethoscope is attached by disposable lightweight tubing to a soft foam compressible ear piece (Kalayjian Enterprises, Chapel Hill,

Chestpieces/precordial stethoscopes

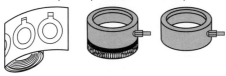

Softear disposable monoscope

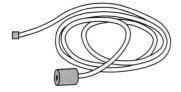

Monoscope reusable ear pieces

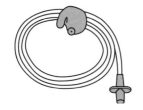

FIGURE 10-7 Precordial stethoscope.

NC).[56] The use of a precordial stethoscope allows the sedation provider the ability to continually monitor changes in heart rate and respiratory status.

Noninvasive pulse oximetry noninvasively measures the arterial oxygen saturation of hemoglobin continuously.[56] The pulse oximeter provides a more reliable warning of hypoxemia in children relative to the capnograph and even changes in clinical signs.[77,78] In fact, the failure to respond to pulse oximeter changes has been implicated in poor sedation outcomes.[2] The AAP recognizes the value of pulse oximeter monitoring in the following principle of pediatric sedation: **All patients sedated for a procedure must be continuously monitored with a pulse oximeter.**[3]

Capnography monitors exhaled carbon dioxide ($ETCO_2$), creating a waveform that can be used to detect changes in ventilatory status.[60,79,80] Capnography waveforms can alert the practitioner to potential hypoventilation, respiratory depression, and hypoperfusion.[60,79,80,81]

> The AAP strongly encourages the use of capnography for monitoring sedated pediatric patients.[3]

Some institutions have included bispectral index monitoring (BIS, Aspect Medical Systems, Newton MA) for procedural sedation. The BIS monitor, introduced in the operating room environment in the late 1990s, uses electrodes attached to the patient's head to monitor cerebral electrical activity and provide a number that correlates to the depth of sedation. BIS monitoring in children correlates well with clinically assessed sedation levels in the intensive care unit.[82] Multiple studies have demonstrated that BIS monitoring reduces total drug administration and produces a faster recovery in pediatric patients undergoing general anesthesia.[83,84] However, acceptance of BIS monitoring for outpatient pediatric sedation remains controversial. Incorporation of this technology has not been accepted into general practice.[85] It is important to incorporate pain and sedation scales into the procedural plan of care and not to rely on ancillary monitors alone.

The JCAHO standards require that health care providers are knowledgeable about pain assessment and management. Facilities are expected to develop policies and procedures supporting the appropriate assessment of pain and the proper use of analgesics. Documentation of pain should include a standardized pediatric-appropriate pain scale such as the Wong Faces of Pain rating scale (Fig. 10-8) for children 3 years of age or older.[87] Box 10-9 illustrates a neonatal/infant pain scale (NIPS) used to evaluate preverbal infants.[88]

A standardized sedation scale should be used to evaluate and document the pediatric patient's level of sedation during the procedure.[86,89] The Ramsay sedation score featured in Chapter 2 evaluates the patients' response to stimuli while sedated and may be used for nonverbal or younger patients.[90,91] The Observer's Assessment of Alertness/

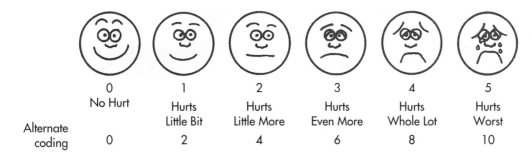

FIGURE 10-8 Wong-Baker FACES Pain Rating Scale. (From Wong DL, Hockenberry-Eaton M, Wilson D, Winkelstein ML, Schwartz P: *Wong's Essentials of Pediatric Nursing,* ed 6, St. Louis, 2001, Mosby, pg 1301.) Copyright Mosby. Reprinted with permission.

BOX 10-9

Neonatal/Infant Pain Scale (NIPS)*

Facial Expression	Pain Assessment
0—Relaxed muscles	Restful face, neutral expression
1—Grimace	Tight facial muscles; furrowed brow, chin, jaw (negative facial expression: nose, mouth, and brow)

Cry	
0—No cry	Quiet, not crying
1—Whimper	Mild moaning, intermittent
2—Vigorous cry	Loud scream; rising, shrill, continuous (*Note:* Silent cry may be scored if infant is intubated as evidenced by obvious mouth and facial movement.)

Breathing Patterns	
0—Relaxed	Usual patterns for this infant
1—Change in breathing	Indrawing, irregular, faster than usual; gagging; breath holding

Arms	
0—Relaxed/ restrained	No muscular rigidity; occasional random movements of arms
1—Flexed/ extended	Tense, straight legs; rigid and/or rapid extension, flexion

Legs	
0—Relaxed/ restrained	No muscular rigidity; occasional random leg movement
1—Flexed/ extended	Tense, straight legs; rigid and/or rapid extension, flexion

State of Arousal	
0—Sleeping/ awake	Quiet, peaceful sleeping or alert random leg movement
1—Fussy	Alert, restless, and thrashing

*Recommended for children younger than 1 year old: a score greater than 3 indicates pain.
Adapted from Lawrence J, et al. The development of a tool to assess neonatal pain. *Neonatal Network.* 1993;12:59-66.

Sedation Scale, also featured in Chapter 2, can be used to evaluate the degree of alertness in patients who are verbal.[91,92] Most sedation scales are relatively easy to use, but they may not detect subtle changes in sedation level.[66]

PEDIATRIC SEDATION TECHNIQUES

The ideal procedural sedation regimen consists of the following inherent characteristics[66]:
◆ Rapid onset
◆ Rapid recovery
◆ Minimal adverse effects
◆ Rapid metabolism to inactive metabolites to prevent cumulative effect

According to the 1992 AAP Committee on Drugs, "Guidelines for Monitoring and Management of Pediatric Patients During and After Sedation for Diagnostic and Therapeutic Procedures," the goals of sedation in the pediatric patient include[3]:
◆ To guard the patient's safety and welfare
◆ To minimize physical discomfort or pain
◆ To minimize negative psychological responses to treatment by providing analgesia and to maximize the potential for amnesia
◆ To control behavior
◆ To return the patient to a state in which safe discharge, as determined by recognized criteria, is possible

The pharmacology of pediatric sedation is complex, and medication choices have increased dramatically. Before selecting a drug regimen, the healthcare provider needs to establish the goals for procedural sedation (analgesia, sedation, amnesia) or simply cooperation. Because no single drug can meet all of these goals, sedatives and analgesics are often combined to achieve the desired effect. Drug combinations utilize synergistic sedative effects and reduce the total amount of each drug administered. Multiple pediatric sedation regimens (Table 10-7) have been attempted, none of which is free from adverse effects.

> Synergism in the diverse pediatric population is not completely predictable and can increase the risk of respiratory depression, hypoxemia, and prolonged sedation.[2,93]

There is no relationship between any one drug class and adverse outcome; however the combination of drugs can be dangerous. **The administration of three or more sedating medications is frequently associated with adverse pediatric outcomes.**[2,93]

Care must be taken to "sedate and wait" in the pediatric patient population. Drugs must be administered in small, incremental doses with adequate time allowed in between doses to assess full pharmacologic effect. **TITRATION IS ESSENTIAL.**

Nonparenteral drugs must be allowed adequate time for full absorption to evaluate complete sedative effect.[93] Repeated assessment of level of consciousness should be recorded while titrating medications to reduce the risk of oversedation.[89]

PHARMACOLOGY

Table 10-8 presents commonly used pediatric sedation routes of administration, dosage guidelines, and pharmacologic reversal agents.

Sedatives/Hypnotics

Chloral hydrate (Somnos) is a commonly administered nonbarbiturate hypnotic in children. Pediatric advantages include ease of oral and rectal administration. Once

Text continued on p. 231

TABLE 10-7

Pediatric Sedation Regimens

DRUG(S)	DOSAGE GUIDELINES	SUCCESS RATE	ADVANTAGES	ADVERSE EVENTS	COMMENTS
Chloral hydrate[1]	PO 78 mg/kg total given in two increments	98%	High success rate No IV needed	>28% Excessive sleeping 68% "unsteady" 15% vomiting	Only 54% resumed normal activity after 4 hr
Pentobarbital[2]	IV 3.75 ± 1.10 mg/kg	97%	High success rate No patients desaturated below 90%		Sedation duration averaged 86 min
Midazolam[3]	IV 0.2 ± 0.03 mg/kg	19% Midazolam alone; 61% with addition of pentobarbital	No patients desaturated below 90%	Poor success rate requiring supplemental pentobarbital	
Thiopental[4]	PR 50 mg/kg <6 mo 35 mg/kg 6-12 mo 25 mg/kg >12 mo	96%	High success rate Rapid onset and offset of action	10% brief desaturation to SaO$_2$ 88% 0.04% prolonged sedation	Average onset time 15 min Mean duration of deep sedation 60.8 ± 27 min
Midazolam + fentanyl[5]	IV midazolam 0.17 ± .08 mg/kg plus IV fentanyl 1.5 ± 0.8 µg/kg	100%	Rapid onset average 11 ± 6.2 min	11% alteration in respiratory status 8.3% oxygen desaturation <90% 0.6% received naloxone 1.2% vomited	Mean discharge time 92 ± 36 min None required assisted ventilation or intubation
Ketamine + midazolam[6]	IV ketamine 1.5 mg/kg plus IV midazolam 0.05 mg/kg plus IV atropine 0.01 mg/kg	More effective than meperidine + midazolam described below	19-min average to therapeutic level 0% reduced respiratory rate	17.7% desaturation 16.6% hypotension	39-min average recovery All patients amnestic for procedure
Meperidine + midazolam[6]	IV meperidine 2 mg/kg plus IV midazolam 0.1 mg/kg	Less effective than ketamine + midazolam described above	24-min average to therapeutic level	82.4% oxygen desaturation 55.6% hypotension 38.9% reduced respiratory rate	74-min average recovery All patients amnestic for procedure
Methohexital[7]	PR 30 mg/kg	96% effective with single rectal dose	IV not required	4% oxygen desaturation 0.3% requiring aggressive airway management	Apnea did not occur in any patients

Continued

TABLE 10-7

Pediatric Sedation Regimens—cont'd

DRUG(S)	DOSAGE GUIDELINES	SUCCESS RATE	ADVANTAGES	ADVERSE EVENTS	COMMENTS
Ketamine[8]	PO 6 mg/kg	More effective than meperidine + promethazine	No oxygen desaturations below 95% Shorter onset and recovery than meperidine and promethazine	Vomiting significantly higher than meperidine + promethazine	Local anesthetic placement better tolerated than meperidine + promethazine Subjective quality of sedation higher
Meperidine + promethazine[8]	IV meperidine 2 mg/kg plus IV promethazine 0.5 mg/kg	Less effective than ketamine PO 6 mg/kg	No oxygen desaturations below 95% Less vomiting than ketamine PO 6 mg/kg	Longer onset than ketamine PO 6 mg/kg	Subjective quality of sedation lower than with ketamine PO 6 mg/kg
Ketamine[9]	IV ketamine 1 mg/kg plus IV glycopyrrolate 0.005 mg/kg	Sedation equally as effective as ketamine and midazolam	Less oxygen desaturations than ketamine plus midazolam technique	1.6% oxygen desaturations 18.7% vomiting 7.1% significant delirium in emergency department 5.7% overall agitation 26.7% emergence delirium at home	Parental and physician satisfaction high
Ketamine + midazolam[9]	IV ketamine 1 mg/kg plus IV glycopyrrolate 0.005 mg/kg plus IV midazolam 0.1 mg/kg	Sedation equally as effective as IV ketamine 1 mg/kg	Less vomiting than IV ketamine 1 mg/kg	7.3% oxygen desaturation 9.6% vomiting 5.7% overall agitation 6.2% significant delirium in emergency department	Parental physician and satisfaction high

Data from:
[1]Kao SC, Adamson SD, Tatman LH, Berbaum KS. A survey of post-discharge side effects of conscious sedation using chloral hydrate in pediatric CT and MR imaging. *Pediatr Radiol.* 1999;29(4):287-290.
[2]Moro-Sutherland DM, Algren JT, Louis PT, et al. Comparison of intravenous midazolam with pentobarbital for sedation for head computed tomography imaging. *Acad Emerg Med.* 2000;7(12):1370-1375.
[3]Alp H, Orbak Z, Guler I, Altinkaynak S. Efficacy and safety of rectal thiopental, intramuscular cocktail and rectal midazolam for sedation in children undergoing neuroimaging. *Pediatr Int.* 2002;44(6):628-634.
[4]Alp H, Guler I, Orbak Z, et al. Efficacy and safety of rectal thiopental: Sedation for children undergoing computed tomography and magnetic resonance imaging. *Pediatr Int.* 1999;41(5):538-541.
[5]Graff KJ, Kennedy RM, Jaffe DM. Conscious sedation for pediatric orthopaedic emergencies. *Pediatr Emerg Care.* 1996;12(1):31-35.
[6]Marx CM, Stein J, Tyler MK, et al. Ketamine-midazolam versus meperidine-midazolam for painful procedures in pediatric oncology patients. *J Clin Oncol.* 1997;15(1):94-102.
[7]Audenaert SM, Montgomery CL, Thompson DE, Sutherland J. A prospective study of rectal methohexital: Efficacy and side effects in 648 cases. *Anesth Analg.* 1995;81(5):957-961.
[8]Alfonzo-Echeverri EC, Berg JH, Wild TW, Glass NL. Oral ketamine for pediatric outpatient dental surgery sedation. *Pediatr Dent.* 1993;15(3):182-185.
[9]Wathen JE, Roback MG, Mackenzie T, Bothner JP. Does midazolam alter the clinical effects of intravenous ketamine sedation in children? A double-blind, randomized, controlled, emergency department trial. *Ann Emerg Med.* 2000;36:579-588.

TABLE 10-8

Pediatric Sedation Techniques

DRUG	ROUTE	ONSET	DURATION	USUAL PEDIATRIC DOSE	COMMENTS
Sedatives/Hypnotics					
Chloral hydrate	PO	40-60 min	4-6 hr	25-75 mg/kg (max of 100 mg/kg or 2 g;	
	PR	40-60 min	4-8 hr	max in neonates of 50 mg/kg	
Pentobarbital	PO/PR	15-60 min	PO/PR/IM: 1-4 hr	PO/PR/IM: 2-6 mg/kg	
	IM	10-15 min		IV: 1-6 mg/kg/dose (max 100	
	IV (slow; no > 50 mg/min)	1-2 min	IV (variable duration)	mg/total dose any route; max IV incremental dose 2 mg/kg)	
Ketamine	IV (slow)	1-2 min	20-30 min	0.5-1 mg/kg	
	IM	2-5 min		2-4 mg/kg	
Benzodiazepines					
Midazolam	IV (slow)	3-5 min	1-2 hr	0.05 mg/kg (max total dose of 0.15 mg/kg or 4 mg; max single dose of 2 mg)	
	IM	5-10 min	1-6 hr	0.05-0.15 mg/kg (max 5 mg)	
	PO	30 min	45 min	0.5 mg/kg (max 15 mg)	
	IN	10-15 min	40 min	0.2 mg/kg (max 5 mg)	
	SL	10-15 min	40 min	0.2 mg/kg (max 5 mg)	
Diazepam	IV'	2-5 min	2-4 hr	0.1-0.3 mg/kg as a single dose (max single dose: 10 mg)	
	PO	30-60 min	2-8 hr		
	IV	3-7 min	6-8 hr	0.025-0.05 mg/kg as a single dose (max 2 mg)	
Lorazepam	IM	20-30 min	6-8 hr		
	PO	20-30 min	6-8 hr	Dilute IV dose; inject <0.05 mg/kg over 2-5 min	
Opioids*					
Fentanyl	IV (slow)	1-5 min	1-2 hr	0.5-1 μg/kg (additional doses prn up to 2 μg/kg or max 100 μg)	
Morphine	IV (slow)	1-2 min	3-4 hr	0.05-0.1 mg/kg, may repeat at 15-min intervals (max 0.2 mg/kg or 10 mg)	
Meperidine	IM	20-60 min	4-5 hr	0.5-1 mg/kg, may repeat at 15-min intervals (max 2 mg/kg or 100 mg)	
	IV (slow)	1-3 min	2-3 hr		
	IM	15-30 min	3-4 hr		

Continued

TABLE 10-8

Pediatric Sedation Techniques—cont'd

DRUG	ROUTE	ONSET	DURATION	USUAL PEDIATRIC DOSE	COMMENTS
Reversal Agents[†]					
Naloxone	IV (slow)	1-2 min	30-60 min	0.005-0.01 mg/kg titrated in incremental doses until desired response is achieved (max 0.1 mg per incremental dose)	Can cause increased blood pressure, increased heart rate, anxiety, ventricular arrhythmias, and pulmonary edema
Flumazenil	IM	2-5 min			Extreme caution in patients taking medications that reduce seizure threshold (e.g., tricyclic antidepressants, theophylline)
	IV (slow) over 15 sec	1-2 min	60 min	0.01 mg/kg IV (max 0.2 mg). Observe child for 45 seconds. If no response, repeat above dose to a max of 1 mg. Re-sedation: Repeat above dose (max dose 3 mg/hr)	May precipitate seizures in patients taking long-term benzodiazepines (e.g., as part of anticonvulsant therapy)

PO, oral; *PR,* rectal; *IM,* intramuscular; *IV,* intravenous; *IN,* intranasal; *SL,* sublingual; *prn,* as needed.

*All sedatives, when used in combination, have significant synergy in producing desired effects (e.g., sedation, hypnosis) as well as adverse effects (e.g., respiratory and cardiac depression). Combinations of narcotics and benzodiazepines are particularly synergistic in producing respiratory depression. Therefore, it may be prudent to reduce doses by 25% when this combination is used.

†Duration of reversal agent may be shorter than the sedative agent; monitor patient and repeat dose as needed. Larger doses of benzodiazepines with long elimination half-lives (e.g., diazepam and lorazepam) necessitate a longer monitoring period after the administration of flumazenil. Use of reversal agents should not be considered a substitute for vigilant airway assessment and management in, for example, the presence of respiratory depression and apnea.

absorbed, the active metabolite trichloroethanol (TCE) depresses the central nervous system.[94,95] The TCE onset of action can occur as soon as 20 minutes, with a duration of action of 4 to 8 hours. However, the half-life is significantly longer, up to 11 hours in children and 48 to 66 hours in neonates.[93,95] A higher dose does not result in earlier onset of sedation or an increase in success rate.[96] Adverse events including respiratory depression and death after patient discharge have been associated with the long half-life of chloral hydrate.[93] Drugs with long half-lives are implicated in numerous cases of serious neurologic outcome and death at home or in the car after pediatric sedation therapy. [93,97] Rigorous recovery and discharge criteria must be met and parents should be educated regarding the potential for prolonged residual sedative effects.

Dissociative Anesthetics

Ketamine is a general anesthetic that induces a cataleptic state with potent analgesic properties. Ketamine is associated with hallucinations, delirium, and nightmares.[95,98] Additional side effects include increased salivary secretions, depressed airway reflexes, and laryngospasm. Ketamine can be administered intramuscularly, orally, and rectally for patients without an intravenous line.[95,98] Healthcare providers administering ketamine must be prepared to rescue the patient from deep sedation or general anesthesia and manage significant airway compromise, which may include laryngospasm.[66,94]

Barbiturates

Methohexital (Brevital) is an ultra-short acting barbiturate used to induce general anesthesia.[95,98] Rectal administration has been used to induce anesthesia in young patients. The use of a pulse oximeter should be used when methohexital is administered rectally, owing to associated upper airway obstruction.[99] **Healthcare providers administering methohexital must be prepared to rescue the patient from any level of sedation, including general anesthesia, and manage significant airway compromise, which may include laryngospasm.[94,95,99]**

Pentobarbital (Nembutal) is a short-acting barbiturate with hypnotic and sedative properties that can be given orally or rectally.[94,95,98] The ease of administration is beneficial to pediatric use.[100]

Alkylphenols (Hypnotic)

Propofol (Diprivan) is a nonbarbiturate general anesthetic associated with anxiolysis and antiemetic properties.[94,95,98] Apnea occurs within 30 seconds of a bolus dose. Long-term pediatric ICU sedation with propofol has been associated with core acidosis and cardiac failure. Propofol is not recommended in children younger than 3 years of age.[95] Healthcare providers administering propofol must be prepared to rescue the patient from any level of sedation, including general anesthesia, and manage significant airway compromise.[94,95,98]

Benzodiazepines

Midazolam (Versed) is a commonly used anxiolytic that provides both sedation and anterograde amnesia.[95,98] Intranasal midazolam is a convenient method for sedating the pediatric patient without an intravenous line. Undiluted intravenous injection (5 mg/mL) provides an adequate concentration for small volume nasal administration.[95] Although irritating to the nasal mucosa, intranasal midazolam may provide a period of anxiolysis to permit intravenous insertion.[37] Intravenous administration induces onset of sedation in only 1 to 5 minutes. The half-life of midazolam in neonates may be prolonged up to 12 hours.[93]

Midazolam administration produces paradoxical reactions in 1% to 2% of all pediatric patients.[101] This is manifested as inconsolable crying, combativeness, disorientation, dysphoria, tachycardia, agitation, and restlessness. Adverse reactions generally dissipate with the administration of the benzodiazepine reversal agent flumazenil.[101]

Opioids

Opioids should be reserved for painful procedures (angiography, cardiac catheterization, skin lacerations) and should not be administered merely to sedate the child for diagnostic procedures.[102]

Morphine is the prototype opioid to which all other opioids are compared. Morphine is more effective for dull aching pain than intermittent sharp pain, which is better alleviated with fentanyl.[103] Morphine is metabolized into active (morphine-6-glucuronide) and inactive (morphine-3-glucuronide) components. Morphine use in infants younger than 3 months of age has been associated with respiratory depression; therefore, doses should be reduced in this age group.[93]

Fentanyl (Sublimaze) is a synthetic opioid 75 to 125 times more potent than morphine.[103] Fentanyl's high lipid solubility creates a rapid onset and short duration of action. Multiple doses or long infusions extend the duration of action. Fentanyl is metabolized into the less pharmacologically active component norfentanyl, which is renally excreted. Bradycardia is more pronounced with fentanyl when compared with morphine. Fentanyl (administered intravenously or transmucosally) has been associated with chest wall and glottic rigidity in pediatric patients, resulting in death or significant neurologic injury.[93,103-104] Fentanyl lollipops delivering transmucosal analgesia in pediatrics are effective pain relievers but are associated with a 50% incidence of vomiting postoperatively.[104,105]

Meperidine (Demerol) is a synthetic opioid that is structurally similar to atropine.[103] Meperidine is one tenth as potent as morphine. The pharmacodynamics of meperidine in children are well defined.[103] Nausea and vomiting are common side effects associated with meperidine use. Meperidine is metabolized into normeperidine, a central nervous system stimulant with a relatively long half-life. Normeperidine has been associated with myoclonus seizures in patients receiving large doses and in patients with impaired renal function.

DPT cocktail is a combination of meperidine (Demerol), promethazine (Phenergan), and chlorpromazine (Thorazine).[102] This combination has been used for more than 20 years as a sedative and analgesic cocktail for pediatric patients. The AAP evaluated the use of this pharmacologic combination in pediatrics and noted that all scientific studies were performed in the adult patient population. The use of DPT cocktail in children has been associated with adverse events such as extended sedation, respiratory depression, and even death.[102] The AAP has published the following recommendations regarding Demerol + Phenergan + Thorazine in pediatric sedation[102]:

1. The risks and potential benefits of DPT cocktail for each patient must be evaluated carefully before it is used. Alternative sedatives/analgesics should be considered.
2. If DPT cocktail is used, all of the guidelines pertaining to deep sedation for monitoring and management of pediatric patients during and after sedation for diagnostic and therapeutic procedures should be followed.
3. Careful monitoring of blood pressure and ventilation should accompany the standard monitoring of oxygen saturation.
4. Additional caution should be exercised when using a lytic cocktail in children with seizure disorders, other central nervous system abnormalities, or congenital heart disease consisting of tetralogy of Fallot–type anatomy or of left ventricular outflow obstruction, such as any type of aortic stenosis.
5. Criteria for discharge from the sedation-monitoring area must be established with full recognition of the "trance-like" state produced by this neuroleptanalgesic technique.

Inhalational Agents

Nitrous oxide is an inhalation agent used as an adjunct to general anesthesia during surgical procedures. Additionally, it is often used in dental and oral-maxillary offices for sedation during invasive dental procedures and emergency departments for repair of lacerations and other painful procedures.[106] Nitrous oxide is delivered via a demand valve mask, which can only be used on children 5 years of age and older. It can be a valuable sedation agent that facilitates painful dental and other procedures.[107,108] A unique side effect profile includes diffusion hypoxia, nausea and vomiting, and sleep-apnea syndrome.[107] Nitrous oxide combined with any other class of sedative medications is frequently associated with adverse outcomes.[109-111] Practitioners administering nitrous oxide sedation should receive competency training beyond the scope of this chapter regarding its safe and proper use.

Local Anesthetics

Even when faced with painful procedures, children may prefer the anxiolysis and amnesia produced by a benzodiazepine to the narcosis produced by a narcotic. When this technique is chosen, the appropriate use of local anesthetics is mandatory.[102] Local anesthesia use is not well established or evaluated in pediatric patients. The dose required to produce a toxic effect has been evaluated rather than the effective dose. Children are equally susceptible to local anesthetic toxicity as adults. Maximum doses of local anesthetics for the pediatric patient are listed in Table 10-9.

FAILED SEDATION

Sedation is inadequate in up to 20% of pediatric patients receiving sedation therapy.[112] In this situation, medications are continually titrated with little or no sedative effect. Midazolam has been associated with paradoxical behavior in up to 2% of pediatric patients.[101] Often the child of failed sedation techniques is restless, combative, and uncooperative. The procedure may need to be rescheduled or referred to the department of anesthesia for general anesthesia administration. Regardless of the level of agitation or of inadequate sedation, the pediatric patient remains at risk for the side effects associated with sedative agents.[93,113-114] Chloral hydrate administered as the sole sedative in recommended doses has been associated with failed sedation in the hospital, only to become difficult to arouse later at

---

TABLE 10-9

Pediatric Local Anesthetic Dosage Guidelines

LOCAL ANESTHETIC	MAXIMUM DOSE (mg/kg)		APPROXIMATE DURATION (min)
	WITHOUT EPINEPHRINE	WITH EPINEPHRINE	
Procaine	7.0	10.0	60-90
2-Chloroprocaine	15.0	20.0	30-60
Tetracaine	1.0	1.5	180-600
Lidocaine	5.0	7.0	90-200
Mepivacaine	5.0	7.0	120-240
Bupivacaine	2.0	3.0	180-600
Ropivacaine	3.0		180-600

From Coté CJ, Strafford MA. *The Principles of Pediatric Sedation.* Boston: Tufts University School of Medicine; 1998.

home.[2,93,96,113] Any patient "failing sedation" must be monitored closely for signs of delayed sedation before discharge home.

RECOVERY

Very rigorous and specific recovery criteria must be met before pediatric patient discharge. The AAP has published the following recommendations regarding discharge criteria in pediatric sedation patients[3]:

◆ Cardiovascular function and airway patency should be satisfactory and stable.
◆ The patient should be easily arousable with intact protective reflexes.
◆ The patient should be able to talk if age and intellect appropriate.
◆ The patient should be able to sit up if age and motor skills allow.
◆ The postsedation level of consciousness should be close to the normal presedation level of consciousness in very young or handicapped patients who do not normally perform the functions addressed in other discharge criteria.
◆ The patient's hydration status should be adequate.

Studies examining adverse events in pediatrics show inadequate recovery time and discharge criteria can increase adverse events in children after receiving sedation.[2,93] All reported deaths and permanent neurologic injuries at home or in the car after a procedure were due to drugs with long half-lives such as chloral hydrate and pentobarbital. Injury has occurred in infants while riding home in car seats after procedural sedation. One hypothesis is the sleeping child's head falls forward, resulting in extreme flexion of the neck, leading to airway obstruction.[93] Oxygen desaturation has been reproduced in healthy infants while riding in car seats who have not received sedation.[114] The infant should be awake enough to spontaneously reposition the head in the presence of obstruction, and the parents should be educated regarding the risk of airway obstruction. Sufficient time (up to 2 hours) should elapse after the last administration of reversal agents (naloxone, flumazenil) to ensure that children do not become re-sedated after reversal effects have abated.[95,98]

Patients should not be discharged if they are actively vomiting, bleeding, experiencing uncontrolled pain, or excessively dizzy. The use of a sedation scoring system to compare the postsedation status with the presedation status is useful. Both the AAP and JCAHO emphasize patient pain control as an integral part of pediatric health care. The AAP states: **Parents of infants and children undergoing operative procedures on an outpatient basis must receive instructions on pain management at home.**[3] Studies reveal pediatric pain is often inadequately managed after ambulatory surgery.[115] Parents should be given written instructions regarding post-procedure diet, medications, activities, and a 24-hour phone number in case of emergency.[3] Instructions regarding signs of infection and dressing care, if applicable, should also be included. If patients are slow to returnto baseline or experience a slower-than-expected recovery, admission to an overnight medical facility may be necessary.[66]

SUMMARY

Pediatric sedation is challenging from a procedural and pharmacologic perspective. The anatomic and physiologic variations associated with pediatric patient care predisposes infants and children to additional morbidity risk. It is imperative that all sedation practitioners are accustomed to the idiosyncracies associated with caring for this specific patient population. Sedation providers must be familiar with the sedative, analgesic, and hypnotic medications and dosages utilized to achieve a state of sedation. Additionally, all healthcare providers must be clinically competent to handle all emergencies that may arise in the pediatric sedation setting.

LEARNER SELF-ASSESSMENT

In order to achieve maximal educational benefit from this chapter, please complete the Learner Self-Assessment' below. This self-assessment tool provides the learner with the ability to identify areas requiring additional review. Reference material for each question is provided in Appendix F.

1. Healthcare practitioner considerations associated with **AAP Guidelines for Monitoring and Management of Pediatric Patients During and After Sedation for Diagnostic and Therapeutic Procedures (American Academy of Pediatrics [AAP] Committee on Drugs [COD]), related to pediatric sedation care** include:

2. The **goals** of pediatric procedural sedation include:

3. The **developmental subsets** of pediatrics include:

4. The **role of the parent** for children receiving sedation includes:

5. The **physiologic response to pain** in the infant includes:

6. **Anatomic and physiologic alterations** in the pediatric patient that may impact on the sedation plan and procedural care include:

7. **Distinct features of the pediatric airway** include:

8. **Airway maneuvers that may improve ventilation** in a pediatric sedation patient include:

9. **The clinical effects associated with hypothermia** in the pediatric patient include:

10. **NPO guidelines** for the sedation patient include:

11. **Pediatric medical problems that may impact on the sedation plan of care** include:

12. **Monitoring methods for the pediatric sedation patient** include:

13. **Sedation scales** used for pediatric sedation include:

14. **Pharmacologic considerations associated with sedative/analgesic agents** for the pediatric patient include:

15. **Care of the "failed sedation" pediatric patient** includes:

16. **Discharge criteria** for the pediatric patient include:

POST-TEST QUESTIONS

Please note: If you are applying for CE credit, you must contact Specialty Health Education, Inc. @ 800-694-8041 for a CE Application Packet.

1. Which of the following pediatric patient populations often require deep levels of sedation for invasive procedures? _____
   A. Healthy teenagers
   B. Children younger than 6 years of age
   C. Children with developmental delays
   D. Both B and C

2. Adverse pediatric procedural sedation events that occur in the _____ setting are more likely to be fatal.
   A. Hospital
   B. Outpatient clinic attached to a hospital
   C. Doctor or dentist office
   D. Intensive care unit

3. Which of the following patient populations has been shown to be at increased risk for adverse anesthesia outcomes? _____
   A. Healthy teenagers
   B. Neonates
   C. Pediatric patients older than 2 years of age
   D. Both B and C

4. The term *neonate* is defined as which of the following: _____
   A. An infant 30 days old or younger
   B. An infant 1 month to 12 months old
   C. An infant younger than 12 months old
   D. Exclusively an infant 1 day old or younger

5. Fears of abandonment and separation anxiety are seen in all phases of pediatric development to some degree. This particular phenomenon, however, is most associated with which of the following age groups: _____
   A. Birth to 1 year of age
   B. One to 3 years of age
   C. Three to 5 years of age
   D. Six to 12 years of age

6. Parental presence during the induction of anesthesia has been shown to be particularly beneficial in which of the following situations: _____
   A. If both parent and child are relatively calm
   B. If the child is older than age 4 years
   C. If the child is younger than age 4 years
   D. Both A and C

7. The infant central nervous system is underdeveloped relative to older children and adults until _____.
   A. Six months of age
   B. One year of age

C. One month of age
D. 18 months to 2 years of age

8. Newborns and infants experience pain similarly to adults characterized by _____.
   A. Tachycardia
   B. Elevated blood pressure
   C. Increased intracranial pressure
   D. All of the above

9. Infants born with hydrocephalus can have _____ due to _____.
   A. Difficult airways, large occiputs
   B. Small occiputs, increased cerebral pressure
   C. Difficult airways, small occiputs
   D. Small occiputs, difficult airways

10. _____ is a leading cause of newborn mortality and morbidity.
    A. Hyperglycemia
    B. Cerebral intraventricular hemorrhage
    C. Hypervolemia
    D. Hypotonia

11. The cerebral metabolic rate for oxygen is higher in children (5 mL/min) than adults (3 to 4 mL/min). Pediatric oxygen metabolic rates are further increased by _____:
    A. Seizures
    B. Fever
    C. Barbiturates
    D. A and B

12. _____ is the primary physiologic factor responsible for changes in pediatric cardiac output:
    A. Blood pressure
    B. Heart rate
    C. Stroke volume
    D. Increased cardiac compliance

13. _____ is the primary cause of bradycardia in infants:
    A. Hypoglycemia
    B. Hypovolemia
    C. Hypoxia
    D. Hyponatremia

14. The parasympathetic nervous system is _____ active in pediatric patients than in adults.
    A. More
    B. Less

C. Equally

D. Similarly

15. Functional closure of the foramen ovale typically occurs _____.

A. Shortly after birth

B. At 4 to 6 weeks of age

C. By 1 year of age

D. By 6 months of age

16. Techniques to avoid intravenous administration of air include _____:

A. Just prior to the child entering the room, inspect the tubing.

B. Before injecting a drug from a syringe intravenously, eject a small amount of drug from the syringe to clear air from the syringe and needle hub.

C. Never leave central lines open to air.

D. All of the above

17. The infants upper airway is characterized by _____.

A. A large tongue, short neck, and narrow nasal passages

B. A small tongue, short neck, and large nasal passages

C. A small occiput, short neck, and narrow nasal passages

D. A large mandible, short neck, and narrow nasal passages

18. Hard plastic oral airways are most appropriate _____.

A. In mildly sedated toddlers

B. In deeply sedated children with upper airway obstruction

C. In wide awake infants

D. In cooperative adolescents

19. Soft nasal airways _____.

A. Are most appropriate in mild or moderately sedated patients

B. Ease ventilation in infants by decreasing resistance of breathing

C. Generally cause less gagging and choking in moderately sedated patients than hard oral airways

D. All of the above

20. The _____ is the narrowest part of the infant lower airway.

A. Vocal cords

B. Cricoid cartilage below the vocal cords

C. Epiglottis

D. Cricoid cartilage above the vocal cords

21. Straight laryngoscope blades are generally used in pediatric patients _____.

A. To manually lift the stiff epiglottis to expose the vocal cords

B. To hyperextend the neck

C. To place the neck in extreme flexion

D. All of the above

22. The pediatric tracheal lumen is _____.

A. Hourglass shaped

B. Shaped like a cylinder

C. Cone shaped

D. Shaped like a box

23. Infants who were premature and required prolonged mechanical ventilation during the neonatal period may be at risk for _____.

A. Supraglottic stenosis

B. Subglottic stenosis

C. The need for a smaller than age-appropriate endotracheal tube

D. B and C

24. The infant breathing pattern of pauses greater than 15 to 20 seconds associated with bradycardia, cyanosis, and pallor is termed _____.

A. Central apnea of infancy

B. Sleep apnea of childhood

C. Irregular apnea

D. Infantile obstructive sleep apnea

25. The age group having the greatest risk for apnea and bradycardia in the first 12 hours after procedural sedation includes _____:

A. Infants (1 to 12 months of age)

B. Infants younger than 45 weeks post conception

C. Toddlers 2 to 5 years old

D. Term infants 3 to 6 months of age

26. Infants have a limited thermoregulatory range due to _____.

A. Small body size

B. Increased surface-to-volume ratio

C. Increased thermal conductance

D. All of the above

27. The amount of infant total body water is _____.

A. 90%

B. 75%

C. 55%

D. 25%

28. The underdeveloped premature and newborn kidney loses which electrolyte via urine? _____

A. Glucose

B. Sodium

C. Magnesium

D. Dextrose

29. Normal blood glucose concentration in full term infants is _____.
    A. 50-90 mg/dL
    B. 100-150 mg/dL
    C. 30-45 mg/dL
    D. 90-120 mg/dL

30. Factors contributing to EMLA use for topical anesthesia and methemoglobin toxicity include _____.
    A. Total surface area in contact with EMLA
    B. The total time EMLA contacts the skin
    C. The total amount of EMLA cream used
    D. All of the above

31. The ASA generally recommends pediatric procedural sedation only be performed by non-anesthesiologists in which of the following patient populations:
    A. ASA III and ASA IV patients only
    B. Any ASA status
    C. ASA I and II only
    D. None of the above

32. Teenage girls should receive which of the following:
    A. A urine pregnancy test
    B. A blood toxicology screen
    C. A blood test to measure hemoglobin
    D. None of the above

33. Most airway disasters have been associated with which of the following:
    A. Failure to use a straight blade for intubation
    B. Failure to anticipate a difficult airway
    C. Failure to use an appropriate-sized mask
    D. Failed sedation

34. Trisomy 21 (Down syndrome) patients have the following characteristics:
    A. Large tongues
    B. Short mandibles
    C. Small oral and nasal passages
    D. All of the above

35. Patients with developmental delay or mental retardation have a _____ response to sedation.
    A. More predictable
    B. Very predictable
    C. Less predictable
    D. Predictable

36. Cerebral palsy is associated with _____.
    A. Gastroesophageal reflux
    B. Seizures
    C. Variable levels of intellect
    D. All of the above

37. Children have on average _____ colds or upper respiratory infections a year.
    A. 1-2
    B. 2-4
    C. 10-12
    D. 3-8

38. The pediatric environment, as defined by the American Academy of Pediatrics, includes _____.
    A. Pediatric-appropriate equipment
    B. Pediatric-appropriate drugs
    C. Personnel comfortable with and knowledgeable about children
    D. All of the above

39. Which of the following is frequently associated with adverse pediatric sedation outcomes: _____
    A. The administration of a single drug with a short to medium half-life
    B. Narcotics
    C. Benzodiazepines
    D. The administration of three or more sedating medications

40. Chloral hydrate has a _____ half life, up to _____ hours in neonates (infants 1 month of age or younger).
    A. Short, 3
    B. Long, 48-66
    C. Quick, 2
    D. Moderate, 5

REFERENCES

1. American Academy of Pediatrics. Guidelines for monitoring and management of pediatric patients during and after sedation for diagnostic and therapeutic procedures (addendum). *Pediatrics.* 2002;110:836-838.

2. Coté CJ, Notterman DA, Karl HW, et al. Adverse sedation events in pediatrics: A critical incident analysis of contributing factors. *Pediatrics.* 2000;105:805-814.

3. American Academy of Pediatrics. Guidelines for monitoring and management of pediatric patients during and after sedation for diagnostic and therapeutic procedures (RE9252). *Pediatrics.* 1992;89:1110-1115.

4. Rackow H, Salanitre E. Modern concepts in pediatric anesthesiology. *Anesthesiology.* 1969;30:208-234.

5. Tiret L, Nivoche Y, Hatton F, et al. Complications related to anaesthesia in infants and children. *Br J Anaesthesiol.* 1988; 61:263-269.

6. Olsson GL, Hallen B. Cardiac arrest during anesthesia: A computerized study. *Acta Anaesthesiol Scand.* 1988;32:653-664.

7. Campling EA, Devlin HB, Lunn JN. *The Report of the National Confidential Enquiry into Perioperative Deaths (NCEPOD) 1989.* London, UK: The Royal College of Surgeons of England; 1990.

8. Cohen MM, Cameron CB, Duncan PG. Pediatric anesthesia morbidity and mortality in the perioperative period. *Anesth Analg.* 1990;70:160-167.

9. Morray JP, Geiduschek JM, Caplan RA, et al. A comparison of pediatric and adult anesthesia closed malpractice claims. *Anesthesiology.* 1993;78:461-467.

10. Holzman RS. Morbidity and mortality in pediatric anesthesia. *Pediatr Clin North Am.* 1994;41:239-256.

11. Geiduschek JM. Registry offers insight on preventing cardiac arrests in children. *Newslett Am Soc Anesthesiologists.* 1998;62:6.

12. American Academy of Pediatrics. Guidelines for the pediatric perioperative anesthesia environment (RE9820). *Pediatrics.* 1999;103:512-515.

13. Steward DJ, Lerman J. *Manual of Pediatric Anesthesia.* Philadelphia: Churchill Livingstone; 2001:3-5.

14. Kost M. *Manual of Conscious Sedation.* Philadelphia: WB Saunders; 1998.

15. Zeev N, Mayes L, Caraminco L, et al. Parental presence during induction of anesthesia: A randomized controlled trial. *Anesthesiology.* 1996;84:1060-1067.

16. Hamid RK, Newfield P. Pediatric neuroanesthesia. In *Handbook of Neuroanesthesia.* Philadelphia: Lippincott Williams & Wilkins; 1994:270-284.

17. Fitzgerald M. Development of pain pathways and mechanisms. In Anand KJS, McGrath PJ (eds). *Pain in Neonates.* Amsterdam: Elsevier; 1993:19-37.

18. Fazzi E, Farinotti L, Scelsa B, et al. Response to pain in a group of healthy term newborns: Behavioral and physiological aspects. *Funct Neurol.* 1996;11:35-43.

19. Krane EJ, Domino K. Anesthesia for neurosurgery. In Motoyama EK, Davis PJ (eds). *Smith's Anesthesia for Infants and Children.* 6th ed. St. Louis: Mosby; 1996:541-570.

20. Steward DJ, Lerman J. *Manual of Pediatric Anesthesia.* Philadelphia: Churchill Livingstone; 2001:12-14.

21. Taddio A, Katz J, Ilersich AL, Koren G. Effect of neonatal circumcision on pain response during subsequent routine vaccination. *Lancet.* 1997;349:599-603.

22. Mattoo TK. Arm cuff in the measurement of blood pressure. *Am J Hypertens* 2002;15(2 Pt 2):67S-68S.

23. Romero T, Covell J, Frieman WF. A comparison of pressure-volume relations of the fetal, newborn, and adult heart. *Am J Physiol.* 1972;222:1285-1290.

24. Lake CL. *Pediatric Cardiac Anesthesia.* 2nd ed. Norwalk, CT: Appleton; 1993:33-42.

25. Motoyama E. Safety and outcome in pediatric anesthesia. In Motoyama EK, Davis PJ (eds). *Smith's Anesthesia for Infants and Children.* 6th ed. St. Louis: Mosby; 1996:897-908.

26. Friedman WF: The intrinsic properties of the developing heart. *Prog Cardiovasc Dis* 1972;15:87-111.

27. Stoelting RK, Dierdorf SK. *Anesthesia and Coexisting Disease.* 3rd ed. Philadelphia: Churchill Livingstone; 1986:581.

28. Levi M, Bharati S. Embryology of the heart and great vessels. In Arcinieges E (ed). *Pediatric Cardiac Surgery.* Chicago: Year Book Medical; 1985:1-12.

29. Hagen PT, Scholtz DG, Edwards WD. Incidence and size of patent foramen ovale during the first 10 decades of life on autopsy study of 965 normal hearts. *Mayo Clin Proc.* 1984;59:17-20.

30. Berry FA. Neonatal anesthesia. In Barash PG, Cullen BF, Stoelting RK (eds). *Clinical Anesthesia,* 3rd ed. Philadelphia: Lippincott-Raven; 1997:1091-1114.

31. Doctor A. Airway and respiratory control. In Krauss B, Brustowicz RN (eds). *Pediatric Procedural Sedation and Analgesia.* Philadelphia: Lippincott Williams & Wilkins; 1999: 3-10.

32. Steward DJ, Lerman J. *Manual of Pediatric Anesthesia.* Philadelphia: Churchill Livingstone; 2001:15-25.

33. Equipment and Monitoring. In Bell C, Zeev N. Kain (eds). *The Pediatric Anesthesia Handbook.* 2nd ed. St. Louis: Mosby; 1997:35-69.

34. Keidan I, Fine G, Kagawa T, et al. Work of breathing during spontaneous ventilation in anesthetized children: A comparative study among the face mask, laryngeal mask, and endotracheal tube. *Anesth Analg.* 2000;91:1381-1388.

35. Mallampati R. Airway management. In Barash PG, Cullen BF, Stoelting RK (eds). *Clinical Anesthesia.* 3rd ed. Philadelphia: Lippincott-Raven; 1997:573-594.

36. Stoelting RK, Dierdorf SK: *Anesthesia and Coexisting Disease.* 3rd ed. Philadelphia. Churchill Livingstone; 1986:579-580.

37. Gronert BJ, Motoyama EK. Induction of anesthesia and endotracheal intubation. In: Motoyama EK, Davis PJ (eds). *Smith's Anesthesia for Infants and Children.* 6th ed. St. Louis: Mosby; 1996:296.

38. Fine GF, Motoyama EK. The effectiveness of controlled ventilation using cuffed vs. uncuffed endotracheal tubes in infants *Anesthesiology.* 2000;A1251.

39. Motoyama EK. Respiratory physiology in infants and children. In Motoyama EK, Davis PJ (eds). *Smith's Anesthesia for Infants and Children.* 6th ed. St. Louis: Mosby; 1996:22-23.

40. Coté CJ, Zaslavsky A, Downes JJ, et al. Postoperative apnea in former preterm infants after inguinal herniorrhaphy: A combined analysis. *Anesthesiology.* 1995;82:809-822.

41. Wellborn LG, Hannallah RS, Luban NLC, et al. Anemia and postoperative apnea in former preterm infants. *Anesthesiology.* 1991;74:1003-1006.

42. Kurth CD, Spitzer AR, Broennie AM, Downes JJ. Postoperative apnea in preterm infants. *Anesthesiology.* 1987;66:483-488.

43. Vassallo SA. Anesthesia for pediatric surgery. In Huford WE, Bailin MT, Davison JK, et al (eds). *Clinical Anesthesia Procedures of the Massachusetts General Hospital.* 5th ed. Philadelphia: Lippincott-Raven; 1998:499-522.

44. Bissionette B, Davis PJ. Thermal regulation: Physiology and perioperative management in infants and children. In Motoyama EK, Davis PJ (eds). *Smith's Anesthesia for Infants and Children.* 6th ed. St. Louis: Mosby; 1996:139-158.

45. Nilsson K. Maintenance and monitoring of body temperature in infants and children. *Pediatr Anaesth.* 1991;91(1):13-20.

46. Vender JS, Gilbert HC. Monitoring the anesthetized patient. In Barash PG, Cullen BF, Stoelting RK (eds). *Clinical Anesthesia,* 3rd ed. Philadelphia: Lippincott-Raven; 1997: 621-641.

47. BH web site: www.bairhugger.com. Accessed May 13, 2003.

48. Information found on web page: http://www.air-ace.dk/Granulab/Granulab.htm#Hazard%20Report. Accessed May 13, 2003.

49. Henderson K, Womack W. Noninvasive monitoring for procedural sedation. In Krauss B, Brustowicz RN (eds). *Pediatric Procedural Sedation and Analgesia.* Philadelphia: Lippincott Williams & Wilkins; 1999:23.

50. Fluid, electrolytes, and transfusion therapy. In Bell C, Kain ZN (eds). *The Pediatric Anesthesia Handbook.* 2nd ed. St. Louis: Mosby; 1997:71-96.

51. Pang LM. Physiologic considerations. In Krauss B, Brustowicz RN (eds). *Pediatric Procedural Sedation and Analgesia.* Philadelphia: Lippincott Williams & Wilkins; 1999:11-16.

52. Dabbagh S, Demetrius E, Gruskin AB. Regulation of fluids and electrolytes in infants and children. In Motoyama EK, Davis PJ (eds). *Smith's Anesthesia for Infants and Children.* 6th ed. St. Louis: Mosby; 1996:105-137.

53. Joint Commission on Accreditation of Health Care Organizations. Sentinel Event Alert. November 30, 2000: Issue 15.

54. Welborn LG, McGill WA, Hannallah RS, et al. Perioperative blood glucose concentrations in pediatric outpatients. *Anesthesiology.* 1986;65:543.

55. Tommasino C. Fluid management. In *Handbook of Neuroanesthesia.* Philadelphia: Lippincott Williams & Wilkins; 1996:379.

56. Cohen IT, Motoyama EK. Intraoperative and postoperative management. In Motoyama EK, Davis PJ (eds). *Smith's Anesthesia for Infants and Children.* 6th ed. St. Louis: Mosby; 1996:313-345.

57. EMLA cream. In *Physicians Desk Reference (PDR).* Montvale, NJ: Thompson PDR; 2003:599-602.

58. Ehrenstrom-Reiz G, Reiz S, Stockman O. Topical anesthesia with EMLA, a new lidocaine-prilocaine cream and the Cusum technique for detection of minimal application time. *Acta Anaesthesiol Scand.* 1983;27:1983.

59. Bjerring P, Anderson PH, Arendt-Nielsen L. Vascular response of human skin after analgesia with EMLA cream. *Br J Anaesth.* 1989;63:655-660.

60. Steven JM, Cohen DE, Sclabassi RJ. Anesthesia equipment and monitoring. In Motoyama EK, Davis PJ (eds). *Smith's Anesthesia for Infants and Children.* 6th ed. St. Louis: Mosby; 1996:229-279.

61. American Society of Anesthesiologists Physical Classification System. http://asahg.org/clinical/physicalstatus.html. Accessed May 13, 2003.

62. Joint Commission on Accreditation of Healthcare Organizations. Standards and Intents for Sedation and Anesthesia Care. In *Revisions to Anesthesia Care Standards, Comprehensive Accreditation Manual for Hospitals.* Oak Brook Terrace, IL: Joint Commission on Accreditation of Healthcare Organizations; 2001.

63. Wadlington JS, Natale M, Crowley N. Anesthesia for obstetrics and gynecology. In Huford WE, Bailin MT, Davison JK, et al (eds). *Clinical Anesthesia Procedures of the Massachusetts General Hospital.* 5th ed. Philadelphia: Lippincott-Raven; 1998:523-546.

64. Dolovich LR, Addis A, Vaillencourt JM, et al. Benzodiazepine use in pregnancy and major malformations of oral cleft: Meta-analysis of cohort and case-control studies. Comment. *BMJ.* 1999;319:918-919.

65. Langried L. Clinical observations in children after prenatal benzodiazepine exposure. *Dev Pharmacol Ther.* 1990;15(3-4):1.

66. O'Donnell JM, Bragg K, Sell S. Procedural sedation: Safely navigating the twilight zone. *Nursing.* 2003;33(4):36-45.

67. Samsoon GLT, Young JRB. Difficult tracheal intubation: A retrospective study. *Anaesthesia.* 1987;42:487.

68. Fincane BT, Santora AH. Evaluation of the airway prior to intubation. In *Principles of Airway Management.* Philadelphia: FA Davis; 1969.

69. King TA, Adams AP. Failed intubation. *Br J Anaesth.* 1990;65:400.

70. Mallampati SR, Gatt SP, Gugino LD, et al. A clinical sign to predict difficult tracheal intubation: A prospective study. *Can Anaesth Soc J.* 1985;32:429.

71. Maxwell LG, Zuckerberg AL, Motoyamo EK, et al. Systemic disorders in pediatric anesthesia. In Motoyama EK, Davis PJ (eds). *Smith's Anesthesia for Infants and Children.* 6th ed. St. Louis: Mosby; 1996:867-868.

72. Barkett PA. Obstructed airway with wired jaws. *Nursing.* 1991;21(12):33.

73. Zuckerberg AL, Yaster M. Anesthesia for orthopedic surgery. In Motoyama EK, Davis PJ, (eds). *Smith's Anesthesia for Infants and Children.* 6th ed. St. Louis: Mosby; 1996: 623-624.

74. Motoyama EK. Anesthesia for ear, nose, and throat surgery. In Motoyama EK, Davis PJ (eds). *Smith's Anesthesia for Infants and Children.* 6th ed. St. Louis: Mosby; 1996:653-676.

75. Litman RS, Kottra JA, Berkowitz RJ, Ward DS: Upper airway obstruction during midazolam/nitrous oxide sedation in children with enlarged tonsils. *Pediatr Dent.* 1998;20:318-320.

76. American Academy of Pediatrics. Guidelines for the pediatric perioperative anesthesia environment (RE9820). *Pediatrics.* 1999;103:512-515.

77. Cote CJ, Rolf N, Liu LMP, Gousouzian NG. A single-blind study of pulse oximetry and capnography in children. *Anesthesiology.* 1991;74:984.

78. Salyer JW. Neonatal and pediatric pulse oximetry. *Respir Care.* 2003;(4):386-398.

79. Woomer JL, Berkheimer DA. Using capnography to monitor ventilation. In O'Donnell JM, Bragg K, Sell S. Procedural Sedation: Safely Navigating the Twilight Zone. *Nursing.* 2003;33:42-43.

80. Miner JR, Heegaard W, Plummer D. End-tidal carbon dioxide monitoring during procedural sedation. *Acad Emerg Med.* 2002;9:275-280.

81. Hart LS, Berns SD, Houck CS, Boenning DA. The value of end-tidal CO2 monitoring when comparing three methods of conscious sedation for children undergoing painful procedures in the emergency department. *Pediatr Emerg Care.* 1997; 13:189-193.

82. Berkenbosch JW, Fichter CR, Tobias JD. The correlation of the bispectral index monitor with clinical sedation scores during mechanical ventilation in the pediatric intensive care unit. *Anesth Analg.* 2002;94:506-511.

83. Bannister CF, Brosius KK, Sigl JC, et al: The effect of bispectral index monitoring on anesthetic use and recovery in children anesthetized with sevoflurane in nitrous oxide. *Anesth Analg.* 2001;92:877-881.

84. Denman WT, Swanson EL, Rosow D, et al. Pediatric evaluation of bispectral index (BIS) monitor and correlation of BIS with end-tidal sevoflurane concentration in infants and children. *Anesth Analg.* 2000;90:872-877.

85. Religa ZC, Wilson S, Ganzberg SI, Casamassimo PS. Association between bispectral analysis and level of conscious sedation of pediatric dental patients. *Pediatr Dent.* 2002;24:221-226.

86. Joint Commission on Accreditation of Healthcare Organizations. Pain Assessment and Management: An Organizational Approach. Oakbrook Terrace, IL: Joint Commission on Accreditation of Healthcare Organizations; 2000.

87. Originally published by Whaley L, Wong D: *Nursing Care of Infants and Children,* Edison, NJ, 1987: 1070. Research reported in Wong D, Baker C: Pain in children: comparison of assessment scales. *Pediatr Nurs.* 1988;14:9-17.

88. Lawrence J, Alcock D, McGrath P, et al. The development of a tool to assess neonatal pain. *Neonatal Network.* 1993;12:59-66.

89. Hofman G, Nowakowski R, Troshynski TJ, et al. Risk reduction in pediatric procedural sedation by application of an American Academy of Pediatrics/American Society of Anesthesiologists process model. *Pediatrics.* 2002;109:236-243.

90. Ramsay MAE, Savege TM, et al. Controlled sedation with alphaxalone-alphadolone. *BMJ.* 1974;ii:66-659.

91. Avramov MN, White PF. Methods for monitoring the level of sedation. *Crit Care Clin.* 1995;11:803-826.

92. Chernik DA, Gillings D, et al. Validity and reliability of the Observer's Assessment of Alertness/Sedation Scale: Study with intravenous midazolam. *J Clin Psychopharmacol.* 1990;10: 244-251.

93. Coté CJ, Karl HW, Notterman DA, et al. Adverse sedation events in pediatrics: Analysis of medications used for sedation. *Pediatrics.* 2000;106:633-644.

94. Malviya S, Voepel-Lewis T. Techniques for pediatric sedation/analgesia. *Anesth Today.* 2000;11(2):5-10.

95. McGhee B, Howrie D, Schmitt C, Dice J (eds). *Children's Hospital of Pittsburgh Pediatric Drug Therapy & Formulary 2002-2003.* Hudson, OH: Lexi-Comp Inc; 2002.

96. Kao SC, Adamson SD, Tatman LH, Berbaum KS. A survey of post-discharge side effects of conscious sedation using chloral hydrate in pediatric CT and MR imaging. *Pediatr Radiol.* 1999;29:287-290.

97. Malviya S, Voepel-Lewis T, Prochaska G, Tait AR. Prolonged recovery and delayed side effects of sedation for diagnostic imaging studies in children. *Pediatrics.* 2000;105:42.

98. Donnelly AJ, Cunningham FE, Baughman VL. *Anesthesiology & Critical Care Handbook.* 2nd ed. Hudson OH: Lexi-Comp Inc; 1999.

99. Audenaert SM, Montgomery CL, Thompson DE, Sutherland J. A prospective study of rectal methohexital: Efficacy and side effects in 648 cases. *Anesth Analg.* 1995;81:957-961.

100. Stain JD, Campbell JB, Harvey LA, Foley LC. IV Nembutal: Safe sedation for children undergoing CT. *AJR Am J Roentgenol.* 1988;151:975-979.

101. Massanari M, Notvitsky J, Reinstein LJ. Paradoxical reactions in children associated with midazolam use during endoscopy. *Clin Pediatr.* 1997;36:681-684.

102. American Academy of Pediatrics. Reappraisal of lytic cocktail/demerol, phenergen, and thorazine (dpt) for the sedation of children (RE9515). *Pediatrics.* 1995;95:598-602.

103. Stoelting RK. *Pharmacology and Physiology in Anesthetic Practice.* Philadelphia: Lippincott-Raven Publishers; 1995.

104. Epstein RH, Mendel HG, Witkowski TA, et al. The safety and efficacy of oral transmucosal fentanyl citrate for preoperative sedation in young children. *Anesth Analg.* 1996; 83:1200-1205.

105. Schechter NL, Weisman SJ, Rosenblum M, et al. The use of oral transmucosal fentanyl citrate for painful procedures in children. *Pediatrics.* 1995;95:335-339.

106. Hulland SA, Freilich MM, Sandor GK. Nitrous oxide-oxygen or oral midazolam for pediatric outpatient sedation. *Oral Surg Oral Med Oral Pathol Oral Radiol Endod.* 2002;93: 643-646.

107. Mason K, Babu K. Nitrous oxide. In Krauss B, Brustowicz RM (eds). *Pediatric Procedural Sedation and Analgesia.* Philadelphia: Lippincott Williams & Wilkins; 1999:83-88.

108. Leelataweewud P, Vann WF Jr, Dilley DC, Lucas WJ: The physiological effects of supplemental oxygen versus nitrous oxide/oxygen during conscious sedation of pediatric dental patients. *Pediatr Dent.* 2000;22:125-133.

109. Litman RS, Kottra JA, Verga KA, et al. Chloral hydrate sedation: the additive sedative and respiratory depressant effects of nitrous oxide. *Anesth Analg.* 1998;86:724-728.

110. Litman RS, Kottra JA, Berkowitz RJ, Ward DS: Breathing patterns and levels of consciousness in children during administration of nitrous oxide after oral midazolam premedication. *J Oral Maxillofac Surg.* 1997;55:1372-1377; discussion 1378-1379.

111. Litman RS, Berkowitz RJ, Ward DS. Levels of consciousness and ventilatory parameters in young children during sedation with oral midazolam and nitrous oxide. *Arch Pediatr Adolesc Med.* 1996;150:671-675.

112. Resek J. Conscious sedation. *Anesth Today.* 2000;11:4-10.

113. Malviya S, Voepel-Lewis T, Prochaska G, Tait AR. Prolonged recovery and delayed side effects of sedation for diagnostic imaging studies in children. *Pediatrics.* 2000;105:E42.

114. Bass JL, Mehta KA. Oxygen desaturation of selected term infants in car seats. *Pediatrics.*1995;96:288-290.

115. Pembrook L. Studies reveal peds' pain inadequately managed after ambulatory surgery. *Anesth News.* 2002;28(11):7, 11.

CHAPTER 11

Postsedation Patient Care, Monitoring, and Discharge Criteria

COMPETENCIES

At the completion of this chapter, the learner shall:

◆ State the purpose of postsedation patient care.

◆ Identify characteristics associated with phase I and phase II perianesthesia nursing practice.

◆ List the recommended patient care equipment that should be maintained in a postsedation patient care area.

◆ List the components of a postsedation patient care report.

◆ Demonstrate the mechanism to assign a postsedation Aldrete score based on 10 objective scoring criteria.

◆ List the objective scoring parameters that comprise the postsedation Aldrete scoring mechanism.

◆ List appropriate discharge criteria for the outpatient postsedation patient.

◆ State components required for effective postsedation teaching.

Joint Commission on Accreditation of Healthcare Organizations Standards for Operative or Other High-Risk Procedures and/or the Administration of Moderate or Deep Sedation or Anesthesia

Standard PC.13.40
Patients are monitored immediately after the procedure and/or administration of moderate or deep sedation or anesthesia.

Elements of Performance for PC.13.40

1. *The patient's status is assessed on arrival in the recovery area.*

2. *Each patient's physiological status, mental status, and pain level are monitored.*

3. *Monitoring is at a level consistent with the potential effect of the procedure and/or sedation or anesthesia.*

4. *Patients are discharged from the recovery area and the hospital by a qualified licensed independent practitioner according to rigorously applied criteria approved by the clinical leaders.*

5. *Patients who have received anesthesia in the outpatient setting are discharged in the company of a responsible, designated adult.*

© Joint Commission: Standards for Operative or Other High-Risk Procedures and/or the Administration of Moderate or Deep Sedation or Anesthesia, January, 2004. Reprinted with permission.

Practice Guidelines for Sedation and Analgesia by Non-Anesthesiologists
American Society of Anesthesiologists Task Force on Sedation and Analgesia by Non-Anesthesiologists

Recommendations. Following sedation/analgesia, patients should be observed in an appropriately staffed and equipped area until they are near their baseline level of consciousness and are no longer at increased risk for cardiorespiratory depression. Oxygenation should be monitored periodically until patients are no longer at risk for hypoxemia. Ventilation and circulation should be monitored at regular intervals until patients are suitable for discharge. Discharge criteria should be designed to minimize the risk of central nervous system or cardiorespiratory depression after discharge from observation by trained personnel.

From American Society of Anesthesiologists Task Force on Sedation and Analgesia by Non-Anesthesiologists. Practice guidelines for sedation and analgesia by non-anesthesiologists. *Anesthesiology.* 2002;96(4):1013. Reprinted with permission.

Postsedation recovery and monitoring after the administration of sedative and analgesic agents depends on a number of variables:

◆ Diagnostic, therapeutic, or surgical procedure performed
◆ Length of procedure
◆ Presedation patient physiologic condition
◆ Presence of procedural complications
◆ Sedative, hypnotic, analgesic medication administered
◆ Quantity of medication administered

The purpose of postsedation monitoring is to ensure the return of physiologic function before discharge or return to the inpatient setting. Additional goals include an opportunity for the healthcare practitioner to increase patient satisfaction, optimize quality patient care, educate patients, and proficiently manage patient complications. The postsedation period provides a time to assess, diagnose, and treat complications associated with the administration of sedation and analgesia. Postsedation monitoring and discharge policies are required by accrediting bodies and recommended by professional practice organizations.[1-3]

> The postsedation period provides a time period for the patient to meet institutionally approved discharge criteria.

The success of any sedation program depends on providing quality presedation and procedural patient care; however, it must also embrace adequate postsedation monitoring and proper discharge planning. **To avoid allegations of premature patient discharge, mechanisms must be in place to assess home readiness or for return to the inpatient setting.** The American Society of Perianesthesia Care Nurses identifies characteristics unique to perianesthesia nursing practice.[4] These characteristics are identified in Box 11-1. Nurses engaged in the postsedation management of patients receiving moderate sedation/analgesia must provide patient care equivalent to those characteristics identified in

postanesthesia phase II as defined by the American Society of Perianesthesia Care Nurses. However, depending on the level of sedation or in the event of an adverse reaction, the nurse must be capable of providing acute emergent care.

Postsedation monitoring may be provided in a variety of settings. Patients may remain monitored in the treatment area or be transferred to a designated postsedation recovery area. The recovery area should be physically conducive to meet the needs of the patient and the caregiver. Postsedation recovery areas must be well lighted and located in a central area with appropriate monitoring and emergency resuscitative equipment available. Recommended equipment and medications required for postsedation patient care are identified in Box 11-2. If the healthcare provider participating in the administration of sedation and procedural patient care does not monitor the patient after the procedure, the patient must be safely transported to a postsedation recovery area. Before transport, the patient should have a stable, patent airway. Oxygen equipment should be available for transport to the postsedation area. The patient is accompanied by the

---

⬛ BOX 11-1

Characteristics Unique to Perianesthesia Nursing Practice

Preanesthesia Phase
Patient preparation (physical and emotional)
Data collection, assessment, planning for postprocedure disposition

Phase I
Implementation of nursing care to provide a safe transition from the fully anesthetized state to a physiologic state requiring less acute care.

Phase II
Implementation of nursing care to prepare the patient for self-care or to be cared for by another.

healthcare provider participating in the procedure who is knowledgeable about the patient's condition. Before the transfer of care to another provider, a verbal report must be given to the healthcare provider assuming care of the patient. It is important for healthcare providers to realize that this transfer of care is a medical legal transfer of patient care, which requires a comprehensive postsedation report. Components of the postsedation report are outlined in Box 11-3. Documentation of the transfer of care should be recorded in the initial assessment area of the postsedation record. To clearly delineate this separate and distinct period of care, various postsedation documentation forms have been developed.

PATIENT ASSESSMENT

If postsedation assessment is not conducted in the same procedural area by the same sedation provider, the patient should be transferred to a designated postsedation clinical setting. The postsedation healthcare provider must perform a complete systems assessment during the first few minutes of the postsedation admission process. Components of a comprehensive postsedation assessment are identified in Box 11-4. **Completion of a comprehensive admission**

BOX 11-2

Recommended Postsedation Equipment and Supplies

1. Mechanism to deliver O_2 to each patient
2. Suction and suctioning equipment
3. Monitoring equipment
   - ECG
   - Blood pressure
   - Sao_2
4. Oxygen-delivery devices and equipment
   - Bag-valve-mask/appropriate size masks
   - Face mask extension and connectors
   - Oropharyngeal airway
   - Nasal airway
   - Endotracheal tubes (age appropriate)
   - Nonrebreather mask
   - Wall oxygen/backup cylinders
   - Yankauer suction tip
   - Laryngoscope/blades
   - Stylets
   - Magill forceps
   - Nasal cannula
5. Defibrillator (cardioversion/transthoracic pacing capability, readily available)
6. Emergency medication resuscitation cart (adult/pediatric)
   - ACLS resuscitative medications
   - Benzodiazepine/opioid reversal agents
7. Intravenous supplies
   - Age-appropriate IV catheters
   - Macro/microdrip tubing
   - IV solutions
   - Dextrose
   - Normal saline solution
   - Lactated Ringer's solution
   - Gloves
   - Alcohol swabs
   - Betadine
   - 4×4-inch gauze pads
   - Tape
   - Central vein catheterization set
8. Methods for:
   - Calling for assistance
   - Ensuring patient privacy

BOX 11-3

Components of Postsedation Report

- Patient's name
- Age
- Diagnostic, therapeutic, or surgical procedure
- Past medical history
- Prescribed, over-the-counter medications, and herbal/homeopathic preparations
- Allergies
- Presedation and procedural vital signs
- Level of consciousness
- Airway status
- Sedative/analgesic/hypnotic medications administered
  - Total dose and frequency of administration
  - Antagonist administered (time)
- Response/reaction to medications
- Adverse response/reaction
  - ECG, blood pressure, Sao_2, respirations
  - Complications
  - Treatment
- Fluid balance
  - Site and size of IV catheters
  - IV solution infused and amount
  - Blood loss
- Postsedation concerns or considerations
  - Review of medical orders
- Location of responsible physician

BOX 11-4

Components of Postsedation Patient Assessment

- Monitor and improve cardiorespiratory function.
- Continue to maintain physical and emotional comfort and provide privacy.
- Assess procedural/surgical site.
- Assess, document, and treat data observed during postsedation assessment.
- Encourage fluids.
- Advise ambulation as tolerated.
- Assess genitourinary status, patient voiding status.
- Review discharge plan with family or responsible adult.
- Review sedation and procedural discharge instructions.
- Provide follow-up as outlined by hospital policy and procedure.

assessment allows the healthcare provider the ability to plan the postsedation phase of patient care. The nursing plan of care in the postsedation setting is derived from the patient history, initial assessment, report from the sedation provider, and utilization of critical thinking skills. Sample patient outcome grids for patients in the postsedation care area are featured in Table 11-1.

POSTSEDATION RECORD AND SCORING MECHANISMS

A postsedation recovery scoring mechanism was introduced into clinical practice in 1970 by Aldrete and Kroulik.[5] Through the evolution of anesthesia and surgery, variations of the Aldrete scoring system have evolved.[6,7] The original Aldrete scoring system was intended for phase I

TABLE 11-1
Postsedation (Phase II) Patient Outcome Grids

POTENTIAL AND ACTUAL PROBLEMS/NURSING DIAGNOSES	OUTCOME GOALS: PATIENT WILL BE ABLE TO:	NURSING INTERVENTIONS	RESOURCES
Altered thought processes and/or memory loss R/T sedation/anesthesia	Display/verbalize appropriate orientation to surroundings and situations Respond lucidly to questions Avoid self-injury R/T altered thought patterns Assume self-care activities within parameters of surgical restrictions Rely on RA who understands nature of patient's temporarily altered thought patterns and responsibility for patient care	Provide frequent affirmations of orientation to time, place, and events Assess patient's orientation Monitor and oversee patient care while patient is vulnerable to environment Provide adequate time for drug clearance before patient discharge Administer medications with caution to avoid further sedation that would greatly alter patient's mental status	Comprehensive report from prior caregivers regarding sedative medications, prior mental status Predetermined discharge criteria that include assessment of mental status and availability of RA to drive and provide home support ASPAN Standards of Perianesthesia Nursing Practice
Ineffective airway clearance Potential for aspiration Ineffective breathing patterns, respiratory depression R/T sedation, anesthesia, positioning, pain, increased respiratory secretions, vomiting, or untoward reactions to medications or local anesthetics	Maintain normal respiratory parameters (rate, depth, ease, clarity of breath sounds) Maintain clear airway Avoid aspiration Maintain adequate oxygenation of tissues Avoid symptoms of hypoxia Perform effective cough and deep breathing exercises	Knowledge of effects of anesthetics, analgesics, sedatives, and muscle relaxants and associated drug interactions Airway maintenance techniques, including suctioning and bag-valve-mask resuscitative techniques as needed Apply stir-up regimen Administer oxygen per protocols Continuous assessment of respiratory status Timely report of untoward symptoms to anesthesiologist/surgeon Provide adequate hydration and safe positioning Identify preexisting respiratory disease and individualize care appropriately	Physiologic monitoring equipment, oxygen, suction and emergency equipment available in unit Crash cart, resuscitator bag, ventilator, airway maintenance supplies, drugs Adequate staffing patterns to ensure proper nurse:patient ratio Immediate access to anesthesia provider Comprehensive anesthesia and/or nursing report before transfer of patient care ASPAN Standards of Perianesthesia Nursing Practice Facility policies regarding interventions for cardiovascular/respiratory problems Intravenous fluids and venipuncture supplies Spirits of ammonia available, especially in bathrooms Emergency call bell system functional

TABLE 11-1

Postsedation (Phase II) Patient Outcome Grids—cont'd

POTENTIAL AND ACTUAL PROBLEMS/NURSING DIAGNOSES	OUTCOME GOALS: PATIENT WILL BE ABLE TO:	NURSING INTERVENTIONS	RESOURCES
Potential alteration in tissue perfusion Cardiovascular instability	Maintain normal cardiovascular parameters, avoiding hypertension and hypotension Demonstrate expected postoperative arousal and mental status Demonstrate normal parameters of peripheral circulation Ambulate without faintness or hypotension	Assess all parameters of vital signs in ongoing fashion, including heart rate and rhythm, blood pressure Assess mental status and progression Assist patient in progressive ambulation within individual patient's abilities Check peripheral pulses, color, and sensory adequacy in ongoing fashion Timely report of untoward symptoms to anesthesiologist/surgeon Maintain adequate fluid balance and hydration	
Altered skin integrity R/T surgical wound Potential for infection at surgical site	Experience appropriate and uncomplicated wound healing Avoid fever	Use aseptic technique and teach to family and patient Enhance circulation of surgical wound site Avoid constricting bandages at surgical site Assess surgical site throughout Phase II stay	Universal precautions PPE and sterile dressing supplies Intravenous fluids Antibiotics, if ordered
Alterations in comfort—pain	Express acceptable comfort level Maintain normal cardiovascular, respiratory parameters	Administer appropriate analgesics, cold therapy Position patient for comfort Provide positive reinforcements and encourage philosophy of wellness throughout process Encourage appropriate pace for increased activities	Physician's orders for analgesics Analgesic medications Knowledge of nursing interventions for comfort—positioning and support of body areas, breathing exercises, positive reinforcement of comfort
Alterations in comfort—nausea and vomiting	Express acceptable comfort level Avoid vomiting and retching	Encourage appropriate pace for oral intake of fluids Administer antiemetics as needed Administer intravenous solutions for hydration as ordered Provide positive reinforcements and encourage philosophy of wellness throughout process	Physician's orders/prescriptions for antiemetics Intravenous fluids Literature R/T reducing gastrointestinal symptoms Appropriate food and beverages—avoid acid producing juices, spicy or difficult-to-digest foods
Self-care deficit	Display sufficient level of alertness and self-care for safe discharge to home with RA	Provide comprehensive nursing care modified to patient's abilities Assess patient for ability to ambulate and call for assistance before discharge Assure availability of RA before discharge	Discharge criteria

Continued

TABLE 11-1

Postsedation (Phase II) Patient Outcome Grids—cont'd

POTENTIAL AND ACTUAL PROBLEMS/NURSING DIAGNOSES	OUTCOME GOALS: PATIENT WILL BE ABLE TO:	NURSING INTERVENTIONS	RESOURCES
Actual or perceived loss of privacy or dignity	Express content at level of privacy provided Maintain dignity and sense of self-esteem	Support patient's right to privacy and dignity Promote unit philosophy that demands support of patient's right to privacy Explain and demonstrate to patient before surgery that privacy and dignity will not be invaded while patient is asleep or sedated Provide privacy—curtains, blankets, clothing that covers patient Allow patient as much decision-making as is possible and encourage RA to do same	Surroundings that are friendly, family focused, private, and apart from view of other patients or staff Patient Bill of Rights Patient linens that provide adequate cover Cubicle curtains
Risk of hemorrhage	Maintain blood volume at normal level Maintain blood pressure at normal levels—avoid hypertension	Ensure availability of intravenous solutions Observe surgical site for signs of bleeding and report to physician Administer anxiolytic and/or antihypertensive medications as ordered Instruct patient on appropriate support of surgical site	Blood bank contract and policies for rapid availability of blood products Antihypertensives Anxiolytic medications Intravenous fluids and supplies
Anxiety R/T fear of home care without nursing support, separation from family, potential diagnosis, etc.	Express lingering fears, questions about home care or other topics Display calm demeanor Verbalize reduced anxiety Rely on RA for support in the home setting	Provide written and verbal information and ongoing explanations regarding care issues within limits of nursing Ensure home support before discharge Encourage questions from patient and RA	Verbal and written discharge instructions that include emergency contact information RA willing and able to provide home support
Potential for injury R/T faintness, weakness, fatigue, prolonged regional block, altered sensory perception	Remains free from injury Ambulates without faintness or injury	Encourage appropriate pace for progression of ambulation Monitor vital signs in relationship to ambulation Reduce obstacles to safe ambulation—wet floors, slippery shoes, improper fit of slings, braces, surgical shoes, crutches, etc. Provide ongoing assessments for potential complications R/T ambulation	Safe environment Nursing attendance during ambulation attempts and while patient is in bathroom Evaluation of patient's home setting during preadmission assessment RA in home setting

ASPAN, American Society of PeriAnesthesia Nurses; *PACU,* postanesthesia care unit; *PPE,* personal protective equipment; *RA,* responsible adult; *R/T,* related to.
From Burden N. *Ambulatory Surgical Nursing.* 2nd ed. Philadelphia: WB Saunders; 2000:483-485.

BOX 11-5

Aldrete Postanesthesia Recovery Scoring System

Activity

Able to move four extremities voluntarily on command	2
Able to move two extremities voluntarily on command	1
Able to move no extremities voluntarily on command	0

Respiration

Able to breathe deeply and cough freely	2
Dyspnic, shallow, or limited breathing	1
Apneic	0

Circulation

Blood pressure ± 20 mm Hg of normal	2
Blood pressure ± 20-50 mm Hg of normal	1
Blood pressure more than ± 50 mm Hg of normal	0

Consciousness

Fully awake	2
Arousable on calling	1
Not responsive	0

O_2 Saturation (color)

Able to maintain O_2 saturation >92% on room air	2
Needs O_2 inhalation to maintain O_2 saturation >90%	1
O_2 saturation <90% even with O_2 supplement	0

Dressing

Dry	2
Wet but stationary	1
Wet but growing	0

Pain

Pain free	2
Mild pain handled by oral medications	1
Pain requiring parenteral medications	0

Ambulation

Able to stand up and walk straight*	2
Vertigo when erect	1
Dizziness when supine	0

Fasting-Feeding

Able to drink fluids	2
Nauseated	1
Nausea and vomiting	0

Urine Output

Has voided	2
Unable to void but comfortable†	1
Unable to void and uncomfortable	0

*May be substituted by Romberg's test or by picking up 12 clips in one hand.

†Aldrete JA, Kroulik D. A post anesthetic recovery score. *Anesth Anal.* 1970;49:924-928.

Data from Aldrete J, Wright A. *Anesthesia News.* 1992; (November):16-17.

postanesthesia care use. Modifications of Aldrete's scoring system, which are more applicable for phase II patient care, are featured in Box 11-5. The modified Aldrete Phase II recovery scoring system assigns a predetermined score to objective clinical criteria, which includes the following parameters:

◆ Activity
◆ Respiration
◆ Circulation
◆ Consciousness
◆ Oxygen saturation
◆ Dressing
◆ Pain
◆ Ambulation
◆ Fasting-feeding
◆ Urine output

A variety of pain assessment tools may be utilized by the postsedation clinician. The NRS, VAS, and ARS pain assessment scales are featured in Figure 11-1. Use of the variables identified in the Aldrete Phase II recovery scoring system (see Box 11-5) provides objective clinical parameters for postsedation assessment. **A postsedation scoring system must be clearly understood by the staff to provide accurate documentation and ensure the safe discharge of the patient when all institutionally approved discharge criteria are met.** Use of a scoring system provides objective parameters related to the patient's postsedation recovery and readiness for discharge. Criteria-based recovery parameters provide a mechanism to objectively assess the needs of the patient. Discharge criteria specific to sedation are highlighted in Box 11-6. These criteria provide objective clinical assessment parameters to ascertain the degree of recovery from sedative/analgesic medications administered.

ACTIVITY

Patients who will be discharged to home after the procedure may generally prepare to ambulate once a postsedation score greater than or equal to 8 (or their presedation Aldrete score) has been achieved. Patients who recover on a gurney or recliner should be placed in a 30- to 40-degree head-up position. Dizziness or light-headedness is assessed, and the patient's activity level is advanced accordingly. If the patient tolerates the head-up position, sitting or dangling the legs for 5-minute increments precedes sitting in a chair and ambulation. Absence of diaphoresis, bradycardia, hypotension, nausea, or vomiting is required before ambulation of the patient. Assisted ambulation is recommended to assess steadiness of gait. Patients may appear alert and prepared to ambulate, only to discover that they are not quite stable enough to enter the bathroom or dressing area. An assisted ambulation method may prevent unexpected falls by patients who overextend their capabilities at any given time.

Patients who have received sedation/analgesia generally retain the ability to tolerate oral fluids without incident. The

Pain Assessment Tools

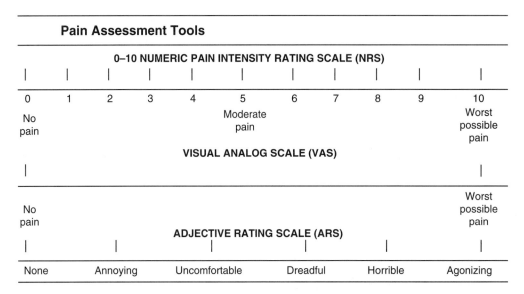

FIGURE 11-1 Pain assessment tools (NRS) (VAS) (ARS). (Reprinted from Acute Pain Management Guidelines Panel. *Acute Pain Management: Operative or Medical Procedures and Trauma. Clinical Practice Guidelines.* AHCPR publication No. 92-0032. Rockville, MD: Agency for Health Care Policy and Research, Public Health Service, US Department of Health and Human Services; February, 1992.)

BOX 11-6

Sedation/Analgesia Discharge Criteria

- **Respiratory assessment**
  - The patient retains the ability to maintain and protect the airway.
  - The patient displays no signs of respiratory distress (snoring, stridor, suprasternal retraction, decreased O_2 saturation, or respiratory rate).
  - The patient demonstrates the ability to cough and tolerates liquids/light nourishment.
  - A minimum of 30 (or 60 depending on hospital policy and procedure) minutes has elapsed after the administration of the last dose of narcotic, sedative, or hypnotic.
  - Patients treated with reversal agents (flumazenil/naloxone) are monitored for a minimum of 120 minutes after the administration of the reversal agent.
- **Level of consciousness, mentation**
  - Fully oriented to time, person, and place or return to baseline mentation and is interested in returning to the inpatient setting or home.
  - Minimal or no nausea; if nausea is present, the patient can ingest and retain oral fluids.
  - Minimal vomiting; if vomiting is present it does not require treatment. If vomiting requires treatment, the patient can ingest and retain oral fluids.

- Minimal dizziness or light-headedness; if present it only occurs when the patient is sitting. The patient can still perform movements that are consistent with age.
- Able to void on instruction; the patient is instructed to contact the physician if no voiding has occurred within 8 hours.
- **Circulation**
  - Stable vital signs for a minimum of 30 to 60 minutes
- **Activity**
  - The patient performs age-appropriate ambulation (walk, sit, stand).
  - The patient demonstrates controlled, coordinated movements.
  - A responsible adult is available for discharge and home environment.
- **Oxygenation and color**
  - The patient maintains Sao_2 greater than 95% on room air or attains presedation oxygen saturation value.
  - Skin color is pink.
- **Procedure site**
  - No bleeding is evident on the dressing and the dressing is dry and intact.
- **Pain**
  - The patient has minimal or no pain before discharge.

encouragement of oral fluids is contraindicated in patients who have received oropharyngeal topical anesthetics. Before oral fluid intake, the presence of a gag reflex and the ability to cough must be documented. Small amounts of oral fluid may then be encouraged before discharge or removal of the intravenous catheter. Oral fluids should not be forced in the presence of nausea and vomiting. Depending on the cause of the nausea and vomiting, patients with nausea or vomiting may benefit from the administration of additional intravenous fluids, gastrokinetic agents, and serotonin antagonists in anticipation of discharge. Medications identified in Table 11-2 have been used in postoperative patients with some success in this patient population.[8-12] **Patients with severe protracted nausea and vomiting require additional observation and should not be discharged.** Specific nursing interventions in this situation include:

◆ Provide positive reinforcement to decrease anxiety.
◆ Avoid signs, smells, and conversations that would provoke nausea and vomiting.
◆ Move or ambulate patient slowly.
◆ Allow the patient to "recover" slowly without aggressive stimulation.
◆ Provide anxiolysis and analgesia if required.
◆ Advance oral intake slowly while avoiding citrus juices and coffee.

TABLE 11-2

Antimetic Medications and Treatment Protocol

GROUP/DRUG	ACTION/USES	DOSAGE RANGES/ROUTES FOR ADULTS	SIDE EFFECTS/SPECIAL NOTES
Phenothiazines			
Prochlorperazine (Compazine)	Patantiemetic, anxiolytic Tranquilizer	PO 5-10 mg IM (deep) 5-10 mg Rectal 25 mg IV 5-10 mg slowly—use great caution to avoid hypotension	Caution with CNS depressants (reduce doses of both), drowsiness, dizziness, hypotension, restlessness, extrapyramidal symptoms. Depressed cough reflex can lead to aspiration.
Chlorpromazine (Thorazine)	Antiemetic, anxiolytic Decreases restlessness	IM (deep) 12.5-25 mg PO 10-25 mg	Caution with other CNS depressants (reduce doses of each). Use caution in cardiovascular or liver disease, asthma, emphysema, drowsiness, sedation, dizziness, faintness, decreased cough reflex, postural hypotension (keep flat for 30 min after injection), extrapyramidal symptoms.
Promethazine (Phenergan)	Antiemetic, sedative, anti–motion sickness, anticholinergic	IM (deep) 12.5-25 mg (reduce with CNS depressants)	Potentiates other CNS depressants, drowsiness, impaired thought patterns, tachycardia, bradycardia, hypotension, extrapyramidal symptoms, caution in patients with heart disease. Never give epinephrine to treat hypotension caused by promethazine because it could further lower blood pressure.
Others			
Trimethobenzamide (Tigan)	Antiemetic—depresses CTZ, sedative, weak antihistamine	PO 250 mg IM (deep) 200 mg, onset in 15 min, lasts 2-3 hr Rectal 200 mg	Drowsiness, sedation, blurred vision, hypotension, extrapyramidal symptoms, disorientation
Benzquinamide (Emete-con)	Antiemetic Depresses CTZ	IM (preferred) 50 mg; onset in 15 min, peak 15 min, lasts 3-4 hr IV 25 mg *very slowly,* decrease dose if patient is taking pressor agent or epinephrine-like drug or in cardiac patient	Drowsiness, sedation, blurred vision, hypotension or hypertension, headache, dry mouth. Dysrhythmias (especially with IV route) include atrial fibrillation, PACs, PVCs. Elevated temperature. Flushing, hepatic metabolism.

Continued

| TABLE 11-2

Antimetic Medications and Treatment Protocol—cont'd

GROUP/DRUG	ACTION/USES	DOSAGE RANGES/ROUTES FOR ADULTS	SIDE EFFECTS/SPECIAL NOTES
Ondansetron (Zofran)	Antiemetic Depresses CTZ and 5-HT$_3$ receptor	PO 16 mg 1 hr before anesthesia induction IV 4 mg undiluted over 2-5 min	Headache, malaise, fatigue, dizziness, sedation. Constipation, diarrhea, abdominal pain. Musculoskeletal pain, chills, urine retention, hypoxia. Drugs that alter hepatic drug-metabolizing enzymes (phenobarbital or cimetidine) may alter pharmacokinetics, but no dosage adjustment is necessary.
Dolasetron mesylate (Anzemet)	Antiemetic Selective serotonin 5-HT$_3$ receptor antagonist	Prevention of postoperative nausea and vomiting: PO 100 mg within 2 hrs prior to anesthesia induction IV 12.5 mg approximately 15 min before cessation of anesthesia Children (2-16 years) PO 1.2 mg/kg within 2 hrs of surgery up to a maximum dose of 100 mg IV 0.35 mg/kg (up to 12.5 mg) approximately 15 min before cessation of anesthesia (injectable formula may be mixed) Headache, dizziness, drowsiness, arrhythmias, hypotension, hypertension, tachycardia	Diarrhea, dyspepsia, abdominal pain, constipation, anorexia. Oliguria, urinary retention. Pruritus, rash. Elevation of liver function tests, chills, fever, pain at injection site. Drugs that prolong ECG intervals. *Drug is not recommended for children younger than 2 years of age.*
Droperidol (Inapsine)	Potent tranquilizer (neuroleptic agent), anxiolytic Potentiates narcotics and CNS depressants	IV 0.625-1.25 mg (reduce doses when given with narcotics or CNS depressants); onset, 3-10 min, peak 30 min, lasts 3-6 hr	Drowsiness, hypotension, anxiety, tachycardia, shivering/chills, extrapyramidal symptoms, laryngospasm, bronchospasm, hepatic metabolism.
Dimenhydrinate (Dramamine)	Antiemetic, anti–motion sickness Depressant action on hyperstimulated labyrinthine function	IM 50 mg IV (dilute) 50 mg in 10 mL slowly over at least 2 min IV infusion 50-100 mg in 500-mL solution	Drowsiness, dizziness, dry mouth, blurred vision, nervousness, restlessness, dysuria, or inability to void, thickened bronchial secretions, tachycardia.
Metoclopramide (Reglan)	Increases gastric motility (gastrokinetic agent) Dopamine antagonist in CTZ	IM 10 mg (range, 5-20), onset 0-15 min, lasts 1-2 hr IV (slowly) dilute 10 mg over at least 15 min; onset, 1-3 min, lasts 1-2 hr	Restlessness, drowsiness, fatigue, extrapyramidal symptoms, hypertension, hypotension. Contraindicated in epileptics, use with caution in hypertensive patients, hepatic metabolism.
Hydroxyzine (Vistaril, Atarax)	Antiemetic, anxiolytic Potentiates narcotics	IM (deep), 25-100 mg decrease up to one half when given with CNS depressants (12.5-50 mg IV) *Do not give IV or SQ*	Potentiates narcotics, barbiturates and other CNS depressants. Drowsiness, dry mouth.
Diphenhydramine (Benadryl)	Anti–motion sickness Competes for H$_1$ receptor site	IM (deep) 10-50 mg IV 10-50 mg PO 25-50 mg	Sedation, hypotension, dizziness, disturbed coordination, thickening bronchial secretions, wheezing. Use with caution in patients with asthma. Increased intraocular pressure, cerebrovascular disease.

TABLE 11-2

Antimetic Medications and Treatment Protocol—cont'd

GROUP/DRUG	ACTION/USES	DOSAGE RANGES/ROUTES FOR ADULTS	SIDE EFFECTS/SPECIAL NOTES
Scopolamine (Transderm Scōp)	Anti–motion sickness Antimuscarinic activity Acts on vestibular pathway and directly on vomiting center	1 patch behind the ear 4 hr before surgery, delivers 0.5 mg over 72 hours	Dry mouth—most common side effect. Dizziness, mydriasis (dilated pupil), blurred vision, drowsiness, confusion/restlessness, bradycardia, photophobia. Avoid in people with glaucoma. Wash hands well after application to avoid getting in eyes. Instruct patient on removal and side effects if discharged with patch in place.

PO, orally; *IM,* intramuscular; *IV,* intravenous; *CNS,* central nervous system; *CTZ,* chemoreception trigger zone; *PAC,* premature atrial contraction; *PVC,* premature ventricular contraction; *5-HT₃,* serotonin; *H₁,* histamine-1.
From Burden N. *Ambulatory Surgical Nursing.* 2nd ed. Philadelphia: WB Saunders; 2000:462-463.

A requirement to have the patient void after the procedure is not universally endorsed. Patients receiving sedation/analgesia may not have urinary retention commonly experienced by postoperative surgical patients, and voiding may not be a problem. However, when opioids are utilized, patients may experience some urinary retention and altered bladder tone. Patients who have not voided before discharge must be instructed to notify or return to the treatment facility in the event of bladder distention or the prolonged inability to void. Outpatients should be discharged in the care of a responsible adult who is capable of[13]:

◆ Assisting the patient
◆ Ensuring patient compliance with postprocedure instruction
◆ Monitoring the patients progress toward recovery

POSTSEDATION TEACHING AND INSTRUCTION

Postsedation teaching should be conducted in the presence of the responsible adult assuming care of the patient on discharge or the healthcare provider accepting care of the patient immediately after the procedure. Written discharge instructions addressing medications, diet, and procedure specific information must be reviewed with each patient and responsible adult. Use of written discharge instructions (procedure and medication) serves both the patient and the facility. The medication discharge form shown in Figure 11-2 identifies medication used, side effects, and specific postsedation guidelines to protect the patient.

Postsedation discharge teaching should take place in an unhurried atmosphere, much like the presedation patient assessment process.

In addition to sedation/analgesia medication instructions, postsedation specific discharge instructions should be reviewed and given to the patient or responsible adult accompanying the patient home. Postsedation discharge instructions featured in Box 11-7 should address medications, activity restriction, diet, procedural side effects, possible complications and symptoms, and access to postsedation or follow-up care. Box 11-8 features key education points for discharge instructions.

POSTPROCEDURE FOLLOW-UP

A mechanism to ascertain postsedation patient status is recommended for patients discharged on the day of the procedure. Inpatient information may be gathered by the sedation practitioner or the physician after the procedure. Methods of gathering additional quality improvement data include the following:

◆ Patient questionnaire
◆ Telephone interview
◆ Satisfaction survey

The purpose of postsedation assessment is to evaluate the following:

◆ Incidence of complications related to the administration of sedation/analgesia
◆ Delayed recovery
◆ Procedural complication rate
◆ Return to function

Follow-up telephone conversations give the nurse the ability to receive direct feedback from the patient. In addition, telephone follow-up allows the clinician the ability to collect quality assurance outcome data.[14] Consistent postsedation assessment is an accurate method to identify complications and ensure the delivery of quality sedation services.

Patient:_____ Date:___/___/_____

Procedure Performed:_____

Medication discharge instructions:

You received the conscious sedation medications indicated below.

☐ Midazolam   ☐ Diazepam

☐ Fentanyl   ☐ Alfentanil

☐ Hydromorphone   ☐ Morphine   ☐ Meperidine

☐ Pentothal   ☐ Methohexital   ☐ Propofol

Common side effects associated with these medications include:

- Drowsiness, dizziness, euphoria, sleepiness or confusion

- Impaired memory recall

- Unsteady gait, loss of fine muscle control and delayed reaction time

- Visual disturbances: difficulty focusing, blurred vision

You may experience some of these side effects or you may not be cognizant of subtle changes in your behavior or reaction time. **Because you received these medications, we are giving you the following instructions.**

- Do not drive for 24 hours

- Do not operate equipment for 24 hours

  ~ Lawnmowers, power tools etc.

  ~ Kitchen accessories: stove, etc.

- Do not consume **any** alcoholic beverages for a minimum of 24 hours

- Do not make important personal or business decisions for 24 hours

- Move slowly and carefully, do not make sudden position changes. Be alert for dizziness or light headedness and move accordingly

- Drink liberal amounts of fluid today. Advance your diet as tolerated (unless you have received specific instructions from your doctor). If you feel nauseated, advance your diet as tolerated

- Do not take any of the following medications unless prescribed by your physician.

  ~ Muscle relaxants

  ~ Sedatives

  ~ Hypnotics

  ~ Mood altering medications

  ~ Narcotics

- Contact your physician or this facility if you have any questions or concerns regarding your postprocedure care.

FIGURE 11-2 Sedation medication discharge instructions.

Contact person:_____ Telephone #:_____

☐ Discharge instructions received

☐ Instructions given to responsible adult:_____

☐ Verbalized understanding

If you report to an emergency room, doctor's office or hospital within 24 hours postprocedure, BRING THIS SHEET WITH YOU and give it to the physician or nurse attending to you.

Date:_____ Time:_____

Responsible Adult:_____ _____
                         Signature   Print Name

Instructions given by:_____
                            Signature

FIGURE 11-2, cont'd

BOX 11-7

Postsedation Discharge Instructions

Physical Activity
- Rest today. If you feel up to it, you may move about but do not overdo it or engage in any strenuous activity.
- You may/may not shower or bathe today. If bathing/showering is prohibited today, you may shower or bathe _____ hours post-procedure. A sponge bath today is permitted.
- Notify your physician if you have not voided within 8 hours of the procedure.
- Advance your diet as tolerated; refer to moderate sedation/analgesia medication discharge instructions.
- You may return to work in _____ hours/days.

Postsedation Medication
- Unless otherwise directed by your physician, you may resume your regularly scheduled medications when you arrive home.
- Take prescribed pain medication as directed by your physician (or acetaminophen tablets every 3 to 4 hrs for minor discomfort).

Procedural Site
- There should be no or minimal bleeding.
- Minimal discomfort may be treated with pain medication prescribed. If severe pain occurs, contact your physician.
- You may remove the dressing within _____ hours.
- Replace dressing with _____.
- If any signs of redness, fever, pus, swelling, or bleeding occur, contact your physician.

Additional Considerations
Contact your physician's office at (   ) ___ - ___ for a follow-up appointment.
    If you have persistent nausea or vomiting, contact your physician. **If you are experiencing complications and cannot contact your physician, report to the hospital emergency department. <u>Please bring your discharge instructions with you.</u>**
RN: _____
Responsible Adult: _____
Date: _____

© 2004, Specialty Health Education, Inc.

BOX 11-8

Key Education Points for Discharge Instructions

Medications
- Note the name, purpose, and dosage schedule for each medication; emphasize the importance of following the directions on the label.
- The patient should resume medications taken before surgery per the physician's order.
- If pain medication is not prescribed, nonprescription, nonaspirin analgesics (e.g., acetaminophen, ibuprofen) may be effective for mild aches and pains.
- Additional pain medication may be ordered by the physician after surgery. The patient should take these medications as directed, preferably with food to prevent gastrointestinal upset.

Activity Restriction
- Advise the patient to take it easy for the remainder of the day after surgery. Dizziness or drowsiness is not unusual after surgery and anesthesia.
- For the next 24 hours, the patient should not:
  - Drive a vehicle or operate machinery or power tools
  - Consume alcohol, including beer
  - Make important personal or business decisions or sign important documents
- Activity level: In specific behavioral terms (e.g., do not lift objects heavier than 20 lb), describe any limitation of activities.

Diet
- Explain any dietary restrictions or instructions.
- If no dietary restriction exists, instruct the patient to progress as tolerated to a regular diet.

Surgical and Anesthesia Side Effects
- Anticipated sequelae of surgery (e.g., bleeding and pain) should be delineated.
- Common side effects associated with anesthesia include dizziness, drowsiness, myalgia, nausea and vomiting, or sore throat.

Possible Complications and Symptoms
- Instruct the patient and responsible adult in pertinent signs and symptoms that could be indicative of postoperative complications.
- The patient should call the responsible physician if he or she develops:
  - Fever >38.3° C (101° F) orally
  - Persistent, atypical pain
  - Pain not relieved by medication
  - Bleeding or unexpected drainage from the wound that does not stop
  - Extreme redness or swelling around the incision site or drainage of pus
  - Urinary retention
  - Continual nausea or vomiting

Treatment and Tests
- Procedures that the patient or responsible adult is expected to perform (e.g., dressing changes or the application of warm moist compresses) should be described in detail.
- A complete list of necessary supplies should be included.
- If any postoperative tests are to be conducted, instructions as to the date, time, test location, and any previsit preparation should be listed.

Access to Postdischarge Care
- Note the telephone number of the responsible and available physician.
- Include the telephone number of the ambulatory center and the hours of operation.
- Note also the name, address, and telephone number of the appropriate emergency care facility.

Follow-up Care
- Identify the date, time, and location of the patient's scheduled return visit to the clinic or surgeon.

From Burden N. *Ambulatory Surgical Nursing.* 2nd ed. Philadelphia: WB Saunders; 2000:506. Modified from Marley RA, Moline BM. Patient discharge from the ambulatory setting. *J Post Anesth Nurs.* 1996;11:41.

SUMMARY

Use of specific discharge criteria in the postsedation recovery period provides the ability to assess, diagnose, and treat complications associated with the administration of sedative/analgesic agents. They also provide the clinician with the ability to verify the patient's return to presedation physiologic status. Postsedation teaching and provision of discharge instructions will prepare the patient to return to the primary care setting or home.

In order to achieve maximal educational benefit from this chapter, please complete the Learner Self-Assessment below. This self-assessment tool provides the learner with the ability to identify areas requiring additional review. Reference material for each question is provided in Appendix F.

1. Healthcare practitioner considerations associated with **JCAHO Standards** related to postsedation patient care include:

2. **Practice Guidelines for Sedation and Analgesia by Non-Anesthesiologists recommendations** promulgated by the ASA Task Force on Sedation **related to postsedation patient care** include:

3. The **purpose of postsedation patient care** includes:

4. Characteristics associated with **phase I and phase II perianesthesia nursing practice** include:

5. **Recommended equipment** that should be maintained in a postsedation patient care area includes:

6. **Components of a postsedation patient care report** include:

7. **Objective parameters that comprise the postsedation Aldrete score** include:

8. **Appropriate discharge criteria for the postsedation patient** include:

9. **Components of effective postsedation teaching** include:

POST-TEST QUESTIONS

Please note: If you are applying for CE credit, you must contact Specialty Health Education, Inc. @800-694-8041 for a CE Application Packet.

1. The primary purpose of postsedation monitoring is to _____.
   A. Ensure the return of physiologic function
   B. Administer additional postsedation medications
   C. Prepare the patient to resume presedation nutrition
   D. Allow time to ambulate the patient immediately post sedation

2. Characteristics unique to Phase II Perianesthesia Nursing Practice include _____.
   A. Patient preparation (physical and emotional)
   B. Implementation of nursing care to provide a safe transition from the fully anesthetized state to a physiologic state requiring less acute care
   C. Implementation of nursing care to prepare the patient for self-care or to be cared for by another
   D. Data collection, assessment, and planning

3. Postsedation "recovery" should be _____.
   A. A minimum of 30 minutes
   B. A minimum of 60 minutes
   C. A minimum of 90 minutes
   D. Completed at the end of the procedure and all patients should be evaluated on an individual basis

4. An assessment tool that incorporates predetermined parameters to objectively assess clinical criteria associated with patient recovery is identified as _____.
   A. Sedation flowsheet
   B. Postsedation scoring mechanism
   C. Mallampati classification system
   D. Subjective scoring mechanism

5. The Aldrete Scoring System assigns a predetermined score to basic objective criteria, which include _____.
   A. Activity level, respiration, circulation, level of consciousness, and oxygenation
   B. Activity level, eye movement, circulation, and level of consciousness
   C. Activity level, respirations, swallowing reflex, and circulation
   D. Respiration, swallowing reflex, circulation, and patient temperature

6. Using the Aldrete Scoring System's circulatory criteria applies a minimum numerical score of _____ for maintenance of the patient's heart rate and blood pressure at ±20% to 50% of presedation values.
   A. Zero
   B. One
   C. Two
   D. Three

7. All of the following statements related to postsedation teaching and instruction are true EXCEPT: _____.
   A. Instructions should be given in an unhurried atmosphere.
   B. Instructions must address medications, diet, activity, and procedure specific information.
   C. Instructions must be given to the patient immediately post sedation.
   D. Instructions should be reviewed in the presence of a responsible adult.

8. Reduction of factors that enhance vagal tone, correction of factors that impair left ventricular function, and pain relief are postsedation treatment protocols for which of the following conditions? _____
   A. Hypertension
   B. Hypoventilation
   C. Airway obstruction
   D. Hypotension

9. Residual sedative effect, preexisting pulmonary disease, and overdose are common etiology in the development of _____ in the postsedation recovery period.
   A. Hypotension
   B. Hypertension
   C. Hypoventilation
   D. Pain

10. Which of the following statements represents "sound" clinical judgment with respect to postsedation patient care? _____
   A. All patients may be discharged 2 hours after the procedure.
   B. Postsedation patient care must be individualized; patients may be discharged after all institutionally approved discharge criteria are met.
   C. Patients who receive oral or intramuscular sedation do NOT require postsedation recovery or observation.
   D. Postsedation recovery is only required when intravenous sedative and analgesic agents are administered.

REFERENCES

1. American Society of Anesthesiologists. Practice guidelines for sedation and analgesia by non-anesthesiologists. *Anesthesiology.* 2002;96:1004-1017.
2. Joint Commission. *Standards for Additional Special Procedures. Standards for Operative or other High-Risk Procedures and/or the Administration of Moderate or Deep Sedation or Anesthesia.* Oakbrook Terrace, IL: Joint Commission on Accreditation of Healthcare Organizations; January, 2004.
3. Association of Operating Room Nurses. *Standards, Recommended Practices, and Guidelines.* Denver: AORN; 2002:185-194.
4. The American Society of Post Anesthesia Nurses. *Standards of Perianesthesia Nursing Practice.* Thoroughfare, NJ: ASPAN; 1998.
5. Aldrete J, Kroulik D. A postanesthetic recovery score. *Anesth Analg.* 1970;49:924.
6. Chung F. Are discharge criteria changing? *J Clin Anesth.* 1992;5:64S.
7. Aldrete A. Postanesthesia recovery score revisited. *J Clin Anesth.* 1995;71.
8. Leeser J, Lip H. Prevention of postoperative nausea and vomiting using ondansetron, a new, selective, 5-HT$_3$ receptor antagonist. *Anesth Analg.* 1991;72:751-755.
9. Lacroix G, Lessard MR, Trepanier CA. Treatment of postoperative nausea and vomiting: Comparison of propofol, droperidol, and metoclopramide. *Can J Anaesth.* 1996;43:115-120.
10. Kovac AL, Scuderi PE, Boerner TF, et al. Treatment of postoperative nausea and vomiting with single intravenous doses of dolasetron mesylate: A multicenter trial. Dolasetron Mesylate PONV Treatment Study Group. *Anesth Analg.* 1997;84:546-555.
11. Madej TH, Simpson KH. Comparison of the use of domperidone, droperidol, and metoclopramide in the prevention of nausea and vomiting following major gynaecological surgery. *Br J Anaesth.* 1986;58:884-887.
12. Palazzo MG, Strunin L. Anaesthesia and emesis. I: Etiology. *Can Anaesth Soc J.* 1984;31:178-187.
13. Marley RA, Moline BM. Patient discharge from the ambulatory setting. *J Post Anesth Nurs.* 1996;11:39-49.
14. Kleinpell RM. Improving telephone follow-up after ambulatory surgery. *J PerAnesth Nurs.* 1997;12:336-340.

Risk Management Strategies

At the completion of this chapter, the learner shall:

◆ Identify JCAHO standards and intents related to performance improvement and sedation patient care.

◆ Define *quality*.

◆ Identify four risk reduction strategies to improve sedation patient care.

◆ Describe practice standards, professional practice recommendations, position statements, and state statutes associated with the administration of sedation/analgesia specifically applicable to your practice setting.

◆ Identify the components of a "sedation" database.

◆ State mechanisms utilized in the successful implementation of a sedation educational program.

◆ Delineate mechanisms of information dissemination within a sedation practice setting.

Joint Commission on Accreditation of Healthcare Organizations Standards for Operative or Other High-Risk Procedures and/or the Administration of Moderate or Deep Sedation or Anesthesia

Because sedation is a continuum, it is not always possible to predict how an individual patient receiving sedation will respond. Therefore, each organization develops specific, appropriate protocols for the care of patients receiving sedation. These protocols are consistent with professional standards and address at least the following:

- Sufficient qualified individuals present to perform the procedure and to monitor the patient throughout administration and recovery.

- Appropriate equipment for care and resuscitation

- Appropriate monitoring of vital signs—heart and respiratory rates and oxygenation

- *Documentation of care*

- *Monitoring of outcomes*

© Joint Commission: Standards for Operative or Other High-Risk Procedures and/or the Administration of Moderate or Deep Sedation or Anesthesia, January, 2004. Reprinted with permission.

Position Statement on the Role of the Registered Nurse (RN) in the Management of Patients Receiving Intravenous Conscious Sedation for Short-Term, Therapeutic, Diagnostic, or Surgical Procedures (Excerpt):

...Demonstrates knowledge of the legal ramifications of administering IV sedation, including the RN's responsibility and liability in the event of an untoward reaction or life threatening complications.

...The institution or practice setting has in place an educational competency validation mechanism that includes a process for evaluating and documenting the individuals who are related to the management of patients receiving IV sedation. Evaluation and documentation of competence occurs on a periodic basis according to institutional policy.

DEVELOPMENT OF A RISK MANAGEMENT STRATEGY

Quality has been broadly defined as the comprehensive positive outcome of a product.[1] Achievement of excellence in healthcare requires quality care and service evaluation. The quality of sedation services is based on compliance with prescribed standards and recommended practice. Implementation of a successful sedation program is based on the delivery of the high-quality technical aspects of care combined with positive outcomes. The delivery of quality sedation services is also dependent on the patient's perception of care rendered. Today consumers are more cognizant than ever of the care they receive. The environment of managed care attempts to create the perception of acceptable value in return for the cost of healthcare.[2] The JCAHO states that *quality* is the "degree to which patient care services increase the probability of undesired outcomes, given the current state of knowledge."[3] To ensure the delivery of high-quality care and reduce patient injury, strategic risk-management programs are designed.

The quality movement in the United States has its conceptual foundation in work done by Demming, whose organizational theory was employed in the business sector in problem-solving techniques and productivity.[4] In 1913, hospitals began outlining requirements to ensure quality of care. Issues addressed at that time included standards for professional staff, case review, audits, medical records, and support services. Thus, the foundation for hospital accreditation was laid. In 1950 the Joint Commission on Accreditation of Hospitals was formed. Standards for quality assurance were established by this organization. Quality assurance programs commenced to determine the level of care being given and received and then take whatever action was required to maintain or improve that care.[5] It is important for hospitals to participate in quality assurance programs and adhere to specific standards of care not only to improve patient care but also to receive Medicare reimbursement. Quality/performance improvement soon followed the quality assurance movement, which focuses on review and evaluation of an organization as a system.

The goal of improving performance is to ensure that an organization designs processes well and systematically monitors, analyzes, and improves its performance to enhance patient outcomes. Examples of improvement efforts include data collection, creating a flowchart for a clinical process, measuring patient outcomes, comparing unit performances, and selecting areas for priority attention.[6] A sedation unit as part of the hospital/facility system must include the following essential performance improvement components:

♦ Designing processes
♦ Monitoring performance through data collection
♦ Analyzing current performance
♦ Improving and sustaining improved performance

Continuous quality improvement accomplishes improvement by measuring process and outcomes, assessing the reasons for current practices and the barriers to change, and intervening to improve current practices.[4] A cause-and-effect diagram used to examine data in a quality improvement process is featured in Figure 12-1. The goal of continuous quality improvement is making improvements in the process of care. Figure 12-2 features a model for improvement. This model summarizes a continuous comprehensive cycle process that:

♦ Identifies or states the "aim"
♦ Identifies measures of improvement
♦ Describes and predicts changes
♦ Plans
♦ Conducts pilot test
♦ Checks and studies results
♦ Acts to improve
♦ Reflects on learning

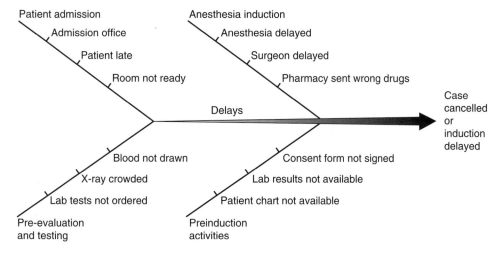

FIGURE 12-1 Cause and effect diagram. (From Foster S, Callahan M. *A Professional Study and Resource Guide for the CRNA.* Park Ridge, IL: American Association of Nurse Anesthetists; 2001:508.)

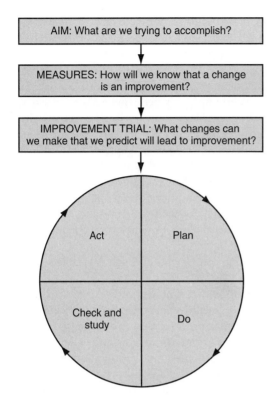

FIGURE 12-2 Model for improvement. (From Foster S, Callahan M. *A Professional Study and Resource Guide for the CRNA.* Park Ridge, IL: American Association of Nurse Anesthetists; 2001:509.)

As emphasized throughout this text, the delivery of sedation and analgesia requires vigilance, clinical competence, proficient monitoring techniques, and assessment skills. Adherence to professional standards, recommended practice guidelines, position statements, and state statutes provides the clinician with parameters and guidelines to provide safe, high-quality sedation services. However, unexpected events and complications may occur as a result of human error, periods of reduced observation, environmental factors (reduced lighting, limited patient access), poor communication, haste, and lack of preparation. When undesirable events occur, they must be rapidly diagnosed with appropriate intervention to restore body homeostasis. **To prevent or reduce the development of adverse events, a risk-reduction strategy should be implemented for all units and personnel engaged in the administration of sedation.** To have an effective performance improvement process and risk reduction strategy requires the support of hospital administration and members of the risk management team.

Individual injury prevention strategies are outlined and include the following:

1. A comprehensive understanding of the goals, definitions, practice standards and guidelines associated with sedation and analgesia (see Chapter 1).

2. Presedation assessment and patient selection (see Chapter 2).
3. Application and demonstrated clinical competence in the use of required monitoring devices (see Chapter 6).
4. Selection of appropriate pharmacologic medications and techniques of administration (see Chapters 3, 4, and 5).
5. Demonstrated clinical competence in airway management skills and rescuing patients from deeper levels of sedation (see Chapters 6 and 7).
6. Postsedation monitoring and discharge planning (see Chapter 11).

Ideally, through implementation of individual risk-reduction strategies, prevention of injury precedes the occurrence of an adverse incident or event.

Application of a risk-management program on a departmental/institution basis requires development and implementation of mechanisms aimed at risk identification, analysis, and control, which are assessed on an ongoing basis. As depicted in Figure 12-3, creation of a sedation database program may complement many of these continuous quality improvement activities. A coordinator (nurse manager, department chairman) guides input into the sedation database. Once the database has been instituted, strategies to implement change are evaluated. The sedation database is an integral component of any performance improvement process.

> Through total staff involvement and commitment, employees are empowered to participate in key components of the performance improvement process.

Institution/Office Policy and Procedure

The development of policies and procedures related to the administration of sedation and analgesia is a multi-disciplinary process. Comprehensive policy development requires consultation and support from members of the administrative, nursing, medical, and anesthesia staff. As outlined throughout this text, policy and procedure development must be derived from current practice standards, recommended practice guidelines, position statements, state statutes, and nurse practice acts promulgated by:

◆ JCAHO
◆ Professional practice organizations
◆ State statutes
◆ Nurse practice acts

JCAHO Standards for sedation and anesthesia are presented in Appendix B. The "Practice Guidelines for Sedation and Analgesia by Non-Anesthesiologists, An Updated Report by the American Society of Anesthesiologists Task Force on Sedation and Analgesia by Non-Anesthesiologists," are featured in Appendix A. The American Nurses Association "Endorsement of Position Statements on the Role of the Registered Nurse (RN) in the Management of Patients Receiving IV Conscious Sedation for Short-Term Therapeutic,

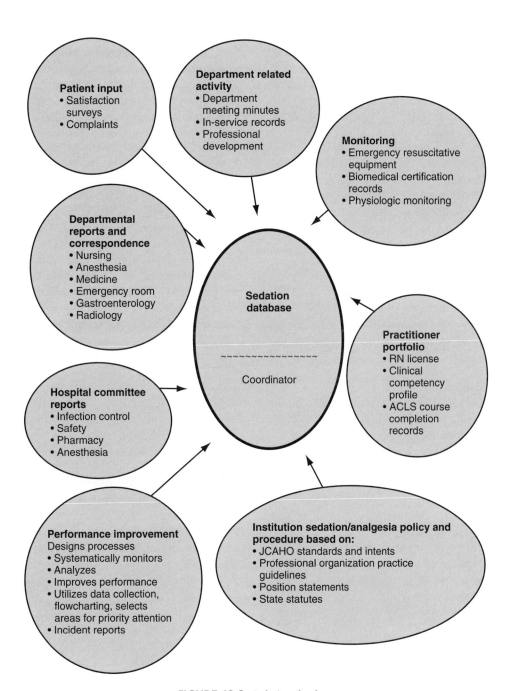

Patient input
• Satisfaction surveys
• Complaints

Department related activity
• Department meeting minutes
• In-service records
• Professional development

Monitoring
• Emergency resuscitative equipment
• Biomedical certification records
• Physiologic monitoring

Departmental reports and correspondence
• Nursing
• Anesthesia
• Medicine
• Emergency room
• Gastroenterology
• Radiology

Sedation database

~~~~~~~~~~~~~~~~

Coordinator

Practitioner portfolio
• RN license
• Clinical competency profile
• ACLS course completion records

Hospital committee reports
• Infection control
• Safety
• Pharmacy
• Anesthesia

Performance improvement
Designs processes
• Systematically monitors
• Analyzes
• Improves performance
• Utilizes data collection, flowcharting, selects areas for priority attention
• Incident reports

Institution sedation/analgesia policy and procedure based on:
• JCAHO standards and intents
• Professional organization practice guidelines
• Position statements
• State statutes

FIGURE 12-3 Sedation database.

Diagnostic, or Surgical Procedures" is featured in Appendix C. Practice standards, recommended practice guidelines, position statements, state board of nursing requirements, and facility policy and procedure must be readily available for review in every practice setting where sedation and analgesia are administered. Each practitioner in the facility must be familiar with these documents before participating in patient care.

Facilities developing or updating sedation policies must address issues that encompass:

Nursing Care

- Professional standards, practice guidelines, position statements, state statutes
- Healthcare provider credentialing and qualifications
- Medication administration, dosage guidelines, techniques of administration
- Monitoring requirements and ongoing clinical competence in monitoring patients
- Patient selection and presedation patient requirements
- Postsedation care and discharge instruction

Patient Care

- Assessment, diagnosis, and intervention
- Protocols, emergent and nonemergent
- Discharge criteria and postsedation care
- Management of procedural and postsedation complications

Institution Administrative Issues

- Professional standards, practice guidelines, position statements, state statutes
- JCAHO performance improvement
- Personnel requirements
- Scheduling practices
- Equipment and supplies
- Emergency preparedness
- Licensed independent practitioner credentialing and clinical competence demonstration

Appropriate policy development must address:
1. A statement of purpose
2. Specific policy development
3. Procedure implementation
4. Evidence of ongoing continuous quality improvement and evaluation

SEDATION DATABASE

The American Society of Anesthesiologist Sedation Model Policy is featured in Chapter 1.

Practitioner Portfolio

A clinical portfolio should be maintained on all personnel engaged in the administration of sedation and analgesia. Components of this portfolio may include the following:
- Registered nursing license or healthcare provider certifications/registrations

- Evidence of Advanced Cardiac Life Support/Basic Cardiac Life Support (ACLS/BCLS) course completion
- Clinical competence profile
- Educational in-service records
- Clinical privilege/position description

The granting of clinical privileges begins by defining the clinical position and role. Box 12-1 features a sample sedation provider position description. Prior clinical experience, educational preparation and training, and the clinical privileges outlined in Figure 12-4 may be granted with or without restriction. Maintenance of a clinical competence profile ascertains the skill level of newly assigned personnel and provides evidence of annual renewal of sedation privileges. A complete clinical competency list is presented in Appendix D.

Monitoring/Emergency Resuscitative Equipment, Biomedical Certification Records

Biomedical certification of medical equipment is recommended on a biannual basis.[7] Preventive maintenance and biomedical certification are used on monitoring and resuscitative equipment to inspect, clean, lubricate, adjust, and replace worn and damaged parts. The purpose of biomedical certification is also to ensure proper functioning of routine monitors and diagnostic and emergency resuscitative equipment. The following equipment requires routine inspection and certification:
- ECG monitors
- Noninvasive blood pressure monitor
- Pulse oximeters
- Defibrillators
- Diagnostic equipment
- Bispectral analysis or capnograph (if utilized)

Documentation and Record Keeping

It is important to maintain a separate file within the sedation database for preventive maintenance, service, and biomedical certification records. Documentation provides a written record of service performed on specific monitoring and resuscitative equipment. Information that should be recorded on the biomedical service sheet includes the following:
- Date of purchase
- Serial number
- Description of device
- Instructions for servicing
- Name, address, and telephone number of manufacturer
- Name, address, and telephone number of biomedical service company

Routine (biannual) maintenance should be documented, including service performed, parts replaced, and the name of the person servicing the equipment. Whether these tasks are performed by in-house or outsourced to biomedical individuals, accurate records must be maintained by the coordinator of the sedation database. Core components

Text continued on p. 266

BOX 12-1

Sample Sedation Provider Position Description

Job Description: Sedation Provider
Supervisor:
The healthcare provider participating in the administration of sedation/analgesia is accountable for the presedation, procedural, and postsedation care as prescribed by the policies, procedures, philosophies, and objectives of this institution. The healthcare provider engaged in the administration of sedation/analgesia works under the direct supervision of the attending physician.

Qualifications
- Graduation from an accredited school of nursing, allied health program, residency program
- ACLS/BCLS course and completion of a dysrhythmia course
- Completion of sedation educational modules as prescribed by this institution
- Hands-on practicum: airway management, monitoring modalities, emergency resuscitative procedures

Direct Patient Care
- Adheres to practice as outlined by state statutes
- Participates in presedation patient assessment
- Implements all aspects of clinical and technical care in accordance with established institution policy and procedure
- Uses universal precautions in all aspects of patient care
- Provides direct 1:1 patient care
- Provides a safe practice environment for patient care
- Uses infection-control practices to decrease the spread of nosocomial infection
- Acts as a patient advocate
- Respects the dignity and confidentiality of all patients
- Provides comprehensive transfer and discharge summary of patient care
- Provides patient education: before, during, and after the procedure

Clinical Competence
Displays clinical competence to:
- Assess the presedation, procedural, and postsedation needs of the patient
- Understand the goals and objectives of sedation/analgesia
- Monitor the patient with no other responsibility that would require the healthcare provider to leave the patient unattended or compromise continuous patient monitoring during the procedure
- Demonstrate function, interpretation, and use of resuscitative medications and monitoring equipment
- Monitor for adverse reactions and physiologic and psychologic changes associated with the administration of sedative/analgesic medications
- Document patient care where sedation/analgesia is administered
- Provide postsedation care and assessment of discharge criteria
- Request physician consultation when indicated
- Participate in the performance improvement process
- Instruct patients using adult learning theories

Leadership
Functions as a role model in:
- Patient care
- Patient education
- Communication
- Attendance

Professional Growth
Maintains a current knowledge base and professional development via:
- Participation in required educational in-service programs
- Attendance at department meetings
- Participation in professional organizations
- Participation in the personal evaluation process
- Maintains ACLS/BCLS course completion
- Shares educational information gathered at seminars with staff members
- Identifies professional and educational needs
- Contributes to organizational goals
- Supports the philosophy, objectives, and goals of the institution
- Participation in patient care, conferences, staff meetings, annual review, revision of goals and objectives, and identification of measures for cost containment

Category: Administration of Sedation-Analgesia

Personal Background Information

Name:_____

                    (Last)   (First)   (Middle Initial)

Home
Address:_____

City:_____ State:_____ Zip Code:_____

Date of Birth:_____/_____/_____ Sex: Male Female

Education:

Practitioner Education: Healthcare Program:_____

                     Date of Graduation:_____/_____/_____ Degree:_____

Additional Education: University:_____

       Address:_____

       City:_____ State:_____

Professional Clinical Experience:

Licensure: State_____ License #_____ Expires:_____

      BCLS Expiration Date: _____/_____/_____ **ACLS** Expiration Date: _____/_____/_____

Employment:

   Institution Name & Address:

      _____

      _____

   Phone Number:_____Supervisor:_____

   Dates of Employment: _____to_____ Reason for Leaving:_____

   Institution Name & Address:

      _____

      _____

   Phone Number:_____Supervisor:_____

   Dates of Employment: _____to_____ Reason for Leaving:_____

   Institution Name & Address:

      _____

      _____

   Phone Number:_____Supervisor:_____

   Dates of Employment: _____to_____ Reason for Leaving:_____

FIGURE 12-4 Application for Clinical Privileges Sedation-Analgesia Services. (© 2004, Specialty Health Education, Inc.)

Continued

References (3):_____

(Name and Address)

_____

(Name and Address)

_____

(Name and Address)

Professional Organization Memberships:

1)_____

2)_____

3)_____

<u>**Clinical Privilege Delineation**</u>

Type of Request　　□　　**Initial**　　　□　　**Annual Renewal**

Name:_____

Please check all clinical procedures for which you are applying:

□ **Presedation assessment**
□ **Intravenous access**
□ **Administration of sedation/analgesia medications listed below:**

　　　_____
　　　_____
　　　_____
　　　_____

Procedural Monitoring	**Administration of oxygen via:**
□ EKG	□ Nasal cannula
□ NIBP	□ Face mask
□ Pulse Oximetry	□ Humidified mask
□ Capnography	□ Bag valve mask
□ Level of Consciousness	

Postprocedure Management:
　　□ Postsedation monitoring
　　□ Discharge assessment
　　□ Postsedation instructions (Procedure and Sedation specific)

Management of Complications:
　　□ Cardiopulmonary resuscitative management
　　□ Respiratory resuscitation

□ Approved　　　　　　　□ With Restriction　　　　　　　□ Denied

_____　　_____
Clinical Manager　　　　　　　　　　Supervisor

Practitioner notified: _____/_____/_____

**Above clinical privileges are granted for a period of one year.

FIGURE 12-4, cont'd. For legend see opposite page.

Completed by:_____ Date of Inspection:____/____/____

Equipment Description:_____

Tag No._____ Location:_____

Next Inspection Date:_____

	OK	Service Required	Service Completed	Date	Initials
1. General Condition					
2. Line Cord, Strain Reliefs					
3. Attachment Plug					
4. Grounding Check____OHMS____					
5. AC Chassis Leakage Properly Grounded On_____ Off_____					
Ungrounded, Correct Polarity On_____ Off_____					
Ungrounded, Reversed Polarity On_____ Off_____					

Additional Information:_____
_____
_____
_____
_____

FIGURE 12-5 Biomedical certification form: AC line-powered equipment.

of a biomedical certification evaluation are identified in Figure 12-5. Service or instruction manuals for all monitoring equipment should be readily available for the clinician's use. Storage of service manuals in the purchasing department or manager's office or removal from the immediate vicinity is not recommended.

Department/Unit-Related Activity

Business and education activity related to the sedation unit must also be documented and stored in the database. Department meeting minutes, in-services, or continuing educational activities should be readily available for staff members who are not able to attend. Continuing education activity reports should be completed by staff members returning from seminars, in-services, or national meetings. This information may then be disseminated at an upcoming staff meeting and available in written form for individual review. An example of a continuing education activity report is featured in Figure 12-6. Through implementation of a brief summary report, unit personnel benefit from a variety of educational seminars and activities attended by clinicians throughout the year.

Effective department meeting strategy includes completion of old business and introduction of new business combined with a mechanism to introduce educational activities. Case reports, journal articles, and professional organization updates are easily coordinated into staff development. Management modalities to assist practitioner clinical and didactic development include the assignment of several staff

Name:

Conference Attended:

Dates of Attendance:

Speaker(s):

Date of Report:

Content of Presentation:

Relevance to Clinical Practice:

Recommendations:

☐ See attached enclosures

☐ See educational articles enclosed

FIGURE 12-6 Continuing education activity report.

members to briefly review medical journals, articles, and professional organization guidelines on a monthly basis. A condensed summary and clinical pertinence report (professional development summary) is presented at each staff meeting. Three or four professional journals pertinent to the unit's activity are reviewed monthly, with selection of appropriate topics for presentation. A professional development summary report is highlighted in Figure 12-7. Implementation of this type of program reduces time and energy expenditure while providing high-quality educational presentations. Documentation of educational activities and minutes of departmental meetings are added to the sedation database by the coordinator or designated representative.

A sample of a departmental meeting summary report is provided in Figure 12-8.

Patient Input

Results of patient satisfaction surveys or questionnaires should be summarized and entered into the database. Areas requiring improvement or those areas consistently addressed by patients require further evaluation. Patient care issues require action to avoid potential injury and improve quality of care. Intangible complaints offered by patients may be difficult to address (e.g., parking, elevators). Presedation preparation strategy should include clear communication and patient instruction. Patients must be given clear

Text continued on p. 271

Title of Article: _____ **Author:** _____

Journal: _____ **Publication Date:** __/__/____

Summary:

Clinical Significance:

Recommendations:

Actions Taken:

Submitted by: _____ **Date:** _____

FIGURE 12-7 Professional development summary report.

Date: ___/___/___

Department:

Recorder/Secretary:

Staff Members Present:

Staff Members Excused:

Meeting Called to Order: _____ AM/PM, By: _____

Old Business:

Actions Taken:

New Business:

Actions Taken:

Professional Development Summary Reports:
Presented by: _____
(See attached reports)

Meeting Adjourned: _____ AM/PM   **By:** _____

FIGURE 12-8 Department meeting summary report.

Memo #: _____

Issued by: _____

Written by: _____

Issue: _____

I have read and understand the contents of Memo #:____

Staff Members:

Name: _____   **Date:** _____   **Initials:** _____

FIGURE 12-9 Staff memo confirmation.

(preferably written) instructions for planned activities. These instructions include the following:

◆ Where to report (building/floor)
◆ What paperwork or insurance information is required
◆ Where to park
◆ What time to report

A user-friendly facility with adequate signs may reduce patient anxiety and complaints. Use of good communication skills and consideration of patient suggestions are required to enhance patient care.

Departmental Reports and Correspondence

Interdisciplinary reports and memos should be readily available for staff review. Nursing, anesthesia, emergency department, gastroenterology, radiology, and all applicable departments interacting with the sedation unit should be posted in an accessible area. Memos, meeting minutes, and reports should be initialed by staff members. A mechanism to ensure that all information has been disseminated to the appropriate personnel is presented in Figure 12-9.

Hospital Committee Reports

Reports and actions of the institution's committee structure must also be disseminated to appropriate unit personnel. A system of communication outlined in Figure 12-10 may facilitate the communication process within the sedation unit.

Performance Improvement

Performance improvement attempts to provide a systematic approach to detection and correction while at the same time improving efficiency in the care that is rendered to patients by healthcare providers. Performance improvement attempts to address all facets of the organization that affect patient outcomes.[8] Continuous performance improvement is a continuous process committed to long-term improvement in patient outcome. JCAHO requires the use of outcome indicators as a basis for quality monitoring. Use of individual specialty indicators attempts to identify deviations in quality of care. An example of indicators used in the sedation setting include:

◆ Presedation status documentation
  • Completion of presedation patient assessment
  • NPO status
  • Allergies
  • Medications
◆ Physician documentation for sedation medications
◆ Physician discharge orders
  • Evidence of postsedation monitoring
  • Satisfaction of discharge criteria
◆ Evidence of continuous monitoring
  • Procedural
  • Postsedation
◆ Documentation of adverse reactions or events

A sample performance indicator report is featured in Figure 12-11.

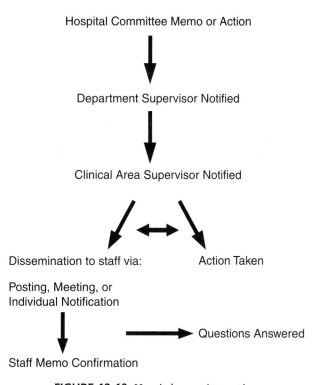

FIGURE 12-10 Hospital committee action.

Patient Identification #_____ Age:_____ Date of Service:____/___/___

Attending Physician: Procedure:

Sedation Nurse: Location:

Monitoring Indicators

A. Continuous ECG monitoring?   ☐ Yes ☐ No

B. Continuous respiratory monitoring?   ☐ Yes ☐ No

C. Continuous blood pressure monitoring?   ☐ Yes ☐ No

D. Continuous pulse oximetry monitoring?   ☐ Yes ☐ No

E. Continuous level of consciousness monitoring?   ☐ Yes ☐ No

F. Continuous patient monitoring by healthcare provider? ☐ Yes ☐ No

Presedation Indicators

☐ Presedation assessment complete

☐ Incomplete informed consent/no signature

☐ Incomplete patient chart

☐ Incomplete labwork

☐ Medical consult required

☐ Noncompliance: NPO status

☐ Noncompliance: presedation medication instructions

Procedural Indicators

☐ Respiratory depression

☐ Respiratory complication: stridor/laryngospasm/arrest

☐ Cardiovascular complications: cardiac arrest/ischemia/CHF/pulmonary edema

☐ Cardiovascular complications: hypotension/hypertension/dysrhythmias

☐ Level of consciousness: unresponsive/obtunded reflexes/agitation

☐ Medication: allergic reaction/wrong medication administered

☐ All medications administered as per facility policy

☐ Reversal agents administered (Flumazenil/Naloxone)

Postsedation Indicators

☐ Prolonged somnolence

☐ Unexpected admission secondary to sedation

☐ Additional reversal agents administered (Flumazenil/Naloxone)

☐ Nausea/Vomiting: _____ times post discharge, current status:

☐ Evidence of postsedation monitoring

☐ Documentation of discharge criteria

☐ Evidence of patient/family dissatisfaction

☐ Postsedation follow-up complete

FIGURE 12-11 Sedation: Performance indicator form. (© 2004, Specialty Health Education, Inc.)

IMPLEMENTATION OF A SEDATION EDUCATIONAL PROGRAM

The administration of sedation and analgesia is both challenging and rewarding. However, the development of a quality-sedation program and the education of clinicians engaged in the administration of sedation involve policy, educational, and operational issues.

Policy Development

As outlined in Chapter 1, policy development is required in any setting where sedation and analgesia are administered. Before inception, any good business sets forth a mission statement to outline the goals and objectives of the organization. A sedation educational program will quickly become derailed if its purpose, objectives, and expectations are not clearly delineated (Box 12-2). Once a mission statement has been established, the scope of services must be delineated. A sedation program scope of services is outlined in Figure 12-12.

As outlined earlier, sedation policies and procedures, practice standards, recommended practice guidelines, position statements, mission statement, and scope of services must be readily available for clinician review in all patient care areas. As outlined in Chapter 1, policy and procedure development must address the following:

- Definitions, goals, objectives
- Presedation patient assessment
- Patient selection criteria
- Monitoring requirements and clinician responsibility
- Methods of recording patient data
- Frequency of patient documentation
- Medications that may be administered by the healthcare provider
- Treatment of complications
- Discharge criteria
- Postsedation instructions

> Policy and procedures must clearly delineate lines of responsibility and accountability. The interdisciplinary development of sedation policy and procedure should attempt to reduce risk factors, provide the highest-quality patient care, and ensure the same level of care throughout the institution.

BOX 12-2

Sedation Setting Purpose, Goals, Objectives Mission Statement

The mission of the sedation program at _____ and the clinicians engaged in the administration of sedation/analgesia in this facility is to provide the highest quality medical care. We will continually attempt to improve the level of care which we provide through clinical service and education. We will develop a system in which the administration of sedation/analgesia services are provided in a stable and supportive environment. Sedation/analgesia will be administered in accordance with practice standards, recommended practice guidelines, professional organization position statements, regulatory agency guidelines, and state statutes.

Sedation Setting Continuing Education Goals, Objectives, and Expectations

I. Purpose
The purpose of the continuing education program is to provide a mechanism for clinical case conference, research, and new product information dissemination to all staff involved in the procedural care of patients receiving sedation/analgesia.

II. Learning Objectives
At the conclusion of the program, participants will:
- Demonstrate an awareness of available literature pertinent to sedation/analgesia.
- Discuss current trends and changes in the administration of sedation/analgesia and care of patients receiving sedation services.
- Demonstrate clear evaluation and review of current literature.
- Discuss scientific principles related to a variety of clinical case scenarios.
- Discuss challenging questions and relate them to the role of performance improvement and risk reduction strategy.
- Present a concise, accurate report and lead a group discussion when applicable.

III. Teaching Methods
Teaching methods include:
- Lecture
- Discussion
- Slides
- Handouts
- Authorized reprints
- Clinical case management synopsis

Department: Sedation Unit

☐ GI Laboratory   ☐ Radiology   ☐ Emergency Room   ☐ ICU/CCU

☐ Operating Room   ☐ Physician's Office   ☐ Short Procedure Unit   ☐ Interventional Radiology

Services Provided: The_____ unit is engaged in the administration of sedation/analgesia to provide a reduced state of anxiety for minor surgical, therapeutic, or diagnostic procedures.

1. Types and ages of patients served (ages, patient groups, frequent diagnostic categories, etc.).
   Sedation/analgesia services will be afforded to all patients within this facility with the exception of (*applicable exceptions*). Clinical services are available for all minor surgical or diagnostic procedures with the exception of (*applicable exceptions*).

2. Methods used to assess and meet patients' care needs (How are patient care or service needs identified and how are they met?):
   Methods used to assess and meet patient needs include:
   - Presedation assessment
   - Procedural monitoring
   - Selection of appropriate pharmacologic medications based on patient assessment
   - Provision of postsedation monitoring, discharge information, and follow-up

3. Scope and complexity of patients' care needs (diagnosis, conditions, etc.):
   The scope of care is dependent on presedation patient assessment, diagnostic or surgical procedure, patient reaction to pharmacologic medications, and recovery from the residual effects of sedatives.

4. Appropriateness, clinical necessity, and timeliness of service provided.
   The appropriateness, clinical necessity, and timeliness of services are provided through periodic review. Mechanisms of review include:
   - Medical chart review
   - Participation in continuous performance-improvement process
   - Management of a risk-management database coordinated by (*individual's name*)

5. Availability of necessary staff (staffing model/assignment methodology, hours of operation, needs related to credentials, age-specific competence, continuing education, etc.):
   Sedation services are provided on a 1:1 basis. Patients will be continuously monitored during the procedure and in the postsedation period.

   Hours of operation: _____ to _____

   On call services are available.

   The following competencies will be evaluated on an annual basis:
   - Knowledge of the goals and objectives of conscious sedation
   - ACLS/BCLS course completion
   - ECG rhythm interpretation
   - Airway evaluation and resuscitation
   - Mechanism of actions; treatment of adverse reactions associated with the administration of sedatives, hypnotics, and narcotics
   - Intravenous insertion skills
   - Sedation/analgesia annual education module examination

   Continuing education and clinical competency records outlined above are maintained in an individual practitioner portfolio. Continuing education in-services are based on patient population, staff needs, technologic advances, and performance appraisals. *Annual competency validation.*

FIGURE 12-12 Scope of service: Clinical departments. (©2004 Specialty Health Education, Inc.)

Continued

6. Extent to which the level of service or care provided meets the patient's needs (treatments, procedures and/or activities provided, patient satisfaction):

The sedation unit (Department of _____) is a _____ bed unit which provides sedation/analgesia for short diagnostic and minor surgical procedures. Patients are provided the highest quality of medical care as promulgated by practice standards, professional organization recommended practice guidelines, position statements, regulatory agencies, and state statutes. Patient satisfaction is assessed via a discharge patient satisfaction survey reviewed by management.

Department Goals for Patient Care:
• Continue to provide the highest medical care to the patient population
• Enhance patient teaching
• Implement programs to improve patient satisfaction

Written: _____ /_____ /_____

Revised: _____ /_____ /_____

FIGURE 12-12, cont'd. For legend see opposite page.

Education

Once the goals and objectives of a sedation program have been outlined, implementation of the service is accomplished through education. Identification of problems that obstruct these goals may include the following:

◆ ACLS training
◆ Interpretation of ECGs and completion of a dysrhythmia course
◆ Pharmacologic education
◆ Personnel requirements
◆ Clinical competency of sedation providers
◆ Provision of monitoring and resuscitative equipment

In an effort to ensure quality patient care, problem areas must be addressed and rectified to the satisfaction of regulatory agencies and state law. Use of a multidisciplinary approach includes education related to presedation, procedural, and postsedation patient care.

SUMMARY

As emphasized throughout this text, identification of variables that affect sedation services, staff education, and patient care issues must be addressed as core components of a sedation program. Policy development, which addresses presedation patient assessment, monitoring, administration of pharmacologic agents, postsedation patient care, and performance improvement methodologies enhances patient care. Credentialing of clinical competencies provides clinicians with the confidence to rapidly assess, diagnose, and intervene when providing sedation services.

> Through proper training and education, the sedation clinician remains confident in his or her ability to effectively stabilize the patient and provide resuscitative care until additional assistance becomes available.

LEARNER SELF-ASSESSMENT

In order to achieve maximal educational benefit from this chapter, please complete the Learner Self-Assessment below. This self-assessment tool provides the learner with the ability to identify areas requiring additional review. Reference material for each question is provided in Appendix F.

1. Healthcare practitioner considerations associated with **JCAHO Standards** related to performance improvement and sedation patient care include:

2. *Quality* is defined as:

3. **Risk reduction strategies to improve sedation** patient care include:

4. **Components of a "sedation" database** applicable to your practice setting include:

5. **Mechanisms utilized in the successful implementation of a sedation educational program** include:

POST-TEST QUESTIONS

Please note: If you are applying for CE credit, you must contact Specialty Health Education, Inc. @ 800-694-8041 for a CE Application Packet.

1. The comprehensive positive outcome of a product is broadly defined as _____.
   A. Excellence
   B. Continuous quality improvement
   C. Risk management
   D. Quality

2. To prevent or reduce the development of adverse events in the sedation setting, sedation units must ensure that they _____.
   A. Screen all patients at least 1 week in advance
   B. Administer only benzodiazepines and opioids to the sedation patient
   C. Participate in risk-reduction strategies
   D. Conduct telephone follow-up with all patients

3. Registered nursing license, ACLS status, and clinical competency profile are components of the _____.
   A. Departmental reports
   B. Continuous quality improvement activity
   C. Practitioner portfolio
   D. Hospital activity reports

4. The ability to assess the presedation, procedural, and postsedation needs of the patient is delineated as _____ in a sedation nurses position description.
   A. Qualifications
   B. Leadership
   C. Professional growth
   D. Clinical competencies

5. Biomedical equipment maintenance is recommended _____.
   A. Monthly
   B. Bimonthly
   C. Quarterly
   D. Biannually

6. The process of _____ attempts to provide a systematic approach to detection and correction while at the same time improving efficiency in the care that is rendered to patients by healthcare providers.
   A. Performance improvement
   B. Leadership
   C. Quality achievement
   D. Information dissemination

7. Examples of continuous quality indicators used in sedation practice include all of the following except _____.
   A. Presedation patient assessment
   B. Monitoring modalities utilized
   C. Patient arrival time
   D. Documentation of adverse reactions

8. Administration of flumazenil (Romazicon) or naloxone (Narcan) to pharmacologically reverse emergent arterial desaturation during a colonoscopy with biopsy should constitute a _____ indicator during retrospective chart review.
   A. Presedation
   B. Procedural
   C. Monitoring
   D. Postsedation

9. Sedation policies and procedures, mission statement, and clinical scope of services _____.
   A. Must be developed separately with no overlap
   B. Are only to be developed by administrators
   C. Require patient input
   D. Must be readily available in all patient care areas where sedation is administered

10. Identification of types and ages of patients served and methods used to assess and meet patient care needs, scope, complexity, and timeliness of services performed for a given sedation location are comprehensively outlined in the practice setting's _____.
    A. Mission statement
    B. Presedation patient instructions
    C. Clinical department scope of services
    D. Hospital handbook

REFERENCES

1. Graham N. *Quality Assurance in Hospitals: Strategies for Assessment and Implementation.* Rockville, MD: Aspen; 1990.
2. Gillen TR. Deming's 14 points and hospital quality: Responding to the consumer's demand for the best value health care. *J Nurs Qual Assur.* 1988;2:70-78.
3. Joint Commission on Accreditation of Healthcare Organizations (JCAHO). *Accreditation Manual for Hospitals.* Oak Terrace, IL: JCAHO; 1997.
4. Foster S, Callahan M. *A Professional Study and Resource Guide for the CRNA.* Park Ridge, IL: American Association of Nurse Anesthetists; 2001:504.
5. Lang N, Marek K. Quality assurance: The foundation of professional care. *J NY State Nurs Assoc.* 1995;26(1):48-50.
6. Joint Commission on Accreditation of Healthcare Organizations (JCAHO). *Accreditation Manual for Hospitals.* Oak Terrace, IL: JCAHO Performance Improvement. CAMH, Update 3, August, 1998.
7. Dorsch J. *Understanding Anesthesia Equipment.* 4th ed. Baltimore: Williams & Wilkins; 2000.
8. Koch MW, Fairley TM. *Integrated Quality Management.* St. Louis: Mosby; 1993.

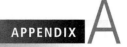

Practice Guidelines for Sedation and Analgesia by Non-Anesthesiologists

(Approved by the House of Delegates on October 25, 1995, and last amended on October 17, 2001)
An Updated Report by the American Society of Anesthesiologists Task Force on Sedation and Analgesia by Non-Anesthesiologists

Developed by the American Society of Anesthesiologists Task Force on Sedation and Analgesia by Non-Anesthesiologists:
Jeffrey B. Gross, M.D. (Chair), Farmington, CT
Peter L. Bailey, M.D., Rochester, NY
Richard T. Connis, Ph.D., Woodinville, WA
Charles J. Coté, M.D., Chicago, IL
Fred G. Davis, M.D., Burlington, MA
Burton S. Epstein, M.D., Washington, DC
Lesley Gilbertson, M.D., Boston, MA

David G. Nickinovich, Ph.D., Bellevue, WA
John M. Zerwas, M.D., Houston, TX
Gregory Zuccaro, Jr., M.D., Cleveland, OH
Correspondence to:
Jeffrey B. Gross, M.D.
Department of Anesthesiology (M/C 2015)
University of Connecticut School of Medicine
Farmington, CT 06030-2015

Supported by the American Society of Anesthesiologists under the direction of James F. Arens, M.D., Chairman, Committee on Practice Parameters. Approved by the House of Delegates, October 17, 2001. A list of the references used to develop these guidelines is available by writing to the American Society of Anesthesiologists.

Reprint Requests to: American Society of Anesthesiologists, 520 N. Northwest Highway, Park Ridge, IL 60068-2573.

Key Words: Conscious sedation; deep sedation; analgesia; practice guidelines; propofol; ketamine

Abbreviated Title: Practice Guidelines for Sedation and Analgesia

Introduction

Anesthesiologists possess specific expertise in the pharmacology, physiology, and clinical management of patients receiving sedation and analgesia. For this reason, they are frequently called upon to participate in the development of institutional policies and procedures for sedation and analgesia for diagnostic and therapeutic procedures. To assist in this process, the American Society of Anesthesiologists has developed these **Guidelines for Sedation and Analgesia by Non-Anesthesiologists.**

Practice guidelines are systematically developed recommendations that assist the practitioner and patient in making decisions about health care. These recommendations may be adopted, modified, or rejected according to clinical needs and constraints. Practice guidelines are not intended as standards or absolute requirements. The use of practice guidelines cannot guarantee any specific outcome. Practice guidelines are subject to revision as warranted by the evolution of medical knowledge, technology, and practice. The guidelines provide basic recommendations that are supported by analysis of the current literature and by a synthesis of expert opinion, open forum commentary, and clinical feasibility data.

This revision includes data published since the Guidelines for Sedation and Analgesia by Non-Anesthesiologists were adopted by the American Society of Anesthesiologists in 1995; it also includes data and recommendations for a wider range of sedation levels than was previously addressed.

A. Definitions

"Sedation and analgesia" comprise a continuum of states ranging from **Minimal Sedation (Anxiolysis)** through **General Anesthesia**. Definitions of levels of sedation/analgesia, as developed and adopted by the American Society of Anesthesiologists, are given in Table A-1. These guidelines specifically apply to levels of sedation corresponding to **Moderate Sedation (frequently called "Conscious Sedation")** and **Deep Sedation,** as defined in Table A-1.

B. Focus

These guidelines are designed to be applicable to procedures performed in a variety of settings (e.g., hospitals, freestanding

TABLE A-1

Continuum of Depth of Sedation
Definition of General Anesthesia and Levels of Sedation/Analgesia

	MINIMAL SEDATION ("ANXIOLYSIS")	MODERATE SEDATION/ANALGESIA ("CONSCIOUS SEDATION")	DEEP SEDATION/ANALGESIA	GENERAL ANESTHESIA
Responsiveness	Normal response to verbal stimulation	Purposeful* response to verbal or tactile stimulation	Purposeful* response following repeated or painful stimulation	Unarousable, even with painful stimulus
Airway	Unaffected	No intervention required	Intervention may be required	Intervention often required
Spontaneous Ventilation	Unaffected	Adequate	May be inadequate	Frequently inadequate
Cardiovascular Function	Unaffected	Usually maintained	Usually maintained	May be impaired

Minimal Sedation (Anxiolysis) is a drug-induced state during which patients respond normally to verbal commands. Although cognitive function and coordination may be impaired, ventilatory and cardiovascular functions are unaffected.

Moderate Sedation/Analgesia ("Conscious Sedation") is a drug-induced depression of consciousness during which patients respond purposefully* to verbal commands, either alone or accompanied by light tactile stimulation. No interventions are required to maintain a patent airway, and spontaneous ventilation is adequate. Cardiovascular function is usually maintained.

Deep Sedation/Analgesia is a drug-induced depression of consciousness during which patients cannot be easily aroused but respond purposefully* following repeated or painful stimulation. The ability to independently maintain ventilatory function may be impaired. Patients may require assistance in maintaining a patent airway, and spontaneous ventilation may be inadequate. Cardiovascular function is usually maintained.

General Anesthesia is a drug-induced loss of consciousness during which patients are not arousable, even by painful stimulation. The ability to independently maintain ventilatory function is often impaired. Patients often require assistance in maintaining a patent airway, and positive pressure ventilation may be required because of depressed spontaneous ventilation or drug-induced depression of neuromuscular function. Cardiovascular function may be impaired.

Because sedation is a continuum, it is not always possible to predict how an individual patient will respond. Hence, practitioners intending to produce a given level of sedation should be able to rescue patients whose level of sedation becomes deeper than initially intended. Individuals administering **Moderate Sedation/Analgesia ("Conscious Sedation")** should be able to rescue patients who enter a state of **Deep Sedation/Analgesia,** while those administering **Deep Sedation/Analgesia** should be able to rescue patients who enter a state of general anesthesia.

*Reflex withdrawal from a painful stimulus is NOT considered a purposeful response.
Developed by the American Society of Anesthesiologists; approved by ASA House of Delegates on October 13, 1999.

clinics, physician, dentist, and other offices) by practitioners who are not specialists in anesthesiology. Because **Minimal Sedation ("Anxiolysis")** entails minimal risk, the guidelines specifically exclude it. Examples of **Minimal Sedation** include peripheral nerve blocks, local or topical anesthesia and either (1) less than 50% N_2O in O_2 with no other sedative or analgesic medications by any route, or (2) a single, oral sedative or analgesic medication administered in doses appropriate for the unsupervised treatment of insomnia, anxiety or pain. The guidelines also exclude patients who are not undergoing a diagnostic or therapeutic procedure (e.g., postoperative analgesia, sedation for treatment of insomnia). Finally, the guidelines do not apply to patients receiving general or major conduction anesthesia (e.g., spinal or epidural/caudal block), whose care should be provided, medically directed, or supervised by an anesthesiologist, the operating practitioner, or another licensed physician with specific training in sedation, anesthesia, and rescue techniques appropriate to the type of sedation or anesthesia being provided.

C. Purpose

The purpose of these guidelines is to allow clinicians to provide their patients with the benefits of sedation/analgesia while minimizing the associated risks. Sedation/analgesia provides two general types of benefit: First, sedation/analgesia allows patients to tolerate unpleasant procedures by relieving anxiety, discomfort, or pain. Second, in children and uncooperative adults, sedation/analgesia may expedite the conduct of procedures which are not particularly uncomfortable but which require that the patient not move. At times these sedation practices may result in cardiac or respiratory depression which must be rapidly recognized and appropriately managed to avoid the risk of hypoxic brain damage, cardiac arrest, or death. Conversely, inadequate sedation/analgesia may result in undue patient discomfort or patient injury because of lack of cooperation or adverse physiological or psychological response to stress.

D. Application

These guidelines are intended to be general in their application and broad in scope. The appropriate choice of agents and techniques for sedation/analgesia is dependent upon the experience and preference of the individual practitioner, requirements or constraints imposed by the patient or procedure, and the likelihood of producing a deeper level of sedation than anticipated. Because it is not always possible to predict how a specific patient will respond to sedative and analgesic medications, practitioners intending to produce a given level of sedation should be able to rescue patients whose level of sedation becomes deeper than initially intended. For moderate sedation, this implies the ability to manage a compromised airway or hypoventilation in a patient *who responds purposefully* following repeated or painful stimulation, while for deep sedation, this implies the ability to manage respiratory or cardiovascular instability in a patient *who does not respond purposefully* to painful or repeated stimulation. Levels of sedation referred to in the recommendations relate to the level of sedation intended by the practitioner. Examples are provided to illustrate airway assessment, preoperative fasting, emergency equipment, and recovery procedures. However, clinicians and their institutions have ultimate responsibility for selecting patients, procedures, medications, and equipment.

E. Task Force Members and Consultants

The ASA appointed a Task Force of 10 members to (a) review the published evidence; (b) obtain the opinion of a panel of consultants including non-anesthesiologist physicians and dentists who routinely administer sedation/analgesia as well as of anesthesiologists with a special interest in sedation/analgesia (see appendix I); and (c) build consensus within the community of practitioners likely to be affected by the guidelines. The Task Force included anesthesiologists in both private and academic practices from various geographic areas of the United States, a gastroenterologist, and methodologists from the ASA Committee on Practice Parameters.

This Practice Guideline is an update and revision of the ASA *Guidelines for Sedation and Analgesia by Non-Anesthesiologists.*[1] The Task Force revised and updated the Guidelines by means of a five-step process. First, original published research studies relevant to the revision and update were reviewed and analyzed; only articles relevant to the administration of sedation by non-anesthesiologists were evaluated. Second, the panel of expert consultants was asked to (a) participate in a survey related to the effectiveness and safety of various methods and interventions which might be used during sedation/analgesia, and (b) review and comment upon the initial draft report of the Task Force. Third, the Task Force held Open Forums at two major national meetings to solicit input on its draft recommendations. National organizations representing most of the specialties whose members typically administer sedation/analgesia were invited to send representatives. Fourth, the consultants were surveyed to assess their opinions on the feasibility and financial implications of implementing the revised and updated Guidelines. Finally, all of the available information was used by the Task Force to finalize the Guidelines.

F. Availability and Strength of Evidence

Evidence-based guidelines are developed by a rigorous analytic process. To assist the reader, the Guidelines make use of several descriptive terms that are easier to understand than the technical terms and data that are used in the actual analyses. These descriptive terms are defined below.

The following terms describe the *strength* of scientific data obtained from the scientific literature:

Supportive: There is sufficient quantitative information from adequately designed studies to describe a statistically significant relationship ($P<0.01$) between a clinical intervention and a clinical outcome, using the technique of meta-analysis.

Suggestive: There is enough information from case reports and descriptive studies to provide a directional assessment of the relationship between a clinical intervention and a clinical outcome. This type of qualitative information does not permit a statistical assessment of significance.

Equivocal: Qualitative data have not provided a clear direction for clinical outcomes related to a clinical intervention and (1) there is insufficient quantitative information or (2) aggregated comparative studies have found no quantitatively significant differences among groups or conditions.

The following terms describe the lack of available scientific evidence in the literature:

Inconclusive: Published studies are available, but they cannot be used to assess the relationship between a clinical intervention and a clinical outcome because the studies either do not meet predefined criteria for content as defined in the "Focus of the Guidelines" or do not provide a clear causal interpretation of findings due to research design or analytic concerns.

Insufficient: There are too few published studies to investigate a relationship between a clinical intervention and clinical outcome.

Silent: No studies that address a relationship of interest were found in the available published literature.

The following terms describe survey responses from the consultants for any specified issue. Responses were solicited on a 5-point scale; ranging from "1" (strongly disagree) to "5" (strongly agree) with a score of "3" being neutral.

Strongly Agree: Median score of "5" (At least 50% of the responses were "5")

Agree: Median score of "4" (At least 50% of the responses were "4" or "5")

Equivocal: Median score of "3" (At least 50% of the scores were "3" or less)

Disagree: Median score of "2" (At least 50% of responses were "1" or "2")

Strongly Disagree: Median score of "1" (At least 50% of responses were "1")

Guidelines

1. Patient Evaluation

There is insufficient published evidence to evaluate the relationship between sedation/analgesia outcomes and the performance of a preoperative patient evaluation. There is suggestive evidence that some pre-existing medical conditions may be related to adverse outcomes in patients receiving either moderate or deep sedation/analgesia. The consultants strongly agree that appropriate pre-procedure evaluation (history, physical examination) increases the likelihood of satisfactory sedation and decreases the likelihood of adverse outcomes for both moderate and deep sedation.

Recommendations: Clinicians administering sedation/analgesia should be familiar with sedation-oriented aspects of the patient's medical history and how these might alter the patient's response to sedation/analgesia. These include: (1) abnormalities of the major organ systems; (2) previous adverse experience with sedation/analgesia as well as regional and general anesthesia; (3) drug allergies, current medications and potential drug interactions; (4) time and nature of last oral intake; and (5) history of tobacco, alcohol or substance use or abuse. Patients presenting for sedation/analgesia should undergo a focused physical examination including vital signs, auscultation of the heart and lungs, and evaluation of the airway. (Refer to Box A-1 for Example I.) Pre-procedure laboratory testing should be guided by the patient's underlying medical condition and the likelihood that the results will affect the management of sedation/analgesia. These evaluations should be confirmed immediately before sedation is initiated.

BOX A-1

Example I: Airway Assessment Procedures for Sedation and Analgesia

Positive pressure ventilation, with or without tracheal intubation, may be necessary if respiratory compromise develops during sedation/analgesia. This may be more difficult in patients with atypical airway anatomy. Also, some airway abnormalities may increase the likelihood of airway obstruction during spontaneous ventilation. Some factors which may be associated with difficulty in airway management are:

History
Previous problems with anesthesia or sedation
Stridor, snoring, or sleep apnea
Advanced rheumatoid arthritis
Chromosomal abnormality (e.g., trisomy 21)

Physical Examination
Habitus: Significant obesity (especially involving the neck and facial structures)
Head and Neck: Short neck, limited neck extension, decreased hyoid-mental distance (<3 cm in an adult), neck mass, cervical spine disease or trauma, tracheal deviation, dysmorphic facial features (e.g., Pierre-Robin syndrome)
Mouth: Small opening (<3 cm in an adult); edentulous; protruding incisors; loose or capped teeth; dental appliances; high, arched palate; macroglossia; tonsillar hypertrophy; non-visible uvula
Jaw: Micrognathia, retrognathia, trismus, significant malocclusion

---

2. Pre-procedure Preparation

The literature is insufficient regarding the benefits of providing the patient (or her/his guardian, in the case of a child or impaired adult) with pre-procedure information about sedation and analgesia. For moderate sedation the consultants agree and for deep sedation the consultants strongly agree that appropriate pre-procedure counseling of patients regarding risks, benefits, and alternatives to sedation and analgesia increases patient satisfaction.

Sedatives and analgesics tend to impair airway reflexes in proportion to the degree of sedation/analgesia achieved. This dependence on level of sedation is reflected in the consultants' opinion: They agree that pre-procedure fasting decreases risks during moderate sedation, while strongly agreeing that it decreases the risk of deep sedation. In emergency situations, when pre-procedure fasting is not practical, the consultants agree that the target level of sedation should be modified (i.e., less sedation should be administered) for moderate sedation, while strongly agreeing that it should be modified for deep sedation. The literature does not provide sufficient evidence to test the hypothesis that pre-procedure fasting results in a decreased incidence of adverse outcomes in patients undergoing either moderate or deep sedation.

Recommendations: Patients (or their legal guardians in the case of minors or legally incompetent adults) should be informed of and agree to the administration of sedation/analgesia including the benefits, risks, and limitations associated with this therapy, as well as possible alternatives. Patients undergoing sedation/analgesia for elective procedures should not drink fluids or eat solid foods for a sufficient period of time to allow for gastric emptying prior to their procedure, as recommended by the American Society of Anesthesiologists "Guidelines for Preoperative Fasting."[2] (Refer to Box A-2 for Example II.) In urgent, emergent, or other situations where gastric emptying is impaired, the potential for pulmonary aspiration of gastric contents must be considered in determining (1) the target level of sedation, (2) whether the procedure should be delayed or (3) whether the trachea should be protected by intubation.

3. Monitoring

Level of consciousness: The response of patients to commands during procedures performed with sedation/analgesia serves as a guide to their level of consciousness. Spoken responses also provide an indication that the patients are breathing. Patients whose only response is reflex withdrawal from painful stimuli are deeply sedated, approaching a state of general anesthesia, and should be treated accordingly. The literature is silent regarding whether monitoring patients' level of consciousness improves patient outcomes or decreases risks. The consultants strongly agree that monitoring level of consciousness reduces risks for both moderate and deep sedation. The members of the Task Force believe that many of the complications associated with sedation and analgesia can be avoided if adverse drug responses are detected and treated in a timely manner (i.e., prior to the

BOX A-2

Example II: Summary of American Society of Anesthesiologists Pre-Procedure Fasting Guidelines[1]

Ingested Material[1]	Minimum Fasting Period[2]
Clear liquids[3]	2 h
Breast milk	4 h
Infant formula	6 h
Non-human milk[4]	6 h
Light meal[5]	6 h

[1]These recommendations apply to healthy patients who are undergoing elective procedures. They are not intended for women in labor. Following the guidelines does not guarantee a complete gastric emptying has occurred.

[2]The fasting periods noted above apply to all ages.

[3]Examples of clear liquids include water, fruit juices without pulp, carbonated beverages, clear tea, and black coffee.

[4]Since non-human milk is similar to solids in gastric emptying time, the amount ingested must be considered when determining an appropriate fasting period.

[5]A light meal typically consists of toast and clear liquids. Meals that include fried or fatty foods or meat may prolong gastric emptying time. Both the amount and type of foods ingested must be considered when determining an appropriate fasting period.

development of cardiovascular decompensation or cerebral hypoxia). Patients given sedatives and/or analgesics in unmonitored settings in anticipation of a subsequent procedure may be at increased risk of these complications.

Pulmonary ventilation: It is the opinion of the Task Force that the primary causes of morbidity associated with sedation/analgesia are drug-induced respiratory depression and airway obstruction. For both moderate and deep sedation, the literature is insufficient to evaluate the benefit of monitoring ventilatory function by observation or auscultation. However, the consultants strongly agree that monitoring of ventilatory function by observation or auscultation reduces the risk of adverse outcomes associated with sedation/analgesia. The consultants were equivocal regarding the ability of capnography to decrease risks during moderate sedation, while agreeing that it may decrease risks during deep sedation. In circumstances where patients are physically separated from the care giver, the Task Force believes that automated apnea monitoring (by detection of exhaled CO_2 or other means) may decrease risks during both moderate and deep sedation, while cautioning practitioners that impedance plethysmography may fail to detect airway obstruction. The Task Force emphasizes that because ventilation and oxygenation are separate though related physiological processes, monitoring oxygenation by pulse oximetry is not a substitute for monitoring ventilatory function.

Oxygenation: Published data suggest that oximetry effectively detects oxygen desaturation and hypoxemia in patients who are administered sedatives/analgesics. The consultants strongly agree that early detection of hypoxemia through the use of oximetry during sedation/analgesia decreases the likelihood of adverse outcomes such as cardiac arrest and death. The Task Force agrees that hypoxemia during sedation and analgesia is more likely to be detected by oximetry than by clinical assessment alone.

Hemodynamics: Although there are insufficient published data to reach a conclusion, it is the opinion of the Task Force that sedative and analgesic agents may blunt the appropriate autonomic compensation for hypovolemia and procedure-related stresses. On the other hand, if sedation and analgesia are inadequate, patients may develop potentially harmful autonomic stress responses (e.g., hypertension, tachycardia). Early detection of changes in patients' heart rate and blood pressure may enable practitioners to detect problems and intervene in a timely fashion, reducing the risk of these complications. The consultants strongly agree that regular monitoring of vital signs reduces the likelihood of adverse outcomes during both moderate and deep sedation. For both moderate and deep sedation, a majority of the consultants indicated that vital signs should be monitored at 5-minute intervals once a stable level of sedation is established. The consultants strongly agree that continuous electrocardiography reduces risks during deep sedation, while they were equivocal regarding its effect during moderate sedation. However, the Task Force believes that electrocardiographic monitoring of selected individuals (e.g., patients with significant cardiovascular disease or dysrhythmias) may decrease risks during moderate sedation.

Recommendations: Monitoring of patient response to verbal commands should be routine during moderate sedation, except in patients who are unable to respond appropriately (e.g., young children, mentally impaired or uncooperative patients), or during procedures where movement could be detrimental. During deep sedation, patient responsiveness to a more profound stimulus should be sought, unless contraindicated, to ensure that the patient has not drifted into a state of general anesthesia. During procedures where a verbal response is not possible (e.g., oral surgery, upper endoscopy), the ability to give a "thumbs up" or other indication of consciousness in response to verbal or tactile (light tap) stimulation suggests that the patient will be able to control his airway and take deep breaths if necessary, corresponding to a state of moderate sedation. Note that a response limited to reflex withdrawal from a painful stimulus is **not** considered a purposeful response and thus represents a state of general anesthesia.

All patients undergoing sedation/analgesia should be monitored by pulse oximetry with appropriate alarms. If available, the variable pitch "beep," which gives a continuous audible indication of the oxygen saturation reading, may be helpful. In addition, ventilatory function should be continually monitored by observation and/or auscultation. Monitoring of exhaled CO_2 should be considered for all patients receiving deep sedation and for patients whose ventilation cannot be directly observed during moderate sedation. When possible, blood pressure should be determined before sedation/analgesia is initiated. Once sedation/analgesia is established, blood pressure should be measured at 5-minute intervals during the procedure, unless such monitoring interferes with the procedure (e.g., pediatric MRI where stimulation from the BP cuff could arouse an appropriately sedated patient). Electrocardiographic monitoring should be used in all patients undergoing deep sedation; it should also be used during moderate sedation in patients with significant cardiovascular disease or those who are undergoing procedures where dysrhythmias are anticipated.

4. Recording of Monitored Parameters

The literature is silent regarding the benefits of contemporaneous recording of patients' level of consciousness, respiratory function or hemodynamics. Consultant opinion agrees with the use of contemporaneous recording for moderate sedation and strongly agrees with its use for patients undergoing deep sedation. It is the consensus of the Task Force that unless technically precluded (e.g., uncooperative or combative patient) vital signs and respiratory variables should be recorded before initiating sedation/analgesia, after administration of sedative/analgesic medications, at regular intervals during the procedure, upon initiation of recovery, and immediately before discharge. It is the opinion of the Task Force that contemporaneous recording (either automatic or manual) of patient data may disclose trends which could prove critical in determining the development or cause of adverse events. Additionally, manual recording ensures that an individual caring for the patient is aware of changes in patient status in a timely fashion.

Recommendations: For both moderate and deep sedation, patients' level of consciousness, ventilatory and oxygenation status, and hemodynamic variables should be assessed and recorded at a frequency which depends upon the type and amount of medication administered, the length of the procedure, and the general condition of the patient. At a minimum, this should be: (1) before the beginning of the procedure; (2) following administration of sedative/analgesic agents; (3) at regular intervals during the procedure; (4) during initial recovery; and (5) just before discharge. If recording is performed automatically, device alarms should be set to alert the care team to critical changes in patient status.

5. Availability of an Individual Responsible for Patient Monitoring

Although the literature is silent on this issue, the Task Force recognizes that it may not be possible for the individual performing a procedure to be fully cognizant of the patient's condition during sedation/analgesia. For moderate sedation, the consultants agree that the availability of an individual other than the person performing the procedure to monitor the patient's status improves patient comfort and satisfaction and that risks are reduced. For deep sedation, the

consultants strongly agree with these contentions. During moderate sedation, the consultants strongly agree that the individual monitoring the patient may assist the practitioner with interruptible ancillary tasks of short duration; during deep sedation, the consultants agree that this individual should have no other responsibilities.

Recommendations: A designated individual, other than the practitioner performing the procedure, should be present to monitor the patient throughout procedures performed with sedation/analgesia. During deep sedation, this individual should have no other responsibilities. However, during moderate sedation, this individual may assist with minor, interruptible tasks once the patient's level of sedation/analgesia and vital signs have stabilized, provided that adequate monitoring for the patient's level of sedation is maintained.

6. Training of Personnel

Although the literature is silent regarding the effectiveness of training on patient outcomes, the consultants strongly agree that education and training in the pharmacology of agents commonly used during sedation/analgesia improves the likelihood of satisfactory sedation and reduces the risk of adverse outcomes from either moderate or deep sedation. Specific concerns may include: (1) potentiation of sedative-induced respiratory depression by concomitantly administered opioids; (2) inadequate time intervals between doses of sedative or analgesic agents resulting in a cumulative overdose; and (3) inadequate familiarity with the role of pharmacological antagonists for sedative and analgesic agents.

Because the primary complications of sedation/analgesia are related to respiratory or cardiovascular depression, it is the consensus of the Task Force that the individual responsible for monitoring the patient should be trained in the recognition of complications associated with sedation/analgesia. Because sedation/analgesia constitute a continuum, practitioners administering moderate sedation should be able to rescue patients who enter a state of deep sedation, while those intending to administer deep sedation should be able to rescue patients who enter a state of general anesthesia. Therefore, the consultants strongly agree that at least one qualified individual trained in basic life support skills (CPR, bag-valve-mask ventilation) should be present in the procedure room during both moderate and deep sedation. In addition, the consultants strongly agree with the immediate availability (1-5 minutes away) of an individual with advanced life support skills (e.g., tracheal intubation, defibrillation, use of resuscitation medications) for moderate sedation and *in the procedure room* itself for deep sedation.

Recommendations: Individuals responsible for patients receiving sedation/analgesia should understand the pharmacology of the agents that are administered, as well as the role of pharmacologic antagonists for opioids and benzodiazepines. Individuals monitoring patients receiving sedation/analgesia should be able to recognize the associated complications. At least one individual capable of establishing a patent airway and positive-pressure ventilation, as well as a means for summoning additional assistance should be present whenever sedation/analgesia are administered. It is recommended that an individual with advanced life support skills be immediately available (within 5 minutes) for moderate sedation and *within the procedure room for deep sedation.*

7. Availability of Emergency Equipment

Although the literature is silent, the consultants strongly agree that the ready availability of appropriately sized emergency equipment reduces the risk of both moderate and deep sedation. The literature is also silent regarding the need for cardiac defibrillators during sedation/analgesia. During moderate sedation, the consultants agree that a defibrillator should be immediately available for patients with both mild (e.g., hypertension) and severe (e.g., ischemia, congestive failure) cardiovascular disease. During deep sedation, the consultants agree that a defibrillator should be immediately available for all patients.

Recommendations: Pharmacologic antagonists as well as appropriately sized equipment for establishing a patent airway and providing positive-pressure ventilation with supplemental oxygen should be present whenever sedation/analgesia is administered. Suction, advanced airway equipment, and resuscitation medications should be immediately available and in good working order (e.g., refer to Box A-3 for Example III). A functional defibrillator should be immediately available whenever deep sedation is administered and when moderate sedation is administered to patients with mild or severe cardiovascular disease.

8. Use of Supplemental Oxygen

The literature supports the use of supplemental oxygen during moderate sedation and suggests the use of supplemental oxygen during deep sedation to reduce the frequency of hypoxemia. The consultants agree that supplemental oxygen decreases patient risk during moderate sedation, while strongly agreeing with this view for deep sedation.

Recommendations: Equipment to administer supplemental oxygen should be present when sedation/analgesia is administered. Supplemental oxygen should be considered for moderate sedation and should be administered during deep sedation unless specifically contraindicated for a particular patient or procedure. If hypoxemia is anticipated or develops during sedation/analgesia, supplemental oxygen should be administered.

9. Combinations of Sedative/Analgesic Agents

The literature suggests that combining a sedative with an opioid provides effective moderate sedation; it is equivocal regarding whether the combination of a sedative and an opioid may be more effective than a sedative or an opioid alone in providing adequate moderate sedation. For deep sedation, the literature is insufficient to compare the efficacy of sedative-opioid combinations with that of a sedative

---

▶ BOX A-3

Example III: Emergency Equipment for Sedation and Analgesia

Appropriate emergency equipment should be available whenever sedative or analgesic drugs capable of causing cardiorespiratory depression are administered. The table below should be used as a guide, which should be modified depending upon the individual practice circumstances. Items in brackets are recommended when infants or children are sedated.

Intravenous Equipment
Gloves
Tourniquets
Alcohol wipes
Sterile gauze pads
Intravenous catheters (24, 22 gauge)
Intravenous tubing (pediatric "microdrip"—60 drops/mL)
Intravenous fluid
Assorted needles for drug aspiration, IM injection (intraosseous bone marrow needle)
Appropriately sized syringes (1 mL syringes)
Tape

Basic Airway Management Equipment
Source of compressed O_2 (tank with regulator or pipeline supply with flowmeter)
Source of suction
Suction catheters (pediatric suction catheters)
Yankauer-type suction
Face masks (infant/child face masks)
Self-inflating breathing bag-valve set (pediatric bag-valve set)
Oral and nasal airways (infant/child sized airways)
Lubricant

Advanced Airway Management Equipment (For Practitioners with Intubation Skills)
Laryngeal mask airways (pediatric laryngeal mask airways)
Laryngoscope handles (tested)
Laryngoscope blades (pediatric laryngoscope blades)
Endotracheal tubes:
    Cuffed 6.0, 7.0, 8.0 mm i.d.
    (Uncuffed 2.5, 3.0, 3.5, 4.0, 4.5, 5.0, 5.5, 6.0 mm i.d.)
Stylet (appropriately sized for endotracheal tubes)

Pharmacologic Antagonists
Naloxone
Flumazenil

Emergency Medications
Epinephrine
Ephedrine
Vasopressin
Atropine
Nitroglycerin (tablets or spray)
Amiodarone
Lidocaine
Glucose (50%) (10% or 25% glucose)
Diphenhydramine
Hydrocortisone, methylprednisolone, or dexamethasone
Diazepam or midazolam

alone. The consultants agree that combinations of sedatives and opioids provide satisfactory moderate and deep sedation. However, the published data also suggest that combinations of sedatives and opioids may increase the likelihood of adverse outcomes, including ventilatory depression and hypoxemia; the consultants were equivocal on this issue for both moderate and deep sedation. It is the consensus of the Task Force that fixed combinations of sedative and analgesic agents may not allow the individual components of sedation/analgesia to be appropriately titrated to meet the individual requirements of the patient and procedure while reducing the associated risks.

Recommendations: Combinations of sedative and analgesic agents may be administered as appropriate for the procedure being performed and the condition of the patient. Ideally, each component should be administered individually to achieve the desired effect (e.g., additional analgesic medication to relieve pain; additional sedative medication to decrease awareness or anxiety). The propensity for combinations of sedative and analgesic agents to cause respiratory depression and airway obstruction emphasizes the need to appropriately reduce the dose of each component as well as the need to continually monitor respiratory function.

10. Titration of Intravenous Sedative/Analgesic Medications

The literature is insufficient to determine whether administration of small, incremental doses of intravenous sedative/analgesic drugs until the desired level of sedation and/or analgesia is achieved is preferable to a single dose based on patient size, weight, or age. The consultants strongly agree that incremental drug administration improves patient comfort and decreases risks for both moderate and deep sedation.

Recommendations: Intravenous sedative/analgesic drugs should be given in small, incremental doses which are titrated to the desired endpoints of analgesia and sedation. Sufficient time must elapse between doses to allow the effect of each dose to be assessed before subsequent drug administration. When drugs are administered by non-intravenous routes (e.g., oral, rectal, intramuscular, transmucosal), allowance should be made for the time required for drug absorption before supplementation is considered. Because absorption may be unpredictable, administration of repeat doses of oral medications to supplement sedation/analgesia is not recommended.

11. Anesthetic Induction Agents Used for Sedation/ Analgesia (Propofol, Methohexital, Ketamine)

The literature suggests that when administered by non-anesthesiologists, propofol and ketamine can provide satisfactory moderate sedation and suggests that methohexital can provide satisfactory deep sedation. The literature is insufficient to evaluate the efficacy of propofol or ketamine administered by non-anesthesiologists for deep sedation. There is insufficient literature to determine whether moderate or deep sedation with propofol is associated with a different incidence

of adverse outcomes than similar levels of sedation with midazolam. The consultants are equivocal regarding whether use of these medications affects the likelihood of producing satisfactory moderate sedation, while agreeing that using them increases the likelihood of satisfactory deep sedation. However, the consultants agree that *avoiding* these medications decreases the likelihood of adverse outcomes during moderate sedation and are equivocal regarding their effect on adverse outcomes during deep sedation.

The Task Force cautions practitioners that methohexital and propofol can produce rapid, profound decreases in level of consciousness and cardiorespiratory function, potentially culminating in a state of general anesthesia. The Task Force notes that ketamine also produces dose-related decreases in level of consciousness culminating in general anesthesia. Although it may be associated with less cardiorespiratory depression than other sedatives, airway obstruction, laryngospasm, and pulmonary aspiration may still occur with ketamine. Furthermore, because of its dissociative properties, some of the usual signs of depth of sedation may not apply (e.g., the patient's eyes may be open while in a state of deep sedation or general anesthesia). The Task Force also notes that there are no specific pharmacological antagonists for any of these medications.

Recommendations: Even if moderate sedation is intended, patients receiving propofol or methohexital by any route should receive care consistent with that required for deep sedation. Accordingly, practitioners administering these drugs should be qualified to rescue patients from any level of sedation including general anesthesia. Patients receiving ketamine should be cared for in a manner consistent with the level of sedation which is achieved.

12. Intravenous Access

Published literature is equivocal regarding the relative efficacy of sedative/analgesic agents administered intravenously as compared to agents administered by non-intravenous routes to achieve moderate sedation; the literature is insufficient on this issue for deep sedation. The literature is equivocal regarding the comparative safety of these routes of administration for moderate sedation and insufficient for deep sedation. The consultants strongly agree that intravenous administration of sedative and analgesic medications increases the likelihood of satisfactory sedation for both moderate and deep sedation. They also agree that it decreases the likelihood of adverse outcomes. For both moderate and deep sedation, when sedative/analgesic medications are administered intravenously, the consultants strongly agree with maintaining intravenous access until patients are no longer at risk for cardiovascular or respiratory depression, because it increases the likelihood of satisfactory sedation and decreases the likelihood of adverse outcomes. In those situations where sedation is begun by non-intravenous routes (e.g., oral, rectal, intramuscular) the need for intravenous access is not sufficiently addressed in the literature. However, initiation of intravenous access after the initial sedation takes effect allows additional sedative/analgesic and resuscitation drugs to be administered if necessary.

Recommendations: In patients receiving intravenous medications for sedation/analgesia, vascular access should be maintained throughout the procedure and until the patient is no longer at risk for cardiorespiratory depression. In patients who have received sedation/analgesia by non-intravenous routes, or whose intravenous line has become dislodged or blocked, practitioners should determine the advisability of establishing or reestablishing intravenous access on a case-by-case basis. In all instances, an individual with the skills to establish intravenous access should be immediately available.

13. Reversal Agents

Specific antagonist agents are available for the opioids (e.g., naloxone) and benzodiazepines (e.g., flumazenil). The literature supports the ability of naloxone to reverse opioid induced sedation and respiratory depression. Practitioners are cautioned that acute reversal of opioid induced analgesia may result in pain, hypertension, tachycardia, or pulmonary edema. The literature supports the ability of flumazenil to antagonize benzodiazepine-induced sedation and ventilatory depression in patients who have received benzodiazepines alone or in combination with an opioid. The consultants strongly agree that the immediate availability of reversal agents during both moderate and deep sedation is associated with decreased risk of adverse outcomes. It is the consensus of the Task Force that respiratory depression should be initially treated with supplemental oxygen and, if necessary, positive-pressure ventilation by mask. The consultants disagree that the use of sedation regimens which are likely to require *routine* reversal with flumazenil or naloxone improves the quality of sedation or reduces the risk of adverse outcomes.

Recommendations: Specific antagonists should be available whenever opioid analgesics or benzodiazepines are administered for sedation/analgesia. Naloxone and/or flumazenil may be administered to improve spontaneous ventilatory efforts in patients who have received opioids or benzodiazepines, respectively. This may be especially helpful in cases where airway control and positive-pressure ventilation are difficult. Prior to or concomitantly with pharmacological reversal, patients who become hypoxemic or apneic during sedation/analgesia should: (1) be encouraged or stimulated to breathe deeply; (2) receive supplemental oxygen; and (3) receive positive-pressure ventilation if spontaneous ventilation is inadequate. Following pharmacological reversal, patients should be observed long enough to ensure that sedation and cardiorespiratory depression does not recur once the effect of the antagonist dissipates. The use of sedation regimens which include routine reversal of sedative or analgesic agents is discouraged.

14. Recovery Care

Patients may continue to be at significant risk for developing complications after their procedure is completed. Decreased procedural stimulation, delayed drug absorption following non-intravenous administration, and slow drug elimination may contribute to residual sedation and cardiorespiratory depression during the recovery period. Examples include intramuscular meperidine-promethazine-chlorpromazine mixtures and oral or rectal chloral hydrate. When sedation/analgesia is administered to outpatients, one must assume that there will be no medical supervision once the patient leaves the medical facility. Although there is not sufficient literature to examine the effects of postprocedure monitoring on patient outcomes, the consultants strongly agree that continued observation, monitoring, and predetermined discharge criteria decrease the likelihood of adverse outcomes for both moderate and deep sedation. It is the consensus of the Task Force that discharge criteria should be designed to minimize the risk for cardiorespiratory depression after patients are released from observation by trained personnel.

Recommendations: Following sedation/analgesia, patients should be observed in an appropriately staffed and equipped area until they are near their baseline level of consciousness and are no longer at increased risk for cardiorespiratory depression. Oxygenation should be monitored periodically until patients are no longer at risk for hypoxemia. Ventilation and circulation should be monitored at regular intervals until patients are suitable for discharge. Discharge criteria should be designed to minimize the risk of central nervous system or cardiorespiratory depression following discharge from observation by trained personnel (e.g., Example IV [refer to Box A-4]).

15. Special Situations

The literature suggests and the Task Force members concur that certain types of patients are at increased risk for developing complications related to sedation/analgesia unless special precautions are taken. In patients with significant underlying medical conditions (e.g., extremes of age; severe cardiac, pulmonary, hepatic or renal disease; pregnancy; drug or alcohol abuse) the consultants agree that pre-procedure consultation with an appropriate medical specialist (e.g., cardiologist, pulmonologist) decreases the risk associated with moderate sedation and strongly agree that it decreases the risks associated with deep sedation. In patients with significant sedation-related risk factors (e.g., uncooperative patients, morbid obesity, potentially difficult airway, sleep apnea) the consultants are equivocal regarding whether pre-procedure consultation with an anesthesiologist increases the likelihood of satisfactory moderate sedation while agreeing that it decreases adverse outcomes; the consultants strongly agree that pre-procedure consultation increases the likelihood of satisfactory outcomes while decreasing the risk associated with deep sedation. The Task Force notes that in emergency situations, the benefits of awaiting pre-procedure consultations must be weighed against the risk of delaying the procedure.

For moderate sedation, the consultants are equivocal regarding whether the immediate availability of an individual

---

BOX A-4

Example IV: Recovery and Discharge Criteria Following Sedation and Analgesia

Each patient-care facility in which sedation/analgesia is administered should develop recovery and discharge criteria which are suitable for its specific patients and procedures. Some of the basic principles which might be incorporated in these criteria are enumerated below.

A. General Principles
1. Medical supervision of recovery and discharge following moderate or deep sedation is the responsibility of the operating practitioner or a licensed physician.
2. The recovery area should be equipped with or have direct access to appropriate monitoring and resuscitation equipment.
3. Patients receiving moderate or deep sedation should be monitored until appropriate discharge criteria are satisfied. The duration and frequency of monitoring should be individualized depending upon the level of sedation achieved, the overall condition of the patient, and the nature of the intervention for which sedation/analgesia was administered. Oxygenation should be monitored until patients are no longer at risk for respiratory depression.
4. Level of consciousness, vital signs and oxygenation (when indicated) should be recorded at regular intervals.
5. A nurse or other individual trained to monitor patients and recognize complications should be in attendance until discharge criteria are fulfilled.
6. An individual capable of managing complications (e.g., establishing a patent airway and providing positive-pressure ventilation) should be immediately available until discharge criteria are fulfilled.

B. Guidelines for Discharge
1. Patients should be alert and oriented; infants and patients whose mental status was initially abnormal should have returned to their baseline. Practitioners and parents must be aware that pediatric patients are at risk for airway obstruction should the head fall forward while the child is secured in a car seat.
2. Vital signs should be stable and within acceptable limits.
3. Use of scoring systems may assist in documentation of fitness for discharge.
4. Sufficient time (up to 2 hours) should have elapsed following the last administration of reversal agents (naloxone, flumazenil) to ensure that patients do not become re-sedated after reversal effects have worn off.
5. Outpatients should be discharged in the presence of a responsible adult who will accompany them home and be able to report any post-procedure complications.
6. Outpatients and their escorts should be provided with written instructions regarding postprocedure diet, medications, activities, and a phone number to be called in case of emergency.

---

with postgraduate training in anesthesiology increases the likelihood of a satisfactory outcome or decreases the associated risks. For deep sedation the consultants agree that the immediate availability of such an individual improves the likelihood of satisfactory sedation and that it will decrease the likelihood of adverse outcomes.

Recommendations: Whenever possible, appropriate medical specialists should be consulted prior to administration of sedation to patients with significant underlying conditions. The choice of specialists depends on the nature of the underlying condition and the urgency of the situation. For severely compromised or medically unstable patients (e.g., anticipated difficult airway, severe obstructive pulmonary disease, coronary artery disease, or congestive heart failure), or if it is likely that sedation to the point of unresponsiveness will be necessary to obtain adequate conditions, practitioners who are not trained in the administration of general anesthesia should consult an anesthesiologist.

Methods and Analyses

The scientific assessment of these Guidelines was based on the following statements, or evidence linkages. These linkages represent directional statements about relationships between obstetrical anesthetic interventions and clinical outcomes.

1. A pre-procedure patient evaluation, (i.e., history, physical examination, laboratory evaluation, consultation):
   a. Improves clinical efficacy (i.e., satisfactory sedation and analgesia).
   b. Reduces adverse outcomes.

2. Pre-procedure preparation of the patient (e.g., counseling, fasting):
   a. Improves clinical efficacy (i.e., satisfactory sedation and analgesia).
   b. Reduces adverse outcomes.

3. Patient monitoring (i.e., level of consciousness, pulmonary ventilation (observation, auscultation), oxygenation (pulse oximetry), automated apnea monitoring (capnography), hemodynamics (ECG, BP, HR):
   a. Improves clinical efficacy (i.e., satisfactory sedation and analgesia).
   b. Reduces adverse outcomes.

4. Contemporaneous recording of monitored parameters (e.g., level of consciousness, respiratory function, hemodynamics) at regular intervals in patients receiving sedation and/or analgesia:
   a. Improves clinical efficacy (i.e., satisfactory sedation and analgesia).
   b. Reduces adverse outcomes.

5. Availability of an individual who is dedicated solely to patient monitoring and safety:
   a. Improves clinical efficacy (i.e., satisfactory sedation and analgesia).
   b. Reduces adverse outcomes.

6a. Education and training of sedation and analgesia providers in the pharmacology of sedation/analgesia agents:
   a. Improves clinical efficacy (i.e., satisfactory sedation and analgesia).
   b. Reduces adverse outcomes.

6b. The presence of an individual(s) capable of establishing a patent airway, positive-pressure ventilation and resuscitation (i.e., advanced life-support skills) during a procedure:
   a. Improves clinical efficacy (i.e., satisfactory sedation and analgesia).
   b. Reduces adverse outcomes.

7. Availability of appropriately sized emergency and airway equipment (e.g., LMA, defibrillators):
   a. Improves clinical efficacy (i.e., satisfactory sedation and analgesia).
   b. Reduces adverse outcomes.

8. The use of supplemental oxygen during procedures performed with sedation and/or analgesia:
   a. Improves clinical efficacy (i.e., satisfactory sedation and analgesia).
   b. Reduces adverse outcomes.

9. Use of sedative agents combined with analgesic agents (e.g., sedative/analgesic cocktails, fixed combinations of sedatives and analgesics, titrated combinations of sedatives and analgesics):
   a. Improves clinical efficacy (i.e., satisfactory sedation and analgesia).
   b. Reduces adverse outcomes.

10. Titration of intravenous sedative/analgesic medications to achieve the desired effect:
   a. Improves clinical efficacy (i.e., satisfactory sedation and analgesia).
   b. Reduces adverse outcomes.

11. Intravenous sedation/analgesic medications specifically designed to be used for general anesthesia (i.e., methohexital, propofol and ketamine):
   a. Improves clinical efficacy (i.e., satisfactory sedation and analgesia).
   b. Reduces adverse outcomes.

12a. Administration of sedative/analgesic agents by the intravenous route:
   a. Improves clinical efficacy (i.e., satisfactory sedation and analgesia).
   b. Reduces adverse outcomes.

12b. Maintaining or establishing intravenous access during sedation and/or analgesia until the patient is no longer at risk for cardiorespiratory depression:
   a. Improves clinical efficacy (i.e., satisfactory sedation and analgesia).
   b. Reduces adverse outcomes.

13. Availability of reversal agents (*naloxone and flumazenil only*) for the sedative and/or analgesic agents being administered:
   a. Improves clinical efficacy (i.e., satisfactory sedation and analgesia).
   b. Reduces adverse outcomes.

14. Post-procedural recovery observation, monitoring, and predetermined discharge criteria reduce adverse outcomes.

15. Special regimens (e.g., pre-procedure consultation, specialized monitoring, *special sedatives/techniques*) for patients with special problems (e.g., uncooperative patients; extremes of age; severe cardiac, pulmonary, hepatic, renal, or central nervous system disease; morbid obesity; sleep apnea; pregnancy; drug or alcohol abuse; emergency/unprepared patients; metabolic and airway difficulties):
   a. Improves clinical efficacy (i.e., satisfactory sedation and analgesia).
   b. Reduces adverse outcomes.

Scientific evidence was derived from aggregated research literature, and from surveys, open presentations and other consensus-oriented activities. For purposes of literature aggregation, potentially relevant clinical studies were identified via electronic and manual searches of the literature. The electronic search covered a 36-year period from 1966 through 2001. The manual search covered a 44-year period of time from 1958 through 2001. Over 3000 citations were initially identified, yielding a total of 1876 non-overlapping articles that addressed topics related to the 15 evidence linkages. Following review of the articles, 1519 studies did not provide direct evidence and were subsequently eliminated. A total of 357 articles contained direct linkage-related evidence.

A directional result for each study was initially determined by a literature count, classifying each outcome as either supporting a linkage, refuting a linkage, or neutral. The results were then summarized to obtain a directional assessment of support for each linkage. Literature pertaining to three evidence linkages contained enough studies with well-defined experimental designs and statistical information to conduct formal meta-analyses. These three linkages were: linkage 8 [supplemental oxygen], linkage 9 [benzodiazepines combined with opioids versus benzodiazepines alone], linkage 13 [naloxone for antagonism of opioids, flumazenil for antagonism of benzodiazepines, and flumazenil for antagonism of benzodiazepine-opioid combinations].

Combined probability tests were applied to continuous data, and an odds-ratio procedure was applied to dichotomous study results. Two combined probability tests were employed as follows: (1) The Fisher Combined Test, producing chi-square values based on logarithmic transformations of the reported *P* values from the independent studies, and (2) the Stouffer Combined Test, providing weighted representation of the studies by weighting each of the standard normal deviates by the size of the sample. An odds-ratio procedure based on the Mantel-Haenszel method for combining study results using 2×2 tables was used with outcome frequency information. An acceptable significance level was set at $P < 0.01$ (one-tailed) and effect size estimates were calculated. Interobserver agreement was established through assessment of interrater reliability testing. Tests for heterogeneity of the independent samples were conducted to assure consistency among the study results. To assess potential publishing bias, a "fail-safe N" value was calculated for each combined probability test. No search for unpublished studies was conducted, and no reliability tests for locating research results were done.

Meta-analytic results are reported in Table A-2. The following outcomes were found to be significant for combined probability tests: (1) *oxygen saturation*—linkage 8 [supplemental oxygen]; (2) *sedation recovery*—linkage 13 [naloxone for antagonism of opioids and flumazenil for antagonism of benzodiazepine-opioid combinations]; (3) *psychomotor recovery*—linkage 13 [flumazenil for antagonism of benzodiazepines], and (4) *respiratory/ventilatory recovery*—linkage 13 [naloxone for antagonism of opioids, flumazenil for antagonism of benzodiazepines, and flumazenil for antagonism of benzodiazepine-opioid combinations]. To be considered acceptable findings of significance, both the Fisher and weighted Stouffer combined test results must agree. Weighted effect size values for these linkages ranged from r = 0.19 to r = 0.80, representing moderate to high effect size estimates.

Mantel-Haenszel odds ratios were significant for the following outcomes: (1) *hypoxemia*—linkage 8 [supplemental oxygen] and linkage 9 [benzodiazepine-opioid combinations versus benzodiazepines alone]; (2) *sedation recovery*—linkage 13 [flumazenil for antagonism of benzodiazepines], and (3) *recall of procedure*—linkage 9 [benzodiazepine-opioid combinations]. To be considered acceptable findings of significance, Mantel-Haenszel odds-ratios must agree with combined test results when both types of data are assessed.

Agreement among Task Force members and two methodologists was established by interrater reliability testing. Agreement levels using a kappa statistic for two-rater agreement pairs were as follows: (1) type of study design, $\kappa = 0.25$ to 0.64; (2) type of analysis, $\kappa = 0.36$ to 0.83; (3) evidence linkage assignment, $\kappa = 0.78$ to 0.89; and (4) literature inclusion for database, $\kappa = 0.71$ to 1.00. Three-rater chance-corrected agreement values were: (1) study design, Sav = 0.45, Var (Sav) = 0.012; (2) type of analysis, Sav = 0.51, Var (Sav) = 0.015; (3) linkage assignment, Sav = 0.81 Var (Sav) = 0.006; (4) literature database inclusion, Sav = 0.84 Var (Sav) =

0.046. These values represent moderate to high levels of agreement.

The findings of the literature analyses were supplemented by the opinions of Task Force members as well as by surveys of the opinions of a panel of Consultants, as described in the text of the Guidelines. The rate of return for this Consultant survey was 78% (N = 51/65). Median agreement scores from the Consultants regarding each linkage are reported in Table A-3.

For moderate sedation, Consultants were supportive of all of the linkages with the following exceptions: linkage 3 (electrocardiogram monitoring and capnography), linkage 9 (sedatives combined with analgesics for reducing adverse outcomes), linkage 11 (avoiding general anesthesia sedatives for improving satisfactory sedation), linkage 13b (routine administration of naloxone), linkage 13c (routine administration of flumazenil), and linkage 15b (anesthesiologist consultation for patients with medical conditions to provide satisfactory moderate sedation). In addition, Consultants were equivocal regarding whether postgraduate training in anesthesiology improves moderate sedation or reduces adverse outcomes.

For deep sedation, Consultants were supportive of all of the linkages with the following exceptions: linkage 9 (sedatives combined with analgesics for reducing adverse outcomes), linkage 11 (avoiding general anesthesia sedatives), linkage 13b (routine administration of naloxone), and linkage 13c (routine administration of flumazenil).

The Consultants were asked to indicate which, if any, of the evidence linkages would change their clinical practices if the updated Guidelines were instituted. The rate of return was 57% (N = 37/65). The percent of responding Consultants expecting *no change* associated with each linkage were as follows: pre-procedure patient evaluation—94%; pre-procedure patient preparation—91%; patient monitoring—80%; contemporaneous recording of monitored parameters—91%; availability of individual dedicated solely to patient monitoring and safety—91%; education and training of sedation/analgesia providers in pharmacology—89%; presence of an individual(s) capable of establishing a patent airway—91%; availability of appropriately sized emergency and airway equipment—94%, use of supplemental oxygen during procedures—100%, use of sedative agents combined with analgesic agents—91%, titration of sedatives/analgesics—97%, intravenous sedation/analgesia with agents designed for general anesthesia—77%, administration of sedative/analgesic agents by the intravenous route—94%, maintaining or establishing intravenous access—97%, availability/use of flumazenil—94%, availability/use of naloxone—94%, observation and monitoring during recovery—89%, special care for patients with underlying medical problems—91%, and special care for uncooperative patients—94%. Seventy-four percent of the respondents indicated that the Guidelines would have *no effect* on the amount of time spent on a typical case. Nine respondents (26%)

Text continued on p. 294

TABLE A-2
Meta-Analysis Summary

LINKAGES	NO. OF STUDIES	FISHER CHI-SQUARE	P	WEIGHTED STOUFFER Zc	P	EFFECT SIZE	MANTEL-HAENSZEL CHI-SQUARE	P	ODDS RATIO	HETEROGENEITY SIGNIFICANCE	HETEROGENEITY EFFECT SIZE
Supplemental Oxygen											
Oxygen saturation[1]	5	71.40	<0.001	5.44	<0.001	0.40	—	—	—	>0.90 (NS)	>0.50 (NS)
Hypoxemia[1]	7	—	—	—	—	—	44.15	<0.001	0.20	—	>0.50 (NS)
Sedatives/Opioids Combined: benzodiazepines + opioids											
Sedation efficacy	7	—	—	—	—	—	3.79	>0.05 (NS)	1.87[4]	—	<0.01
Recall of procedure	6	—	—	—	—	—	18.47	<0.001	2.16[4]	—	<0.01
Hypoxemia	5	—	—	—	—	—	11.78	<0.001	2.37	—	>0.05 (NS)
Naloxone for Opioids											
Sedation recovery at 5 min[1,2,3]	5	38.36	<0.001	3.13	<0.001	0.23	—	—	—	>0.30 (NS)	>0.02 (NS)
Respiration/ventilation[1,2,3]	5	38.72	<0.001	3.97	<0.001	0.33	—	—	—	>0.10 (NS)	<0.001
Flumazenil for Benzodiazepines											
Sedation recovery at 5 min	6	—	—	—	—	—	104.76	<0.001	8.15	—	>0.10 (NS)
Psychomotor recovery											
At 15 min	5	41.80	<0.001	1.69	0.046 (NS)	0.20	—	—	—	>0.70 (NS)	>0.50 (NS)
At 30 min	5	43.02	<0.001	3.36	<0.001	0.19	—	—	—	>0.90 (NS)	>0.50 (NS)
Respiration/ventilation[2,3]	6	53.25	<0.001	5.03	<0.001	0.80	—	—	—	<0.01	<0.001
Flumazenil for Benzodiazepine-Opioid Combinations											
Sedation recovery at 5 min	5	72.12	<0.001	6.76	<0.001	0.37	—	—	—	<0.001	<0.001
Respiration/ventilation[2,3]	6	55.06	<0.001	5.11	<0.001	0.25	—	—	—	>0.10 (NS)	<0.001
Nausea/vomiting	5	—	—	—	—	—	0.28	>0.80 (NS)	1.22	—	>0.70 (NS)

[1] Non-randomized comparative studies are included.
[2] Studies in which anesthesiologist administered benzodiazepines, opioids, or reversal agents are included.
[3] Studies in which subjects consist of intensive care unit patients, postoperative patients, or volunteers with no procedures are included.
[4] Der Simonian-Laird random-effects odds ratio.

TABLE A-3

Consultant Survey Summary

LINKAGE/INTERVENTION	OUTCOME	MODERATE SEDATION		DEEP SEDATION	
		N	MEDIAN* OR PERCENT	N	MEDIAN* OR PERCENT
1. Pre-procedure patient evaluation	Satisfactory sedation	51	5	51	5
	Adverse outcomes	51	5	51	5
2. Pre-procedure fasting	Satisfactory sedation	51	4	51	5
	Adverse outcomes	51	4	51	5
3. Monitoring					
a. Level of consciousness	Satisfactory sedation	51	5	49	5
	Adverse outcomes	51	5	50	5
b. Breathing (observation/auscultation)	Satisfactory sedation	51	5	49	5
	Adverse outcomes	51	5	50	5
c. Pulse oximetry	Satisfactory sedation	51	5	50	5
	Adverse outcomes	51	5	50	5
d. Blood pressure/heart rate	Satisfactory sedation	50	4	49	5
	Adverse outcomes	50	5	49	5
e. Electrocardiogram	Satisfactory sedation	51	3	50	4
	Adverse outcomes	51	3	49	5
f. Capnography	Satisfactory sedation	50	3	48	4
	Adverse outcomes	50	3	49	4
4. Contemporaneous recording	Satisfactory sedation	51	4	50	5
	Adverse outcomes	51	4	50	5
5. Individual for patient monitoring	Satisfactory sedation	49	4	48	5
	Adverse outcomes	49	4	48	5
6a. Education and training	Satisfactory sedation	50	5	49	5
	Adverse outcomes	50	5	49	5
6b. Individual with basic life support skills present in room		50	5	49	5
6b. Availability of advanced life support skills					
In procedure room		2	4.2%	39	79.6%
Immediate vicinity (1-5 min)		27	56.2%	8	16.3%
Same building (5-10 min)		14	29.2%	2	4.1%
Outside provider		5	10.4%	0	0.0%

Item	Category	N	Median	N	Median
7. Emergency intravenous and airway equipment	Adverse outcomes	51	5	49	5
8. Supplemental oxygen	Adverse outcomes	50	4	49	5
9. Sedatives combined with analgesics	Satisfactory sedation	50	4	49	4
10. Titration	Adverse outcomes	50	3	49	3
	Satisfactory sedation	51	5	50	5
11. Avoiding general anesthetic sedatives	Adverse outcomes	51	5	50	5
	Satisfactory sedation	50	3	49	2
12a. IV sedatives	Adverse outcomes	50	4	49	3
	Satisfactory sedation	51	5	50	5
12b. IV access	Adverse outcomes	51	4	50	4
	Satisfactory sedation	50	4	49	5
13a. Immediate availability of naloxone or flumazenil	Adverse outcomes	51	5	49	5
13b. Routine administration of naloxone	Satisfactory sedation	37	5	37	5
	Adverse outcomes	37	2	37	2
13c. Routine administration of flumazenil	Satisfactory sedation	37	2	37	2
	Adverse outcomes	37	1	37	2
14. Observation, monitoring and discharge criteria	Adverse outcomes	50	2	49	5
15a. Med specialist consult, med conditions	Satisfactory sedation	50	5	49	5
	Adverse outcomes	50	4	49	5
15b. Anesthesiologist consultation, patients with underlying medical conditions	Satisfactory sedation	51	4	50	4
	Adverse outcomes	51	3	50	5
15c. Anesthesiologist consultation, patients with significant sedation risk factors	Satisfactory sedation	51	4	50	5
	Adverse outcomes	51	4	50	5
16. Postgraduate training in anesthesiology	Satisfactory sedation	51	4	50	4
	Adverse outcomes	51	3	50	4
17. In emergency situations, sedate patients less deeply	Adverse outcomes	51	4	51	5

*Strongly Agree: Median score of "5" (At least 50% of the responses were "5")
Agree: Median score of "4" (At least 50% of the responses were "4" or "5")
Equivocal: Median score of "3" (At least 50% of the scores were "3" or less)
Disagree: Median score of "2" (At least 50% of responses were "1" or "2")
Strongly Disagree: Median score of "1" (At least 50% of responses were "1")

indicated that there would be an increase in the amount of time they would spend on a typical case with the implementation of these Guidelines. The amount of increased time anticipated by these respondents ranged from 1-60 minutes.

Readers with special interest in the statistical analyses used in establishing these Guidelines can receive further information by writing to the American Society of Anesthesiologists: 520 North Northwest Highway, Park Ridge, Illinois 60068-2573. *Anesthesiology* 2002;96:1004-1017. © 2002 American Society of Anesthesiologists, Lippincott Williams & Wilkins, Inc.

REFERENCES

1. American Society of Anesthesiology, *Anesthesiology* 1996; 84:459-471, Lippincott William and Wilkins, Inc.
2. American Society of Anesthesiology. *Anesthesiology* 1999; 90:896-905. Lippincott Williams and Wilkins.

JCAHO Standards for Operative or Other High-Risk Procedures and/or the Administration of Moderate or Deep Sedation or Anesthesia

Operative or other procedures and the administration of sedation or anesthesia often occur simultaneously. However, procedures do occur without sedation, and sedation or anesthesia is administered for noninvasive procedures (hyperbaric treatment, CT scan, MRI). Therefore, the following standards address both operative or other procedures and/or the administration of moderate or deep sedation or anesthesia.

Whenever an operative or other procedure is conducted, whether or not sedation or anesthesia is administered, appropriate patients must be involved in planning for and providing care to the patient. All procedures carry risk, but that risk is increased when sedation or anesthesia is administered.

The standards for sedation and anesthesia care apply when patients in any setting receive, for any purpose by any route, the following:

◆ General, spinal, or other major regional sedation and anesthesia or

◆ Sedation (with or without analgesia) that, in the manner used, may be reasonably expected to result in the loss of protective reflexes

Because sedation is a continuum, it is not always possible to predict how an individual patient receiving sedation will respond. Therefore, each hospital develops specific, appropriate protocols for the care of patients receiving sedation. These protocols are consistent with professional standards and address at least the following:

◆ Sufficient qualified individuals present to perform the procedure and to monitor the patient throughout administration and recovery

◆ Appropriate equipment for care and resuscitation

◆ Appropriate monitoring of vital signs—heart and respiratory rates and oxygenation

◆ Documentation of care

◆ Monitoring of outcomes

Definitions of four levels of sedation and anesthesia include the following:

◆ **Minimal sedation (anxiolysis).** A drug-induced state during which patients respond normally to verbal commands. Although cognitive function and coordination may be impaired, ventilatory and cardiovascular functions are unaffected.

◆ **Moderate sedation/analgesia ("conscious sedation").** A drug-induced depression of consciousness during which patients respond purposefully to verbal commands, either alone or accompanied by light tactile stimulation. No interventions are required to maintain a patent airway and spontaneous ventilation is adequate. Cardiovascular function is usually maintained.

◆ **Deep sedation/analgesia.** A drug-induced depression of consciousness during which patients cannot be easily aroused but respond purposefully after repeated or painful stimulation. The ability to independently maintain ventilatory function may be impaired. Patients may require assistance in maintaining a patent airway and spontaneous ventilation may be inadequate. Cardiovascular function is usually maintained.

◆ **Anesthesia.** Consists of general anesthesia and spinal or major regional anesthesia. It does not include local anesthesia. General anesthesia is a drug-induced loss of consciousness during which patients are not arousable, even by painful stimulation. The ability to independently maintain ventilatory function is often impaired. Patients often require assistance in maintaining a patent airway, and positive pressure ventilation may be required because of depressed spontaneous ventilation or drug-induced depression of neuromuscular function. Cardiovascular function may be impaired.

Standard PC.13.10

Not applicable

Standard PC.13.20

Operative or other procedures and/or the administration of moderate or deep sedation or anesthesia are planned.

Rationale for PC.13.20

Because the response to procedures is not always predictable and sedation-to-anesthesia is a continuum, it is not always possible to predict how an individual patient will respond. Therefore, qualified individuals are trained in professional standards and techniques to manage patients in the case of a potentially harmful event.

Elements of Performance for PC.13.20

1. Sufficient numbers of qualified staff are available* to evaluate the patient, perform the procedure, monitor, and recover the patient.

2. Individuals administering moderate or deep sedation and anesthesia are qualified† and have the appropriate credentials to manage patients at whatever level of sedation or anesthesia is achieved, either intentionally or unintentionally.

3. A registered nurse supervises perioperative nursing care.

4. Appropriate equipment to monitor the patient's physiologic status is available.

5. Appropriate equipment to administer intravenous fluids and drugs, including blood and blood components, is available as needed.

6. Resuscitation capabilities are available.

Before operative and other procedures or the administration of moderate or deep sedation or anesthesia:

7. Patient acuity is assessed to plan for the appropriate level of postprocedure care.

8. Preprocedural education, treatments, and services are provided according to the plan for care, treatment, and services.

9. The site, procedure, and patient are accurately identified and clearly communicated, using active communication techniques, during a final verification process, such as "time out," prior to the start of any surgical or invasive procedure.

10. A presedation of preanesthesia assessment is conducted.

11. Before sedating or anesthetizing a patient, an LIP with appropriate clinical privileges plans or concurs with the planned anesthesia.

12. The patient is reevaluated immediately before moderate or deep sedation and before anesthesia induction.

---

*For hospitals providing obstetric or emergency operative services, this means they can provide anesthesia services as required by law and regulation.

†**Qualified** The individuals providing moderate or deep sedation and anesthesia have at a minimum had competency-based education, training, and experience in the following:
1. Evaluating patients before moderate or deep sedation and anesthesia.
2. Performing the moderate or deep sedation and anesthesia, including rescuing patients who slip into a deeper-than-desired level of sedation or analgesia. This includes the following:
   a. *Moderate* sedation – are qualified to rescue patients from deep sedation and are competent to manage a compromised airway and to provide adequate oxygenation and ventilation.
   b. *Deep* sedation – are qualified to rescue patients from general anesthesia and are competent to manage an unstable cardiovascular system as well as a compromised airway and inadequate oxygenation and ventilation.

Standard PC.13.30
Patients are monitored during the procedure and/or administration of moderate or deep sedation or anesthesia.
Elements of Performance for PC.13.30

1. Appropriate methods are used to continuously monitor oxygenation, ventilation, and circulation during procedures that may affect the patient's physiological status.

2. The procedure and/or the administration of moderate or deep sedation or anesthesia for each patient are documented in the medical record.

Standard PC.13.40
Patients are monitored immediately after the procedure and/or administration of moderate or deep sedation or anesthesia.
Elements of Performance for PC.13.40

1. The patient's status is assessed on arrival in the recovery area.

2. Each patient's physiological status, mental status, and pain level are monitored.

3. Monitoring is at a level consistent with the potential effect of the procedure and/or sedation or anesthesia.

4. Patients are discharged from the recovery area and the hospital by a qualified LIP or according to rigorously applied criteria approved by the clinical leaders.

5. Patients who have received anesthesia in the outpatient setting are discharged in the company of a responsible, designated adult.

Standard PC.13.50
Electroconvulsive therapy is used with adequate justification, documentation, and regard for patient safety.
Elements of Performance for PC.13.50

1. Written policies regulate electroconvulsive therapy.

2. Whenever electroconvulsive therapy is used, the procedure is adequately justified and documented in the patient's medical record.

3. Before initiating electroconvulsive therapy for a child or youth, two qualified, experienced child psychiatrists who are not directly involved in treating the child or youth do the following:
   • Examine the child or youth
   • Consult with the psychiatrists responsible for the child or youth
   • Document their concurrence with the treatment in the child's or youth's medical record

4. Written consent for any electroconvulsive therapy is obtained from the patient and documented in the clinical/case record.

Standard PC.13.60
Psychosurgery or other surgical treatments for emotional, mental, or behavioral disorders are performed with adequate justification, documentation, and regard for patient safety.

Endorsement of Position Statement on the Role of the Registered Nurse (RN) in the Management of Patients Receiving IV Conscious Sedation for Short-Term Therapeutic, Diagnostic, or Surgical Procedures

Policy/Position: The Board of Directors endorsed the Position Statement on the Role of the Registered Nurse (RN) in the Management of Patients Receiving IV Conscious Sedation for Short-Term Therapeutic, Diagnostic, or Surgical Procedures. This was a result of the joint work of ANA and several specialty nursing organizations to develop position statements (see endorsements).

A. Definition of IV Conscious Sedation

Intravenous conscious sedation is produced by the administration of pharmacologic agents. A patient under conscious sedation has a depressed level of consciousness but retains the ability to independently and continuously maintain a patent airway and respond appropriately to physical stimulation and/or verbal command.

B. Management and Monitoring

It is within the scope of practice of a registered nurse to manage the care of patients receiving IV conscious sedation during therapeutic, diagnostic, or surgical procedures provided the following criteria are met:

1. Administration of IV conscious sedation medications by non-anesthetist RNs is allowed by state laws and institutional policy, procedures, and protocol.

2. A qualified anesthesia provider or attending physician selects and orders the medications to achieve IV conscious sedation.

3. Guidelines for patient monitoring, drug administration, and protocols for dealing with potential complications or emergency situations are available and have been developed in accordance with accepted standards of anesthesia practice.

4. The registered nurse managing the care of the patient receiving IV conscious sedation shall have no other responsibilities that would leave the patient unattended or compromise continuous monitoring.

5. The registered nurse managing the care of patients receiving IV conscious sedation is able to:
   a. Demonstrate the acquired knowledge of anatomy, physiology, pharmacology, cardiac arrhythmia recognition and complications related to IV conscious sedation and medications.
   b. Assess total patient care requirements during IV conscious sedation and recovery. Physiologic measurements should include, but not be limited to, respiratory rate, oxygen saturation, blood pressure, cardiac rate and rhythm, and patient's level of consciousness.
   c. Understand the principles of oxygen delivery, respiratory physiology, transport and uptake, and demonstrate the ability to use oxygen delivery devices.
   d. Anticipate and recognize potential complications of IV conscious sedation in relation to the type of medication being administered.
   e. Possess the requisite knowledge and skills to assess, diagnose and intervene in the event of complications or undesired outcomes and to institute nursing interventions in compliance with orders (including standing orders) or institutional protocols or guidelines.
   f. Demonstrate skill in airway management resuscitation.
   g. Demonstrate knowledge of the legal ramifications of administering IV conscious sedation and/or monitoring patients receiving IV conscious sedation, including the RN's responsibility and liability in the event of an untoward reaction or life-threatening complication.

6. The institution or practice setting has in place an educational/competency validation mechanism that includes a process for evaluating and documenting the individuals' demonstration of the knowledge, skills, and abilities related to the management of patients receiving IV conscious sedation. Evaluation and documentation of competence occurs on a periodic basis according to institutional policy.

C. Additional Guidelines

1. Intravenous access must be continuously maintained in the patient receiving IV conscious sedation.

2. All patients receiving IV conscious sedation will be continuously monitored throughout the procedure as well as the recovery phase by physiologic measurements including, but not limited to, respiratory rate, oxygen saturation, blood pressure, cardiac rate and rhythm, and patient's level of consciousness.

3. Supplemental oxygen will be immediately available to all patients receiving IV conscious sedation and administered per order (including standing orders).

4. An emergency cart with a defibrillator must be immediately accessible to every location where IV conscious sedation is administered. Suction and a positive-pressure breathing device, oxygen, and appropriate airways must be in each room where IV conscious sedation is administered.

5. Provisions must be in place for back-up personnel who are experts in airway management, emergency intubation, and advanced cardiopulmonary resuscitation if complications arise.

Endorsed by:

American Association of Critical-Care Nurses
American Association of Neuroscience Nurses
American Association of Nurse Anesthetists
American Association of Occupational Health Nurses
American Association of Spinal Cord Injury Nurses
American Nephrology Nurses' Association
American Nurses Association
American Radiological Nurses Association
American Society of Pain Management Nurses
American Society of Plastic and Reconstructive Surgical Nurses
American Society of Post Anesthesia Nurses
American Urological Association
Allied Association of Operating Room Nurses
Association of Pediatric Oncology Nurses
Association of Rehabilitation Nurses
Dermatology Nurses Association
NAACOG, The Organization for Obstetric, Gynecologic & Neonatal Nurses
National Association of Orthopaedic Nurses
National Flight Nurses Association
National Student Nurses Association
Nurse Consultants Association, Inc.
Nurses Organization of Veterans Affairs
Nursing Pain Association

Clinical Competencies for Sedation/Analgesia

The practitioner demonstrates knowledge related to the **goals, definitions, practice standards, and guidelines** related to procedural sedation.

COMPETENCY	REMEDIATION/GOALS	DATE/INITIALS
Identifies JCAHO standards related to the administration of sedation by qualified providers. Defines minimal sedation, moderate sedation, deep sedation, and general anesthesia. Identifies goals and objectives of moderate sedation/analgesia. States the clinical endpoints of moderate sedation/analgesia. Lists regulatory, statutory, and recommended practice guidelines associated with the administration of sedation. Identifies applicable standards and intents promulgated by the Joint Commission on Accreditation of Healthcare Organizations as they relate to the administration of sedation/analgesia by healthcare providers. Compare and contrast practice standards, practice guidelines, and position statements related to sedation care.		

© 2004, Specialty Health Education, Inc.

The practitioner demonstrates knowledge related to **presedation assessment and patient selection** related to procedural sedation.

COMPETENCY	REMEDIATION/GOALS	DATE/INITIALS
Identifies JCAHO standards related to presedation patient assessment. Lists the goals of presedation patient assessment. Identifies methods utilized to calculate ideal body weight. States the components of the patient's medical history and its impact on procedural care. Lists specific physiologic alterations in the cardiovascular, pulmonary, hepatic, renal, neurologic, and endocrine systems identified in the presedation patient assessment and their implications for procedural patient care. States the implications for the sedation plan of care based on the patient's past surgical/anesthesia history.		

Continued

COMPETENCY	REMEDIATION/GOALS	DATE/INITIALS
Lists the treatment protocol for an allergic reaction. Identifies the sedation patient population which requires presedation laboratory testing. States the sedation patient care considerations associated with positive findings on social history including: • Tobacco use • Alcohol consumption • Substance abuse • Herbal product use • Pregnancy States the current recommended NPO guidelines for sedation patients. Defines assault and battery as it relates to informed consent. Utilizes the ASA Physical Status Classification System to assign a numerical summary assessment at the conclusion of the presedation patient interview.		

© 2004, Specialty Health Education, Inc.

The practitioner demonstrates knowledge of **pharmacologic concepts** as they relate to the administration of procedural sedation.

COMPETENCY	REMEDIATION/GOALS	DATE/INITIALS
States the clinical considerations in the procedural sedation setting for the following pharmacologic terminology: • Synergism • Potency • Tachyphylaxis Defines pharmacokinetics as it relates to procedural sedation. Lists the patient care considerations associated with each of the following pharmacokinetic processes including absorption, distribution, metabolism, and excretion. States the role of the cytochrome P-450 system in the biotransformation of sedative and analgesic medications. Defines pharmacodynamics as it relates to procedural sedation. States the role of agonist and antagonist activity at pharmacologic receptor sites.		

© 2004, Specialty Health Education, Inc.

The practitioner demonstrates knowledge related to **sedation/analgesia medications and techniques of administration.**

COMPETENCY	REMEDIATION/GOALS	DATE/INITIALS
Lists the ideal pharmacologic characteristics of sedative, analgesic, and hypnotic medications. States the pharmacokinetic and pharmacodynamic considerations and end organ effects associated with the following medications: • Benzodiazepines • Opioids • Sedatives • Hypnotics		

Continued

COMPETENCY	REMEDIATION/GOALS	DATE/INITIALS
• Barbiturates • Dissociative anesthetics • Local anesthetic solutions Lists the advantages, disadvantages, and patient care considerations associated with: • Titration to clinical effect technique • Bolus technique • Continuous-infusion technique Lists medications utilized in the sedation setting that are contraindicated in the presence of specific disease states. Identifies the indications, side effects, and clinical pharmacology associated with sedative, hypnotic, and analgesic medications. States the cardiovascular, respiratory, and central nervous system effects associated with medications utilized to achieve a sedate state.		

© 2004, Specialty Health Education, Inc.

The practitioner demonstrates knowledge related to **procedural patient monitoring requirements** for the patient presenting for sedation services.

COMPETENCY	REMEDIATION/GOALS	DATE/INITIALS
Identifies JCAHO standards and intents related to physiologic monitoring requirements for patients presenting for procedural sedation. Identifies the rationale, advantages, and disadvantages associated with the following monitoring parameters utilized during procedural sedation: • ECG • Blood pressure • Pulse oximetry • Level of consciousness • End-tidal carbon dioxide • Bispectral index analysis States the ECG lead positions that are best utilized in the detection of dysrhythmias versus ischemia. Identifies types of dysrhythmias that may impact on the patient's physiologic status during procedural sedation. Lists factors that contribute to the development of hypotension and hypertension. Outlines treatment protocols for hypotension and hypertension in the sedation setting. States the advantages associated with the use of end-tidal carbon dioxide monitoring during procedural sedation. Identifies the pharmacokinetic profile associated with sedative, analgesic, and hypnotic medications utilized in the sedation setting. Lists medications utilized in the sedation setting that are contraindicated in the presence of specific disease states. Identifies the indications, side effects, and clinical pharmacology associated with sedative, hypnotic, and analgesic medications. States the cardiovascular, respiratory, and central nervous system effects associated with medications utilized to achieve a sedate state.		

© 2004, Specialty Health Education, Inc.

The practitioner demonstrates knowledge related to **airway management and management of respiratory complications** which may occur during procedural sedation.

COMPETENCY	REMEDIATION/GOALS	DATE/INITIALS
Identifies the components of a presedation airway evaluation. States the clinical signs and symptoms associated with respiratory insufficiency and airway obstruction. Lists treatment modalities designed to relieve airway obstruction and restore air flow in the sedated patient. States the proper technique for nasal and oral airway insertion. Demonstrates the proper application of a face mask for positive-pressure ventilation. Identifies the components and treatment modalities associated with the "Sedation Airway Algorithm."		

© 2004, Specialty Health Education, Inc.

The practitioner demonstrates knowledge related to **intravenous insertion techniques and intravenous solutions** utilized during procedural sedation.

COMPETENCY	REMEDIATION/GOALS	DATE/INITIALS
States the principles of intravenous therapy. Lists the methods of intravenous cannula insertion required for procedural sedation. Identifies systemic complications associated with intravenous catheter placement. States the common intravenous solutions utilized during procedural sedation. States the presedation, procedural and postprocedural care associated with intravenous therapy.		

© 2004, Specialty Health Education, Inc.

The practitioner demonstrates knowledge related to **sedation considerations for the geriatric patient.**

COMPETENCY	REMEDIATION/GOALS	DATE/INITIALS
Defines the term *geriatric*. Identifies the cardiorespiratory, renal, hepatic, and central nervous system physiologic alterations which impact on geriatric patient care. Lists pharmacodynamic/pharmacokinetic considerations associated with the aging process. States specific procedural considerations associated with administering benzodiazepines, opioids, and sedative/hypnotics to the geriatric patient population. States airway management considerations associated with caring for the "aged" patient.		

© 2004, Specialty Health Education, Inc.

The practitioner demonstrates knowledge related to **postsedation patient care, monitoring and discharge criteria.**

COMPETENCY	REMEDIATION/GOALS	DATE/INITIALS
States the purpose of postsedation patient care.		
Identifies characteristics associated with phase I and phase II perianesthesia nursing practice.		
Lists the recommended patient care equipment that should be maintained in a postsedation patient care area.		
Lists the components of a postsedation patient care report.		
Demonstrates the mechanism to assign a postsedation Aldrete score based on ten objective scoring criteria.		
Lists objective scoring parameters which comprise the postsedation Aldrete scoring mechanism.		
Lists appropriate discharge criteria for the outpatient postsedation patient.		
States the components required for effective postsedation teaching.		

© 2004, Specialty Health Education, Inc.

The practitioner demonstrates knowledge related to the **risk management strategies** related to procedural sedation.

COMPETENCY	REMEDIATION/GOALS	DATE/INITIALS
Identifies risk reduction strategies to improve sedation patient care.		
Describes practice standards, professional practice recommendations, position statements, and state statutes associated with the administration of sedation/analgesia applicable to your practice setting.		
Identifies the components of a "sedation" database.		
States mechanisms utilized in the successful implementation of a sedation educational program.		
Delineates mechanisms of information dissemination within a sedation practice setting.		

© 2004, Specialty Health Education, Inc.

The practitioner demonstrates knowledge related to **sedation considerations for the pediatric patient.**

COMPETENCY	REMEDIATION/GOALS	DATE/INITIALS
States the goals of pediatric procedural sedation.		
Defines the developmental subsets of pediatrics and states examples of developmentally appropriate rapport.		
States the role of the parents or primary caregivers of children receiving procedural sedation.		
Lists the infant's physiologic response to pain.		
States characteristics of the infant central nervous system.		
States the relationship of the parasympathetic vs. sympathetic nervous system in children younger than 1 year of age.		
Lists significant differences between the cardiovascular system of a small child vs. an adult.		
States the primary cause of bradycardia in infants.		

Continued

COMPETENCY	REMEDIATION/GOALS	DATE/INITIALS
Identifies methods to avoid air administration via pediatric intravenous catheters.		
Lists distinct features of the infant's upper airway.		
Lists distinct features of the infant's lower airway.		
Explains the significance of subglottic edema in children.		
States methods to determine the appropriate-sized pediatric endotracheal tube.		
States specific airway maneuvers which may improve ventilation in the pediatric patient.		
Lists the clinical effects associated with hypothermia in the pediatric patient.		
Identifies correct NPO guidelines for the sedation patient.		
Identifies pediatric medical problems which may impact on the sedation plan of care.		
Identifies monitoring methods for the pediatric sedation patient.		
Identifies sedation scales utilized for the pediatric sedation patient.		
States pharmacologic considerations associated with sedative/analgesic agents for the pediatric patient.		
Lists specific discharge criteria for the pediatric sedation patient.		

American Association of Nurse Anesthetists Latex Allergy Protocol

Introduction

In recent years, latex allergy has been recognized as a significant problem for both specific patient and provider populations. The incidence of latex allergy throughout the general population has been estimated between 1% and 6% while certain pediatric populations may experience an incidence as high as 73% (spina bifida and related pathologies). Healthcare workers who are regularly exposed to latex-containing devices and products maintain an incidence of allergic response that ranges from 8% to 17%.

Latex allergy is an immunologic reaction to natural rubber latex, processed from the *Hevea Brasiliensis* tree indigenous to Central and South America. Newer rubber medical supplies, particularly very soft "dipped" products, contain the greatest proportion of low molecular weight soluble proteins thought to be responsible for the allergic response.

The more recent appearance and recognition of latex allergy as a serious medical concern has resulted from the incorporation of increased barrier precautions in preventing the transmission of infectious bloodborne pathogens. The increase in the number of medical gloves imported to the United States increased awareness among providers. Improved methods in diagnosing latex allergy also accounts for the recent rise in the number of reported cases.

Immediate hypersensitivity reactions to latex vary from contact urticaria to systemic anaphylaxis and laryngeal edema that require lifesaving intervention. Allergic contact dermatitis can also occur and is a delayed hypersensitivity which mimics a poison ivy-type skin reaction. No immunotherapy or desensitization currently exists for latex allergy. Each systemic reaction occurs with less provocation and presentation of a greater magnitude.

Anaphylactic reactions have complicated a variety of common medical procedures including surgery (particularly of the genitourinary tract) and anesthesia, barium enemas, as well as oral, vaginal, and rectal examinations utilizing latex gloves. In most cases, there has been contact between latex products and mucous membranes. However, in some exquisitely sensitive individuals, exposure through inhalation of aerosolized latex or through intravenous administration has led to severe reactions. This type of reaction is similar to immediate drug reactions or stinging insect venom and may be associated with rapidly progressive anaphylaxis and death.

Populations at Risk for Developing Latex Allergy

A complete and thorough medical history remains as the most reliable screening test to predict the likelihood of an anaphylactic reaction. Individuals (particularly in the pediatric population) who are most likely to exhibit a sensitivity to latex that may result in varying degrees of reactivity include:

- Those who possess a known or suspected allergy to latex by having exhibited an allergic or anaphylactic reaction, positive skin testing, or positive IgE antibodies against latex.
- Those with documented history of intraoperative anaphylaxis of unknown etiology.
- Those with neural tube defects including:
  - Spina bifida
  - Myelomeningocele/meningocele
  - Lipomyelomeningocele
- Those who have experienced some interaction between their central nervous and immune systems.
- Those who have had multiple operations, particularly as a neonate.
- Those who require chronic bladder catheterizations as a result of:
  - Spinal cord trauma
  - Exstrophy of the bladder
  - Neurogenic bladder
- Those who possess some history of atopy and multiple allergies including food products. Particular allergies to fruits and vegetables including bananas, avocado, celery, fig, chestnut, papaya and passion fruit are most significant.
- Children with a strong or confirmed allergy to bananas should be considered to be allergic to latex.

Individuals who have experienced a significant degree or repeated exposure to latex products are more likely to develop a latex allergy. These situations may include treatment that involves:

- Occupational exposure to latex (i.e., latex industry, healthcare workers).

- Repeat surgical procedures
- Surgical procedures involving mucosal membranes
- Repeated placement of ventriculoperitoneal shunts (i.e., cerebral palsy)
- Repeated or chronic intravenous and urinary catheterizations
- A history of allergic reaction after touching balloons, rubber gloves or powder from rubber gloves, dental dams, latex consumer products, and medical devices; especially atopic patients.
- Healthcare providers or other workers who give a history of mild latex glove eczema rarely have anaphylactic events. However, a history of severe or worsening latex glove–induced eczema, urticaria, or work-related conjunctivitis, rhinitis, asthma, or urticaria may indicate allergic sensitization and increase the risk for more severe reactions in the future.

Latex Avoidance Precautions

By touching any latex object, the healthcare worker can transmit the allergen by hand to the patient. Caution should be taken to keep the powder from the gloves away from the patient, as the powder will act as a carrier for the latex protein. Therefore, in order to reduce the possibility of the latex protein becoming airborne, care must be taken not to snap gloves on and off.

Patients should be identified as being *latex sensitive.* The room should be labeled *latex free* to avoid personnel from bringing rubber products (wrist bands, chart labels, room signs, etc.) into the room. A master list of latex-free devices and products is readily available from several internet web sites, including:

Kendall's Healthcare Products

Search their Latex-Free Database:
www.kendall-ltp.com

Hudson RCI

Latex-free respiratory care and anesthesia products:
www.hudsonrci.com/

Establish a latex consultant in your institution; an allergist is recommended. Develop programs to educate healthcare workers in the care of *latex-sensitive* patients. Develop educational programs for patients and their families in the care and precautions that should be taken to prevent latex exposure. This should encompass a first aid protocol in the event a severe reaction should arise. Encourage latex-sensitive patients to obtain and carry with them, at all times, some type of identification such as a medical alert bracelet and to have an epinephrine auto-injection kit if warranted.

Resource articles on latex allergy and a sample letter to manufacturers requesting latex information and resource articles are available in a *Latex Packet* from the Practice Department, American Association of Nurse Anesthetists, 222 South Prospect Avenue, Park Ridge, IL 60068-4001. Phone: (847) 692-7050.

Recommendations for Patient Care
Patients with Latex Allergy or Latex Risk

Schedule *latex-allergy* and/or *latex-risk* patients as the first case(s) in the morning. This will allow later dust (from the previous day) to be removed overnight.

The Operating Room

- Remove all latex products from the operating room.
- Bring a *latex-free* cart (if available) into the room.
- Use a *latex-free* reservoir bag, airways and endotracheal tubes, and laryngeal mask airways.
- Use a *non-latex* breathing circuit with plastic mask and bag.
- Ventilator must have a *non-latex* bellows.
- Place all monitoring devices, cords/tubes (oximeter, blood pressure, electrocardiograph wires) in stockinet and secure with tape to prevent direct skin contact. Items sterilized in ethylene oxide must be rinsed before use. Residual ethylene oxide reacts and can cause an allergic response in a latex-allergic patient.

Intravenous Line Preparation

- Use intravenous (IV) tubing without latex ports; utilize stopcocks if available.
- If unable to obtain IV tubing without latex ports, cover latex ports with tape.
- Cover all rubber injection ports on IV bags with tape and label in the following way: ***Do not inject or withdraw fluid through the latex port.*** Note: Pulmonary artery catheters (especially the balloon), central venous catheters, and arterial lines may all contain latex components!

Operating Room Patient Care

- Use non-latex gloves. (Use caution when selecting non-latex gloves. Not all substitutes are equally impermeable to bloodborne pathogens; care and investigation should be taken in the selection of substitute gloves.)
- Use *non-latex* tourniquets or use *non-latex* examination gloves or polyvinyl chloride tubing.
- Draw medication directly from opened multidose vials (remove stoppers) if medications are not available in ampules.
- Draw up medications immediately prior to the beginning of the case or their administration. The rubber allergen could leach out of the plunger of the syringe causing a reaction. The intensity of this reaction appears to increase over time.
- Utilize *latex-free* or glass syringes.
- Use stopcocks to inject drugs rather than latex ports.
- Minimize mixing/agitating lyophilized drugs in multidose vials with rubber stoppers.
- Notify Pharmacy and Central Supply that the patient you are caring for is latex sensitive so that these departments can use appropriate procedures when preparing preparations and instruments for the patient. Also notify radiology, respiratory therapy, housekeeping, food service and postoperative care units so the appropriate precautions can be made to protect the patient.

◆ Place clear and readily visible signs on the doors of the operating room to inform all who enter that the patient has a latex allergy.

Signs and Symptoms of Allergic Reactions to Latex

Symptoms usually occur within 30 minutes following anesthesia induction; however, the actual onset can range from 10 to 290 minutes.

Awake Patient
◆ Itchy eyes
◆ Generalized pruritus
◆ Shortness of breath
◆ Feeling of faintness
◆ Feeling of impending doom
◆ Unexplained restlessness and crying
◆ Agitation
◆ Nausea
◆ Vomiting
◇ Abdominal cramping
◆ Diarrhea
◆ Wheezing

Anesthetized Patient
◆ Tachycardia
◆ Hypotension
◆ Wheezing
◆ Bronchospasm
◆ Cardiorespiratory arrest
◆ Flushing
◆ Facial edema
◆ Laryngeal edema
◆ Urticaria

Emergency Response and Management

◆ Removal of all latex-containing products and agents, if possible. Do not delay immediate emergency therapy.
◆ Inform the surgical team to stop treatment/abort procedure.
◆ Assess and sustain ABCs of resuscitation.
◆ Maintain the airway and administer 100% oxygen.
◆ Discontinue inhalational halogenated agents (they are cardiovascular depressants which sensitize the myocardium to catecholamines which may be required for therapy.)
◆ Start intravascular volume expansion with Ringer's lactate or normal saline (10 to 50 mL/kg if hypotension is present and the patient has no history of congestive heart failure or any volume-related contraindication).
◆ Treat pharmacologically as indicated by presentation and clinical course. Administer epinephrine; start with a 0.5 to 1 µg/kg bolus (10 µg/mL dilution). Escalate to higher doses depending upon the patient's response. If an IV has not been established, epinephrine can be given subcutaneously in doses larger than would be administered intravenously (10 µg/kg dose). Endotracheal dosage may be necessary if IV access has not been established.

Secondary pharmacologic treatment may include the following:
◆ Hydrocortisone, 0.25 to 1 g, or methylprednisolone, 1 mg/kg IV.
◆ Diphenhydramine, 0.5 to 1 mg/kg (maximum dose 50 mg).
◆ Epinephrine infusion (2 to 4 µg/min or more, titrate to effect).
◆ Aminophylline (5 to 6 mg/kg over 20 minutes for persistent bronchospasm).
◆ Ranitidine, 0.5 to 2 mg/kg IV (maximum dose 150 mg).
◆ Sodium bicarbonate (0.5 to 1 mEq/kg for persistent hypotension with acidosis diagnosed with laboratory confirmation).

Nonpharmacologic considerations should include:
◆ Obtain allergy, pulmonary, pediatric consults as indicated.
◆ Draw and send a blood sample for IgE RAST testing and tryptase level (1 hour post reaction).
◆ Report incident to appropriate institutional entities (e.g., pharmacy, therapeutics, UR, QOC, etc.)
◆ Document events thoroughly and succinctly to examine at morbidity and mortality review at a later date.

Postreaction stabilization should include appropriate monitoring by dedicated providers well versed in managing post-anaphylaxis patients. The pediatric, intensive or special care area should be used when appropriate.

Pretreatment

Debate regarding the efficacy of premedication agents to treat patients with confirmed latex allergy remains somewhat controversial. Individual consideration for each patient undergoing elective operations or diagnostic and therapeutic procedures who has a known latex allergy should be initiated with the involvement of their primary care or allergy specialist provider. Premedication with steroids, antihistamines, and H_2 blockers prior to general anesthesia or deep sedation may be preferred for children with a known and documented latex allergy. While these agents will not **prevent** an allergic reaction they may attenuate such a response by lessening the severity of a reaction. The patient's regular provider or specialist managing their allergy should consult to recommend appropriate pretreatment when warranted.

Latex Avoidance and Alternative Management Options

Common latex medical devices used in perioperative areas include:
◆ Mattresses on stretchers
◆ Rubber gloves
◆ Adhesive tape (porous)
◆ Urinary catheters and drainage systems
◆ Electrode pads
◆ Wound drains
◆ Eyeshields
◆ Stomach and intestinal tubes
◆ Chest tubes and drainage systems
◆ Condom urinary collection devices

◆ Protective sheets
◆ Enema tubing kits
◆ Instrument pads
◆ IV solutions and tubing systems
◆ Fluid-circulating thermal blankets
◆ Hemodialysis equipment
◆ Ambu (bag-valve) masks
◆ Medication syringes
◆ Bulb syringes
◆ Elastic bandages, wraps
◆ Medication vial stoppers (multi-dose)
◆ Stethoscope tubing
◆ Band-Aids and other similar bandage products
◆ Gloves: examination and sterile
◆ Dental dams
◆ Surgical drapes
◆ Patient-controlled analgesia syringes
◆ Tourniquets

Anesthesia equipment and products containing latex include:

◆ Stethoscope tubing
◆ Rubber masks
◆ Electrode pads (e.g., electrocardiogram, peripheral nerve stimulator, contact pads)
◆ Head straps
◆ Rubber tourniquets, Esmarch bandages
◆ Rubber, oral, nasal; pharyngeal airways
◆ Teeth guards, eyeshields, bite blocks
◆ Blood pressure cuffs (inner bladder, and tubing)
◆ Breathing circuits containing rubber
◆ Reservoir breathing bags, disposable oxygen masks, nasal cannulae
◆ Rubber ventilator hoses and bellows
◆ Rubber endotracheal tubes
◆ Latex cuffs on plastic endotracheal tubes

◆ Latex injection ports on intravenous tubing, stopcocks
◆ Certain epidural catheter injection adapters
◆ Multidose vial stoppers
◆ Patient-controlled analgesia syringes
◆ Rubber suction catheters, specimen traps
◆ IV solutions and tubing systems (injection ports)

SUGGESTED READINGS

Dormans JP, Templeton JJ, Edmonds C, et al. Intraoperative ana-phylaxis due to exposure to latex (natural rubber) in children. *J Bone Joint Surg [Am]*. 1994;76:1688-1691.

Freeman GL. Co-occurrence of latex and fruit allergies. In *Allergy and Asthma Proceedings*. March–April, 1997, vol 18, II.

Holzman R. *Latex-Free Environment Precautions for Patients with a Latex Allergy/Patients at High Risk for Latex Allergy*. Boston: Boston Children's Hospital (Departmental Policy); 1992.

Kelly KJ, Kurup VP, Reijula KE, Fink JN. The diagnosis of natural rubber latex allergy. *J Allergy Clin Immunol*. 1994;93:813-816.

Latex Allergies: Anesthesia concerns. *AANA NewsBulletin/ Anesthesia Quality Plus*. 1992;46(9 Suppl):3.

Pasquariello CA, Lowe DA, Schwartz RE. Intraoperative anaphy-laxis to latex. *Pediatrics*. 1993;91:983-986.

Porri F, Pradal M, Lemiere C, et al. Association between latex sensi-tization and repeated latex exposure in children. *Anesthesiology*. 1997;86:599-602.

Theissen U, Theissen JL, Mertes N, Brehler R. IgE-mediated hyper-sensitivity to latex in childhood. *Allergy*. 1997;52:655-669.

Turjanmaa K, Alenius H, Makinen-Kiljunen S, et al. Natural rubber latex allergy. *Allergy*. 1996;51:593-602.

Vessey JA, McVay CJ, Holland CV, et al. Latex allergy: A threat to you and your patients? *Pediatr Nurs*. 1993;19:517-520.

Developed in 1993 by the Infection and Environmental Control Task Force. Revised by the Occupational Safety and Hazard Committee and approved by the AANA Board of Directors on July 31, 1998.

Learner Self-Assessment References

The following reference information is provided to enhance your ability to identify areas which require additional review.

CHAPTER 1 Goals, Definitions, Practice Standards, and Guidelines

1. Healthcare practitioner considerations associated with **JCAHO Standards** related to the administration of sedation by qualified personnel include:
Chapter 1, pages 1-2.

2. As outlined in the **"Continuum of Sedation,"** the following states of sedation and anesthesia are defined as:
   a. Minimal sedation

   b. Moderate sedation/analgesia

   c. Deep sedation/analgesia

   d. Anesthesia

   Chapter 1, page 4.

3. The **goals and objectives** associated with the administration of moderate sedation/analgesia include:
   Chapter 1, pages 4-5.
   a.

   b.

   c.

4. The **clinical endpoints** associated with a state of "moderate sedation" include:
   Chapter 1, pages 4-5.
   a.

   b.

5. Identify specific **legal scope-of-practice issues** related to the administration of sedation/analgesia by non-anesthesia personnel as they relate to:
   a. Practice standards

   b. Practice guidelines

   c. Position statements

   Chapter 1, pages 5-12.

CHAPTER 2 Presedation Assessment and Patient Selection

1. Healthcare practitioner considerations associated with **JCAHO Standards** related to presedation patient assessment for moderate sedation include:
Chapter 2, pages 21-22.

2. **Practice Guidelines for Sedation and Analgesia by Non-Anesthesiologists** promulgated by the ASA Task Force on Sedation **related to presedation patient assessment** include:
Chapter 2, pages 22-23.

3. **Goals** of presedation patient assessment include:
   a.

   b.

   c.

   d.

   Chapter 2, page 23.

4. Two **methods utilized to calculate ideal body weight** include:

   a.

   b.

   Chapter 2, page 25.

5. The **components of the patient's medical history** and its impact on planned procedural care include:

   a.

   b.

   c.

   d.

   e.

   f.

   g.

   Chapter 2, pages 24-60.

6. Specific alterations in the **cardiovascular, pulmonary, hepatic, renal, neurologic, and endocrine systems** identified in the presedation patient assessment and their implications for procedural patient care include:

   a. Cardiac

   b. Pulmonary

   c. Hepatic

   d. Renal

   e. Neurologic

   f. Endocrine

   Chapter 2, pages 24-44.

7. Implications for the sedation plan of care **based on the patient's past surgical and anesthetic history** include:
   Chapter 2, pages 44-45.

8. Treatment protocol for an **allergic reaction** during a sedation procedure include:
   Chapter 2, pages 45-46.

9. The sedation patient population, which requires **presedation laboratory testing** includes:
   Chapter 2, pages 48-53.

10. Patient care considerations associated with positive findings on the **presedation social history** include:
    a. Tobacco use

    b. Alcohol consumption

    c. Substance abuse

    d. Herbal product use

    e. Pregnancy

    Chapter 2, pages 46-60.

11. **Current NPO guidelines** for sedation patients include:
    a. Solids

    b. Liquids

    Chapter 2, page 61.

12. The **ASA Physical Classification System** summarizes physiologic status, which includes:
    a. ASA I

    b. ASA II

    c. ASA III

    d. ASA IV

    e. ASA V

    Chapter 2, pages 62-63.

CHAPTER 3 Pharmacologic Concepts

1. Healthcare practitioner considerations associated with **JCAHO Standards** related to sedation/analgesia medication administration include:
Chapter 3, pages 70-71.

2. **Practice Guidelines for Sedation and Analgesia by Non-Anesthesiologists** promulgated by the ASA Task Force on Sedation **related to sedation/analgesia medication administration** include:
Chapter 3, pages 71-72.

3. What **patient care considerations** arise with regard to the following pharmacologic definitions?
   a. Synergism

   b. Potency

   c. Tachyphylaxis

   Chapter 3, page 72.

4. **What patient care considerations are associated with the pharmacokinetic profile** of sedative and analgesic medications?
   a. Absorption

   b. Distribution

   c. Metabolism

   d. Excretion

   Chapter 3, pages 73-76.

5. What role does the **cytochrome P-450 system play in the biotransformation** of sedative and analgesic medications?
Chapter 3, page 74.

6. The **pharmacodynamic effects associated** with benzodiazepine and opioid use include:
Chapter 3, page 76.

7. The **clinical pertinence** associated with the utilization of pharmacologic agonists and antagonists in the sedation setting include:
Chapter 3, pages 76-77.

CHAPTER 4 Sedation/Analgesia Medication and Techniques of Administration

1. Healthcare practitioner considerations associated with **JCAHO Standards and Intents** related to sedation/analgesic medications and techniques of administration include:
Chapter 4, pages 81-82.

2. **Practice Guidelines for Sedation and Analgesia by Non-Anesthesiologists** promulgated by the ASA Task Force on Sedation **related to sedation/analgesic medications and techniques of administration** include:
Chapter 4, pages 82-83.

3. **Healthcare practitioner considerations associated with the pharmacokinetic, pharmacodynamic and end organ effects** associated with the following sedation/analgesic medications include:
   a. Benzodiazepines

   b. Opioids

   c. Sedative/hypnotics

   d. Butyrophenones

   e. Barbiturates

   f. Dissociative anesthetics

   g. Local anesthetic solutions

   Chapter 4, pages 83-92.

4. The **advantages, disadvantages, and patient care considerations** associated with the following techniques of administration include:
   a. Single-dose titration technique

   b. Bolus technique

   c. Continuous-infusion technique

   Chapter 4, pages 93-95.

CHAPTER 5 Sedation/Analgesia Pharmacologic Profile

1. Healthcare practitioner considerations associated with **JCAHO Standards** related to sedation/analgesic medication administration include:
Chapter 5, pages 99-100.

2. **Practice Guidelines for Sedation and Analgesia by Non-Anesthesiologists** promulgated by the ASA Task Force on Sedation **related to sedation/analgesic medication administration** include:
Chapter 5, pages 100-101.

3. The **pharmacokinetic profile** associated with sedative, analgesic, and hypnotic medications utilized in the sedation setting include:
Chapter 5, pages 102-123.

4. The **pharmacodynamic profile** associated with sedative, analgesic, and hypnotic medications utilized in the sedation setting include:
Chapter 5, pages 102-123.

5. **Indications, side effects, contraindications, and clinical pharmacology** associated with sedative, hypnotic, and analgesic medications include:
Chapter 5, pages 102-123.

6. **Cardiovascular, respiratory, and central nervous system effects** associated with sedative, hypnotic, and analgesic medications include:
Chapter 5, pages 102-123.

CHAPTER 6 Procedural Patient Monitoring

1. Healthcare practitioner considerations associated with **JCAHO Standards** related to physiologic monitoring requirements for sedation/analgesia patients include:
Chapter 6, pages 127-128.

2. **Practice Guidelines for Sedation and Analgesia by Non-Anesthesiologists recommendations** promulgated by the ASA Task Force on Sedation **related to physiologic**

monitoring of the patient presenting for sedation/analgesia clinical services include:
Chapter 6, pages 129-130.

3. **The rationale, advantages, and disadvantages associated with ECG, blood pressure, pulse oximetry, and level of consciousness monitoring** utilized during sedation procedures include:
Chapter 6, pages 131-159.

4. **Which ECG lead positions are best utilized in the detection of dysrhythmias versus ischemia?**
Chapter 6, page 131.

5. **Which rhythm disturbances may impact on the patient's physiologic status** during sedation/analgesia procedures?
Chapter 6, pages 137-145.

6. **Recommended treatment protocols for hypertension/hypotension** and their prescribed treatment protocols include:
Chapter 6, pages 146-147.

7. **Advantages associated with use of end-tidal carbon dioxide monitoring** during sedation/analgesia procedures include:
Chapter 6, pages 148-151.

8. **Required components of the sedation/analgesia record** include:
Chapter 6, pages 155-159.

CHAPTER 7 Airway Management and Management of Respiratory Complications

1. Healthcare practitioner considerations associated with **JCAHO Standards** related to airway management, oxygenation, and ventilation associated with sedation/analgesia include:
Chapter 7, pages 164-165.

2. **Practice Guidelines for Sedation and Analgesia by Non-Anesthesiologists recommendations** promulgated by the ASA Task Force on Sedation **related to airway management, oxygenation, ventilation, focused physical examination, and oxygen delivery devices** associated with the administration of sedation/analgesia include:
Chapter 7, pages 165-166.

3. **Components of the presedation airway evaluation** include:

   a.

   b.

   c.

   d.

   e.

Chapter 7, pages 167-170.

4. **Clinical signs and symptoms associated with respiratory insufficiency and airway obstruction** include:
Chapter 7, page 171.

5. **Treatment modalities designed to relieve airway obstruction and restore air flow** include:

   a.

   b.

   c.

   d.

   e.

Chapter 7, pages 172-177.

6. **The proper technique for nasal and oral airway insertion** includes:
   a. Nasal insertion

   b. Oral insertion

Chapter 7, pages 172-176.

7. Considerations for **proper application of a face mask for positive-pressure ventilation** include:
Chapter 7, pages 175-177.

8. Components of the **"Sedation Airway Algorithm"** include:
Chapter 7, page 172.

CHAPTER 8 Intravenous Insertion Techniques/ Intravenous Solutions

1. Healthcare practitioner considerations associated with intravenous fluids and drugs include:
Chapter 8, pages 185-186.

2. Practice Guidelines for Sedation and Analgesia by Non-Anesthesiologists recommendations promulgated by the ASA Task Force on Sedation related to intravenous medications and vascular access include:
Chapter 8, page 186.

3. The **principles of intravenous therapy** include:
Chapter 8, page 186.

4. List methods of **intravenous cannula insertion** required for moderate sedation patients.
Chapter 8, pages 188-189.

5. Identify **systemic complications** associated with intravenous catheter placement.
Chapter 8, pages 190-192.

6. State **common intravenous solutions** utilized during the administration of moderate sedation/analgesia.
Chapter 8, pages 194-196.

7. State the **presedation, procedural, and postsedation care** associated with intravenous therapy.
Chapter 8, pages 185-197.

CHAPTER 9 Geriatric Patient Care

1. **Practice Guidelines for Sedation and Analgesia by Non-Anesthesiologists recommendations** promulgated by the ASA Task Force on Sedation **related to geriatric patient care** include:
   Chapter 9, page 201.

2. The term *geriatric* is defined as:
   Chapter 9, page 202.

3. **Cardiorespiratory, renal, hepatic, and central nervous system physiologic alterations** that impact geriatric patient care include:
   Chapter 9, pages 202-204.

4. **Pharmacodynamic and pharmacokinetic considerations** associated with the aging process include:
   Chapter 9, pages 204-205.

5. Specific **procedural considerations** associated with administering benzodiazepines, opioids, and sedative hypnotics to the geriatric patient include:
   Chapter 9, page 205.

6. **Airway management issues** associated with caring for the geriatric sedation patient include:
   Chapter 9, page 205.

CHAPTER 10 Pediatric Patient Care

1. Healthcare practitioner considerations associated with **Guidelines for Monitoring and Management of Pediatric Patients During and After Sedation for Diagnostic and Therapeutic Procedures: American Academy of Pediatrics (AAP), Committee on Drugs (COD), related to pediatric sedation care** include:
   Chapter 10, page 210.

2. The **goals of pediatric procedural sedation** include:
   Chapter 10, page 211.

3. The **developmental subsets of pediatrics** include:
   Chapter 10, page 211.

4. The **role of the parent for children receiving sedation** includes:
   Chapter 10, pages 211-212.

5. The **physiologic response to pain in the infant** includes:
   Chapter 10, page 212.

6. **Anatomic and physiologic alterations** in the pediatric patient that **may impact on the sedation plan and procedural care include:**
   Chapter 10, pages 212-213.

7. **Distinct features of the pediatric airway that must be appreciated by the healthcare provider administering sedation** to the pediatric patient include:
   Chapter 10, pages 213-214.

8. **Airway maneuvers that may improve ventilation** in a pediatric sedation patient include:
   Chapter 10, pages 215-218.

9. **The clinical effects associated with hypothermia** in the pediatric patient include:
   Chapter 10, pages 218-219.

10. **NPO guidelines** for the sedation patient include:
    Chapter 10, page 221.

11. **Pediatric medical problems** that may impact the sedation plan of care include:
    Chapter 10, pages 223-224.

12. **Monitoring methods for the pediatric sedation patient** include:
    Chapter 10, pages 224-226.

13. **Sedation scales** used for pediatric sedation include:
    Chapter 10, pages 225-226.

14. **Pharmacologic considerations associated with sedative/analgesic agents** for the pediatric patient include:
    Chapter 10, pages 226-232.

15. **Care of the "failed sedation" pediatric patient** includes:
    Chapter 10, pages 232-233.

16. **Discharge criteria** for the pediatric patient include:
    Chapter 10, page 233.

CHAPTER 11 Postsedation Patient Care, Monitoring, and Discharge Criteria

1. Healthcare practitioner considerations associated with **JCAHO Standards** related to postsedation patient care include:
   Chapter 11, page 241.

2. **Practice Guidelines for Sedation and Analgesia by Non-Anesthesiologists recommendations** promulgated by the ASA Task Force on Sedation **related to postsedation patient care** include:
   Chapter 11, page 242.

3. **The purpose of postsedation patient care** includes:
   Chapter 11, page 242.

4. Characteristics associated with **phase I and phase II perianesthesia nursing practice** include:
   Chapter 11, page 242.

5. **Recommended patient care equipment** that should be maintained in a postsedation patient care area includes:
   Chapter 11, page 243.

6. **Components of a postsedation patient care report** include:
   Chapter 11, page 243.

7. **Objective parameters that compromise the postsedation Aldrete score** include:
   Chapter 11, page 247.

8. **Appropriate discharge criteria for the postsedation patient** include:
   Chapter 11, page 248.

9. **Components of effective postsedation teaching** include:
   Chapter 11, page 254.

CHAPTER 12 Risk Management Strategies

1. Healthcare practitioner considerations associated with **JCAHO Standards** related to performance improvement and sedation patient care include:
   Chapter 12, page 258.

2. *Quality* is defined as:
   Chapter 12, page 259.

3. **Risk reduction strategies to improve sedation patient care** include:
   Chapter 12, pages 259-260.

4. **Components of a "sedation" database** applicable to your practice setting include:
   Chapter 12, page 261.

5. **Mechanisms utilized in the successful implementation of a sedation educational program** include:
   Chapter 12, pages 273-275.

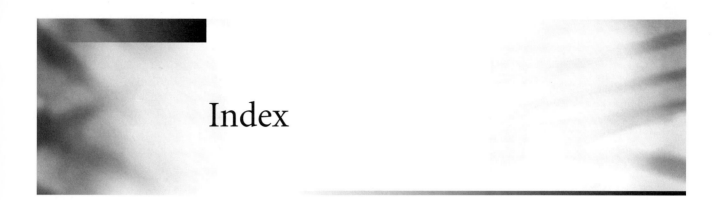

Index

Note: Page numbers followed by b indicate boxes; f, figure, and t, tables.